BASIC CLINICAL PHARMACOKINETICS

Fourth Edition

Michael E. Winter, Pharm.D.

Professor of Clinical Pharmacy, School of Pharmacy
University of California, San Francisco

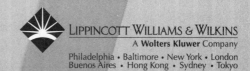

LIPPINCOTT WILLIAMS & WILKINS
A **Wolters Kluwer** Company

Philadelphia • Baltimore • New York • London
Buenos Aires • Hong Kong • Sydney • Tokyo

Editor: David B. Troy
Managing Editor: Matthew J. Hauber
Marketing Manager: Samantha S. Smith
Production Editor: Caroline Define
Designer: Doug Smock
Compositor: Graphic World
Printer: R.R. Donnelley & Sons

351 West Camden Street
Baltimore, MD 21201

530 Walnut Street
Philadelphia, PA 19106

The publisher is not responsible (as a matter of product liability, negligence, or otherwise) for any injury resulting from any material contained herein. This publication contains informa-tion relating to general principles of medical care that should not be construed as specific in-structions for individual patients. Manufacturers' product information and package inserts should be reviewed for current information, including contraindications, dosages, and pre-cautions.

Printed in the United States of America

Library of Congress Cataloging-in-Publication Data

Winter, Michael E.
    Basic clinical pharmacokinetics / Michael E. Winter.--4th ed.
        p. ; cm.
    Includes bibliographical references and index.
    ISBN 0-7817-4147-5
    1. Pharmacokinetics. 2. Pharmacokinetics--Problems, exercises, etc. I. Title.
    [DNLM: 1. Pharmacokinetics. 2. Pharmacology, Clinical QV 38 W786b 2003]
    RM301.5.W56 2003
    615'.7--dc21   2003054516

The publishers have made every effort to trace the copyright holders for borrowed mater-ial. If they have inadvertently overlooked any, they will be pleased to make the necessary arrangements at the first opportunity.

To purchase additional copies of this book, call our customer service department at **(800) 638-3030** or fax orders to **(301) 824-7390**. International customers should call **(301) 714-2324**.

Visit Lippincott Williams & Wilkins on the Internet: *http://www.LWW.com*. Lippincott Williams & Wilkins customer service representatives are available from 8:30 am to 6:00 pm, EST.

04 05 06 07 08
1 2 3 4 5 6 7 8 9 10

NOTICE TO READER

CONTRIBUTORS

Betsy L. Althaus, Pharm.D.
National Comprehensive Cancer Center
University of California
San Francisco, California

Peter J. Ambrose, Pharm.D.
Clinical Professor
Department of Clinical Pharmacy
School of Pharmacy
University of California
San Francisco, California

Amir Aminimanizani, Pharm.D.
Assistant Professor of Clinical Pharmacy
USC School of Pharmacy
Los Angeles, California

Paul Beringer, Pharm.D.
Associate Professor of Clinical Pharmacy
and Clinical Medicine
USC School of Pharmacy
Los Angeles, California

Maureen S. Boro, Pharm.D.
Pharmacokinetics Specialist
Department of Veterans Affairs
Associate Clinical Professor
Department of Clinical Pharmacy
School of Pharmacy
University of California
San Francisco, California

Melissa M. L. Choy, Pharm.D.
Assistant Clinical Professor
Department of Clinical Pharmacy
School of Pharmacy
University of California
San Francisco, California

Patrick R. Finley, Pharm.D., BCPP
Associate Clinical Professor
Department of Clinical Pharmacy
School of Pharmacy
University of California
San Francisco, California

John E. Murphy, Pharm.D.
Professor and Head
Department of Pharmacy Practice and
Science
The University of Arizona College of
Pharmacy
Tucson, Arizona

Kevin Y. Ohara, Pharm.D.
Inpatient Pharmacist Specialist
Inpatient Pharmacy
Kaiser Permanente
Los Angeles, California

David J. Quan, Pharm.D.
Associate Clinical Professor
Department of Clinical Pharmacy
School of Pharmacy
University of California, San Francisco
San Francisco, California

Jeanne Hawkins Van Tyle, Pharm.D., M.S.
Butler College of Pharmacy and Health
Sciences
Indianapolis, Indiana

Mark D. Watanabe, Pharm.D., Ph.D.
Assistant Clinical Professor
Department of Clinical Pharmacy
School of Pharmacy
University of California, San Francisco
San Francisco, California

Michelle M. Wheeler, Pharm.D.
Clinical Assistant Professor
College of Pharmacy
University of Utah
Salt Lake City, Utah

Michael E. Winter, Pharm.D.
Professor of Clinical Pharmacy
Department of Clinical Pharmacy
School of Pharmacy
University of California
San Francisco, California

PREFACE

Since the publication of the first edition of *Basic Clinical Pharmacokinetics*, the use of serum drug concentrations as a guide for monitoring drug therapy has continued to gain increased acceptance. The use of pharmacokinetic and biopharmaceutic principles in predicting plasma drug concentrations, as well as the changes in plasma drug concentrations that accrue over time, are now widely accepted as useful adjuncts in patient care. With the continued advancement of analytical technology, every health care institution and practitioner has ready access to drug concentration assays, and for some drugs (e.g., aminoglycosides, cyclosporine, digoxin, phenytoin), monitoring serum drug concentrations has become the standard of practice. As we gain more knowledge about both the limitations and application of drug concentrations and their correlation with either efficacy or toxicity, concentration sampling strategies change. Appropriate use of serum drug concentrations, however, continues to be a major problem in the clinical setting. Basic pharmacokinetic principles must be applied rationally to specific patients. The trend in patient care is towards cost containment. This includes everything from minimizing and streamlining drug therapy and laboratory testing to the increased use of automation. The use of serum drug concentrations is not immune to the pressure to do more with less. It is my hope that this fourth edition of *Basic Clinical Pharmacokinetics* will help the clinician in the rational application of pharmacokinetics and therapeutic drug monitoring to patient care and help to ensure that drug concentration monitoring is focused in an optimal way on the most appropriate patients.

The book is divided into two parts: Part One reviews basic pharmacokinetic principles, and Part Two illustrates the clinical application of pharmacokinetics to specific drugs through the presentation and solution of common clinical problems. As in previous editions, Part One is divided into sections that describe major pharmacokinetic parameters and their clinical applications. Equations that express the relationships between the various parameters and the resultant plasma concentrations are presented and discussed. A number of physiological and mathematical assumptions have been made. This is a common practice in the clinical setting, and an attempt has been made to alert the reader to these assumptions. There are a large number of texts and articles that present a much more detailed and in-depth analysis and explanation of the pharmacokinetic principles being discussed. It is not the intent of this book to explore all of these issues. Rather, it is the goal of this book to simplify pharmacokinetics so that it can be understood and visualized by practitioners, and consequently, the use of pharmacokinetic principles can become part of their professional practice. In this fourth edition, I have attempted to maintain a simple clinical approach to the application of pharmacokinetic principles to patient care. A number of sections in Part One have been expanded. For example, the section on Interpretation of Plasma Drug Concentrations still contains a discussion to help the reader understand how and why to choose a pharmacokinetic revision model. In the discussion on how to evaluate the usefulness or validity of the pharmacokinetic predictions, a brief discussion on Bayesian analysis as a pharmacokinetic analysis tool has been included to help put into perspective the advantages and limitations of computer-generated pharmacokinetic data. In addition to peritoneal and standard hemodialysis, the section on Dialysis of Drugs now contains a brief review of high-flux or high-efficiency hemodialysis and continuous renal replacement therapy and their impact on drug therapy in patients with compromised renal function. The reader is strongly urged to read each section in the order that it appears in the text because many of the concepts discussed in the latter portions of the text are based on an understanding of those presented earlier.

Many individuals feel overwhelmed by the apparent complexity of some of the equations used to describe pharmacokinetic behavior of drugs. Therefore, extensive explanations that emphasize major concepts accompany the more complex equations. Figures are provided to help the reader visualize the concepts that are being reviewed. The principles discussed in Part One will give the clinician the basis for manipulating the dosing regimens and interpreting plasma drug concentrations for the drugs discussed in Part Two of this text.

The drugs discussed in Part Two were selected because they represent the most commonly monitored drugs in the clinical setting, assays are widely available, and an understanding of their pharmacokinetic and biopharmaceutic properties can substantially aid clinicians in dosing these drugs more rationally and safely. Some drugs have been deleted because their use and therapeutic monitoring are uncommon (e.g., primidone and quinidine) or are currently limited to overdose/toxicology cases (e.g., salicylates). The updates include new information on the clinical use of serum drug concentrations, and where appropriate, new cases and examples have been added to further expand and exemplify the use of pharmacokinetics in clinical practice (e.g., aminoglycosides and high-dose once daily regimens). The chapter formerly titled Cyclosporine is now titled Immunosuppressants because it has been expanded to include sirolimus and tacrolimus in addition to cyclosporine.

For each of the drugs, examples of the most common pharmacokinetic manipulations, such as calculation of a loading dose and maintenance dose, are presented. An example of the process used to interpret a reported plasma concentration is also given. In addition, pathophysiologic factors that influence the pharmacokinetics of these drugs and their significance are considered. Examples of the most common problems encountered in clinical practice are also given to help the reader recognize when caution should be used in making patient care decisions based upon serum drug concentrations and pharmacokinetic principles. Ultimately, it is hoped that the reader will be able to recognize the fundamental principles that are being applied to each of the drugs. As you develop confidence and skill in using pharmacokinetics as a clinical tool, you will be able to apply these same principles to new drugs.

Although plasma drug concentrations are useful in evaluating drug therapy, they constitute only one source of information. They should not, therefore, be used as the sole criterion on which treatment is based. Pharmacokinetic calculations should be considered only as an adjunctive guide to the determination of dosing regimens.

If a calculated dosing regimen seems unreasonable, re-evaluation is essential since mathematical error is always a possibility. Another problem inherent in these calculations is that the pharmacokinetic parameters utilized may be inappropriate for the patient under consideration. Many of the pharmacokinetic parameters available in the literature are based upon small numbers of patients or normal volunteers. Therefore, values obtained from these experimental data are, at best, estimates for any given patient. If the basic underlying pharmacokinetic assumptions are not applicable to the particular patient, even the most elegant calculation is invalid.

Review articles and some texts commonly list pharmacokinetic parameters for a number of drugs and are a good initial source of pharmacokinetic information. However, the reader is encouraged to seek out the original literature to evaluate the methodology and data from which this information was derived. Some factors that should be considered in scrutinizing these studies include the number and type of subjects, type and specificity of drug assay, degree of inter- and intra-subject variability, statistical analysis of the data, and whether the drug was studied prospectively or retrospectively. The potential problems associated with using literature data to predict disposition of a drug within a specific patient emphasize the need to obtain accurate plasma level measurements. Clearly, the literature can serve as a guide to make initial a priori clinical decisions, but even with the best predictions, significant variance does exist. Therefore, only with appropriate drug sampling, accurate and specific assay procedures, and logical pharmacokinetic analysis can patient-specific parameters be derived that will be useful adjuncts to providing optimal patient care and improving clinical outcomes.

ACKNOWLEDGMENT

The completion of the fourth edition of *Basic Clinical Pharmacokinetics* would not have been possible without the support of my family, friends, and colleagues. I thank Dean Mary Anne Koda-Kimble and Department Chair Lloyd Young for their support, guidance, and inspiration throughout the years. I am also grateful to the highly professional co-authors who lent their expertise, knowledge, and skill to update the individual drug chapters.

I would also like to recognize and thank the many students, residents, and colleagues who have provided me with feedback about what helps them understand and apply pharmacokinetics to their professional practice.

Finally, I thank my family for their continued encouragement and support.

CONTENTS

APPENDICES

PART ONE

Basic Principles

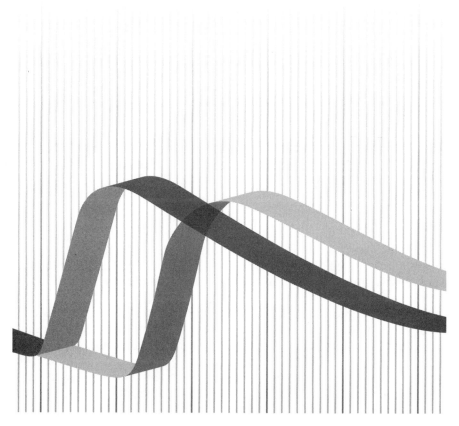

Bioavailability (F)

DEFINITION

Bioavailability is the percentage or fraction of the administered dose that reaches the systemic circulation of the patient. Examples of factors that can alter bioavailability include the inherent dissolution and absorption characteristics of the administered chemical form (e.g., salt, ester), the dosage form (e.g., tablet, capsule), the route of administration, the stability of the active ingredient in the gastrointestinal (GI) tract, and the extent of drug metabolism before reaching the systemic circulation. Drugs can be metabolized by GI bacteria, by the GI mucosa, and by the liver before reaching the systemic circulation.

To calculate the amount of drug absorbed, the administered dose should be multiplied by a bioavailability factor, which is usually represented by the letter "F." For example, the bioavailability of digoxin (Lanoxin) is estimated to be 0.7 for orally administered tablets.[1-3] This means that if 250 μg (0.25 mg) of digoxin is given orally, the effective or absorbed dose can be calculated by multiplying the administered dose by F:

$$\text{Amount of Drug Absorbed or Reaching the Systemic Circulation} = (F)(Dose) \qquad \text{[Eq. 1]}$$

$$\text{Amount of Drug Absorbed or Reaching the Systemic Circulation} = (F)(Dose)$$

$$= (0.7)(250\ \mu g)$$

$$= 175\ \mu g$$

It should be emphasized that this factor does not take into consideration the rate of drug absorption; it only estimates the extent of absorption. Although the rate of absorption can be important when rapid onset of pharmacologic effects is required, it is not usually important when a drug is administered chronically. The rate of absorption is important only when it is so slow that it limits the absolute bioavailability of the drug, or when it is so rapid that too much drug is absorbed. "Dose dumping" can occur under certain conditions with some sustained-release preparations.[4,5] In addition, incomplete absorption of sustained-release dosage forms should be considered in patients who have a short GI transit time. GI transit times of 24 to 48 hours are probably average, but patients with bowel disease may have transit times of only a few hours. A lower-than-average bioavailability should be considered in these patients, especially when the duration of absorption is extended.

DOSAGE FORM

As noted previously, bioavailability can vary among different formulations and dosage forms of a drug. For example, digoxin elixir has a bioavailability of approximately 80% (F = 0.8), whereas the soft gelatin capsules have a bioavailability of 100% (F = 1.0). This is in contrast to the tablets, which have a bioavailability of 70% (F = 0.7).[2,6,7] When drugs are administered parenterally, the bioavailability is usually considered to be 100% (F = 1.0). By rearranging Equation 1, this principle can be used to calculate equivalent doses of a drug when a patient is to receive a different dosage form of the same drug.

$$\frac{\text{Dose of New}}{\text{Dosage Form}} = \frac{\text{Amount of Drug Absorbed From Current Dosage Form}}{\text{F of New Dosage Form}} \qquad [\text{Eq. 2}]$$

For example, if a patient who has been receiving digoxin 250 μg (0.25 mg) in the tablet dosage form, with a bioavailability of 0.7, needs to receive digoxin elixir, an equivalent dose of the elixir would be calculated as follows:

$$\text{Dose of Elixir} = \frac{(0.7)(250 \ \mu g)}{0.8}$$

$$= \frac{175 \ \mu g}{0.8}$$

$$= 219 \ \mu g$$

If the soft gelatin capsules of digoxin were to be administered, the bioavailability or F of the new dosage form would have been 1.0 and the equivalent dose would have been 175 μg.

The bioavailability of parenterally administered drugs is usually assumed to be 1.0. Drugs which are administered as inactive precursors that must then be converted to an active product are an exception to this rule. If some of the inactive precursor is eliminated from the body (renally excreted or metabolized to an inactive compound) before it can be converted to the active compound, the bioavailability will be <1.0. For example, parenteral chloramphenicol is given as the succinate ester, and this chloramphenicol ester must be hydrolyzed to the active compound. The bioavailability of the parenterally administered chloramphenicol succinate ranges from 55% to 95%, because from 5% to 45% of the chloramphenicol ester is eliminated renally before it can be converted to the active compound.[8] Generally, for those drugs with nearly complete absorption (F > 0.8) bioavailability is usually consistent. For those drugs with a low oral bioavailability (F < 0.5) there is often a large variation in the extent of absorption. This is not a hard and fast rule as any drug under the right conditions can have an altered bioavailability.

CHEMICAL FORM (S)

The chemical form of a drug must also be considered when evaluating bioavailability. For example, when a salt or ester of a drug is administered, the bioavailability factor (F) should be multiplied by the fraction of the total molecular weight that the active drug represents. If "S" represents the fraction of the administered dose that is the active drug, then the amount of drug absorbed from a salt or ester form can be calculated as follows:

$$\text{Amount of Drug Absorbed or Reaching the Systemic Circulation} = (S)(F)(\text{Dose}) \qquad \text{[Eq. 3]}$$

The "S" factor should be included in all bioavailability equations as a constant reminder of its importance in assessing bioavailability of the active drug form. When a drug is administered in its parent or active form, the "S" for that drug is 1.0.

Equation 2 can now be expanded to consider the salt factor and the bioavailability when calculating the dose of a new dosage form:

$$\frac{\text{Dose of New}}{\text{Dosage Form}} = \frac{\text{Amount of Drug Absorbed From Current Dosage Form}}{(S)(F) \text{ of New Dosage Form}} \qquad \text{[Eq. 4]}$$

Aminophylline and phenytoin are examples of this principle (Fig. 1). Aminophylline is the ethylenediamine salt of the pharmacologically active moiety, theophylline. Eighty to eighty-five percent (by weight) of this salt is theophylline, so that the "S" for aminophylline is approximately 0.8. Uncoated aminophylline tablets are considered to be completely (100%) bioavailable; the bioavailability factor (F) for this dosage form is, therefore, 1.0. It is important to consider the salt form in determining the amount of theophylline absorbed from an aminophylline tablet. When Equation 3 is applied to this situation, it can be demonstrated that 160 mg of theophylline is absorbed from a 200 mg aminophylline tablet:

$$\text{Amount of Drug Absorbed or Reaching the Systemic Circulation} = (S)(F)(\text{Dose})$$

$$= (0.8)(1)(200 \text{ mg Aminophylline})$$

$$= 160 \text{ mg Theophylline}$$

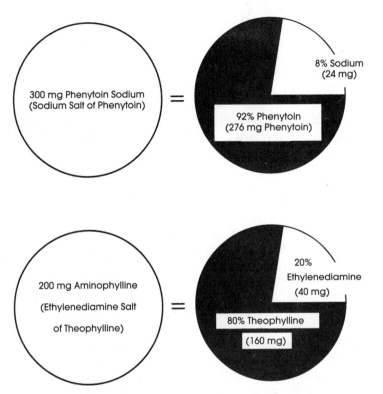

FIGURE 1. The effect of the chemical drug form on bioavailability. The examples above emphasize the importance of considering the chemical form when calculating the amount of active drug actually administered. The amount of active drug administered may represent only a fraction (S) of the salt, ester, or other chemical form of the drug contained in the formulation. The bioavailability (F) of the dosage form itself must also be considered when drugs are administered by the oral route.

Similarly, 300 mg of phenytoin sodium with an S of 0.92 represents only 276 mg of phenytoin reaching the systemic circulation, assuming complete absorption (F = 1).

$$\frac{\text{Amount of Drug Absorbed or}}{\text{Reaching the Systemic Circulation}} = \text{(S)(F)(Dose)}$$

$$= \text{(0.92)(1)(300 mg Phenytoin Sodium)}$$

$$= \text{276 mg Phenytoin}$$

In some cases the labeled amount of drug has already taken into account the amount of active drug. Valproate sodium, the sodium salt of valproic acid, is manufactured and labeled with the amount of valproic acid and therefore, a value of 1 would be appropriate for S. Fosphenytoin sodium is the sodium salt of the phosphate ester of phenytoin. Although fosphenytoin sodium is only 61% phenytoin, the manufacturers have labeled the drug as phenytoin sodium equivalents or P.E. Therefore, to calculate the amount of phenytoin in 100 mg of Fosphenytoin P.E., an S value of 0.92 would be used.

The important concept is to understand and be able to calculate the amount of the labeled drug that will be available to the patient as active drug. To do this, both the fraction of the dose that is active drug (S) and the bioavailability or fraction of administered dose that will reach the systemic circulation (F) needs to be considered when calculating doses and dosing regimens.

FIRST-PASS EFFECT

Because orally administered drugs are absorbed from the GI tract into the portal circulation, some drugs may be extensively metabolized by the liver before reaching the systemic circulation. The term "first pass" refers to metabolism by the liver as the drug passes through the liver via the portal vein following absorption. This "first-pass effect" can substantially decrease the amount of active drug reaching the systemic circulation and thus its bioavailability (Fig. 2).

Propranolol is an example of a drug that has a significant portion of an orally administered dose that does not reach the systemic circulation because it is metabolized as it passes through the liver following absorption from the GI tract. Because of this "first-pass effect," oral bioavailability is low and orally administered doses are much larger than doses administered intravenously. However, the propranolol issue is further complicated by the fact that one of the metabolites, 4-hydroxy-propranolol, is pharmacologically active.[9] Lidocaine is an example of a drug with a first-pass effect that is so great that oral administration is not practical as a route of administration if systemic effects are desired.[10] In addition, some drugs are extensively metabolized by cytochrome enzymes, primarily CYP 3A4, that are located in the gut wall. As an example, the low and variable bioavailability ($F \approx 0.3$) of cyclosporine is in part due to metabolism by CYP 3A4 in the gut wall.[11]

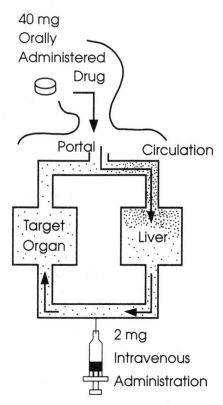

FIGURE 2. First-pass effect. When drugs with a high "first-pass effect" are administered orally, a large amount of the absorbed drug is metabolized before it reaches the systemic circulation. If the drug is administered intravenously, the liver is bypassed and the fraction of the administered dose that reaches the circulation is increased. Parenteral doses of drugs with a high "first-pass" are much smaller than oral doses necessary to produce equivalent pharmacologic effects.

Administration Rate (R_A)

The administration rate is the average rate at which absorbed drug reaches the systemic circulation. This is usually calculated by dividing the amount of drug absorbed (see Equation 3) by the time over which the drug was administered (dosing interval). The dosing interval is usually represented by the symbol, tau (τ).

$$\text{Administration Rate } R_A = \frac{(S)(F)(Dose)}{\tau} \qquad \text{[Eq. 5]}$$

When drugs are administered as a continuous infusion, the dosing interval can be expressed in any convenient time unit. For example, the theophylline administration rate resulting from aminophylline infused at a rate of 40 mg/hr is calculated from Equation 5 as follows:

$$\text{Administration Rate } R_A = \frac{(S)(F)(Dose)}{\tau}$$

$$= \frac{(0.8)(1)(40\ mg)}{1\ hr}$$

$$= 32\ mg/hr$$

or

$$\text{Administration Rate } R_A = \frac{(S)(F)(Dose)}{\tau}$$

$$= \frac{(0.8)(1)(40\ mg)}{60\ min}$$

$$= 0.53\ mg/min$$

When drugs are administered at fixed dosing intervals, the calculated administration rate is an average value. For example, the average administration rate of digoxin resulting from an oral dose of 250 µg of digoxin given orally as tablets every day would be calculated using Equation 5 as follows:

$$\text{Administration Rate } R_A = \frac{(S)(F)(Dose)}{\tau}$$

$$= \frac{(1)(0.7)(250\ \mu g)}{1\ day}$$

$$= 175\ \mu g/day$$

or

$$\text{Administration Rate } R_A = \frac{(S)(F)(Dose)}{\tau}$$

$$= \frac{(1)(0.7)(250 \ \mu g)}{24 \ hr}$$

$$= 7.29 \ \mu g/hr$$

Although each digoxin tablet is actually absorbed over 1 to 2 hours, the average "administration rate" is calculated over the entire dosing interval. Although the administration rate of 7.29 µg/hr and 175 µg/day are equivalent, most clinicians think of the dosing rate that is consistent with how the drug is administered. In this case, the usual interval would be 1 day because digoxin is most commonly administered once each day. In the section on clearance, we will consider how the drug administration rate, drug clearance, and the usually reported units for drug concentration all need to be consistent for the purposes of performing pharmacokinetic calculations.

Desired Plasma Concentration (C)

PROTEIN BINDING

Most clinical laboratory reports of drug concentrations in plasma (C) represent drug that is bound to plasma protein plus drug that is unbound or free. It is the free or unbound drug that is in equilibrium with the receptor site and is, therefore, the pharmacologically active moiety. Thus, in the case of a drug with significant plasma binding, the reported plasma drug concentration indirectly reflects the concentration of free or active drug (Fig. 3).

Some disease states are associated with decreased plasma proteins or with decreased binding of drugs to plasma proteins.[12–15] In these situations, drugs that are usually highly protein bound have a larger percentage of free or unbound drug present in plasma. Therefore, a greater pharmacologic effect can be expected for any given drug concentration in plasma (C). Clinicians must always consider altered protein binding and whether the fraction of free drug concentration or fraction unbound (fu) is altered when interpreting or establishing desired plasma drug concentrations.

$$fu = \frac{\text{Free Drug Concentration}}{\text{Total Drug Concentration}}$$

$$fu = \frac{C\ free}{C\ bound + C\ free} \qquad \text{[Eq. 6]}$$

The fraction of drug that is unbound (fu) does not vary with the drug concentration for most drugs that are bound primarily to albumin. This is because the number of protein binding sites far exceeds the number of drug molecules available for binding. When the plasma concentrations for drugs bound to albumin exceed 25 to 50 mg/L, however, albumin binding sites can start to become saturated. As a result, fu, or the fraction of drug that is free, will change with the plasma drug concentration. For example, salicylates and valproic acid (Depakote) can saturate plasma protein binding sites, and both of these drugs frequently have plasma concentrations exceeding 25 to 50 mg/L.[16,17] For those drugs that do not reach serum concentrations capable of saturating protein-binding sites, the plasma protein concentration (in many cases, this is albumin) and the binding affinity of the drug for the plasma protein are the two major factors that control the fraction unbound (fu).

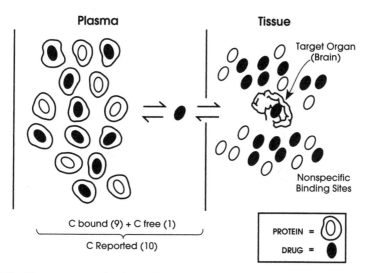

FIGURE 3. Plasma concentration of a highly protein-bound drug: normal plasma protein concentration. The plasma drug concentration reported by the laboratory represents a total of both "bound" and "free" drug. It is the "free" drug that is in equilibrium with the target organs and is the pharmacologically active moiety. In this illustration, fu (or the fraction of free drug to total drug concentration) is 0.1.

LOW PLASMA PROTEIN CONCENTRATIONS

Low plasma protein concentrations decrease the plasma concentration of bound drug (C bound); however, the concentration of free drug (C free) generally is unaffected. Therefore, the fraction of drug that is free (fu) increases as plasma protein concentrations decrease. Free or unbound drug concentrations are not significantly increased, because the free drug that is released into plasma secondary to low plasma protein concentrations equilibrates with the tissue compartment (compare Fig. 4 with Fig. 3). Therefore, if the volume of distribution (V) is relatively large (e.g., phenytoin 0.65 L/kg), only a minor increase in C free will result (also see Volume of Distribution).

The relationship between the plasma drug concentration and the plasma protein concentration can be expressed as follows:

$$\frac{C'}{C_{\text{Normal Binding}}} = (1 - fu)\left[\frac{P'}{P_{\text{NL}}}\right] + fu \qquad \text{[Eq. 7]}$$

This equation can be used to estimate the degree to which an altered plasma protein concentration will affect the desired therapeutic drug concentration. C' represents the patient's plasma drug concentration, and P' represents the patient's plasma protein concentration. $C_{\text{Normal Binding}}$ is the plasma drug concentration that would be expected if the patient's plasma

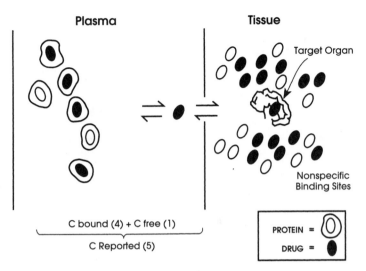

FIGURE 4. Effect of decreased plasma protein concentration on plasma drug concentration. Compare this figure with Figure 3. The decreased protein concentration decreases the plasma drug concentration reported by the laboratory. In this situation, the concentration of free, or active, drug remains the same because free drug that is released as a result of the lowered plasma protein concentration is taken up by nonspecific tissue binding sites and/or cleared from the body. For this reason, the pharmacologic effect, which can be expected from the reported C of 5, will be the same as that produced by the reported C of 10 in Figure 3. In this illustration, fu (or the fraction of free drug to total drug concentration) is increased to 0.2.

protein concentration were normal (P_{NL}). Note that fu is the free fraction associated with "normal plasma protein binding." The $C_{Normal\ Binding}$ for any given drug can be calculated by rearranging Equation 7:

$$C_{Normal\ Binding} = \frac{C'}{(1 - fu)\left[\dfrac{P'}{P_{NL}}\right] + fu} \qquad [Eq.\ 8]$$

For example, a patient with a low serum albumin of 2.2 gm/dL (normal albumin, 4.4 gm/dL) and an apparently low plasma phenytoin concentration of 5.5 mg/L still has a therapeutically acceptable plasma drug concentration when it is adjusted for the low serum albumin. When the normal free fraction (fu) for phenytoin of 0.1 is substituted into Equation 8, an adjusted phenytoin plasma concentration of 10 mg/L is calculated.

$$C_{\text{Normal Binding}} = \cfrac{C'}{(1 - fu)\left[\cfrac{P'}{P_{NL}}\right] + fu}$$

$$= \cfrac{5.5 \text{ mg/L}}{(1 - 0.1)\left[\cfrac{2.2 \text{ gm/dL}}{4.4 \text{ gm/dL}}\right] + 0.1}$$

$$= \cfrac{5.5 \text{ mg/L}}{(0.9)(0.5) + 0.1}$$

$$= 10 \text{ mg/L}$$

The phenytoin concentration that would have been reported from the laboratory if the patient's albumin concentration was "normal" would be approximately 10 mg/L. This calculation is based on the assumption that phenytoin is primarily bound to albumin and that an average normal albumin concentration is 4.4 gm/dL (range, 3.5 to 5.5 gm/dL). While Equation 8 could be used to adjust for any drug significantly bound to albumin, the degree to which the drug concentration will be adjusted or "normalized" for the alteration in serum albumin between 3.5 to 5.5 gm/dL will be minimal and is generally unwarranted.

Many other drugs are bound primarily to globulin rather than albumin. Adjustments of plasma drug concentrations for these drugs based on serum albumin concentrations would, therefore, be inappropriate. Unfortunately, adjustments for changes in globulin binding are difficult because drugs usually bind to a specific globulin that is only a small fraction of total globulin concentration. In general, acidic drugs (e.g., phenytoin, most of the anti-epileptic drugs, and some neutral compounds) bind primarily to albumin; basic drugs (e.g., lidocaine and quinidine) bind more extensively to globulins.[13,18–21]

ELEVATED PLASMA PROTEIN CONCENTRATIONS

The fu value (fraction of total drug concentration which is free or unbound) for selected drugs is provided in Table 1. Because increases in serum albumin are uncommon in the clinical setting, the use of Equation 8 for high serum albumin would be rare. Many basic drugs, however, are bound to the acute phase reactive protein,[22,23] alpha$_1$-acid glycoprotein (AAG). This plasma protein has been known to be significantly decreased and increased under certain clinical conditions. For example, increases in plasma quinidine concentrations have been observed following surgery or trauma.[18,24] The change in the quinidine concentration is the result of increased concentrations of the plasma binding proteins (alpha$_1$-acid glycoproteins) and increased bound concentrations of quinidine. There appears to be little or no change in the free quinidine level because re-equilibration with the larger

TABLE 1   **Drugs and fu Values for Plasma Protein Binding**

Drug	fu Value
Amitriptyline	0.04[a]
Carbamazepine	0.2
Chlordiazepoxide	0.05
Chlorpromazine	0.04[a]
Cyclosporine	< 0.1[c]
Diazepam	0.01
Digoxin	0.70
Digitoxin	0.10
Ethosuximide	1.0
Gabapentin	0.97
Gentamicin	0.9
Imipramine	0.04[a]
Lidocaine	0.30[a]
Lithium	1.0
Methadone	0.13[a]
Methotrexate	0.5
Nafcillin	0.10
Nelfinavir	0.02
Phenobarbital	0.5
Phenytoin	0.10
Procainamide	0.84
Propranolol	0.06[a]
Quinidine	0.20[a]
Salicylic Acid	0.16[b]
Valproic Acid	0.15[b]
Vancomycin	0.9
Warfarin	0.03

[a]Basic drugs that are bound significantly to plasma proteins other than albumin.[12,18,19,33]
[b]Concentration-dependent plasma protein binding (see Salicylate and Valproic Acid chapters).
[c]Bound to lipoproteins and other blood elements.[34,35]

tissue stores occurs. In this situation, there would be a decrease in unbound free fraction (fu), and the therapeutic levels of free or unbound drug should correlate with higher-than-usual drug concentration (bound plus free). Other basic compounds with significant binding to alpha$_1$-acid glycoproteins would be expected to be similarly affected. Unfortunately, alpha$_1$-acid glycoprotein concentrations are almost never assayed in the clinical setting, making it difficult to evaluate the relationship between the total drug concentration and the unbound or free fraction. For this reason, evaluation of plasma levels for basic drugs that are significantly protein bound is often difficult. A careful evaluation of the patient's clinical response to a measured drug level, as well as an evaluation of any concurrent medical problems (such as surgery, trauma, or inflammatory disease) that could influence plasma protein concentrations and drug binding, is required.

Patients with cirrhosis vary considerably in their plasma protein binding characteristics. Some patients have significantly elevated binding capabilities, whereas others have significantly decreased binding capabilities. This variation probably reflects the fact that some cirrhotic patients have a strong stimulus for the production of alpha$_1$-acid glycoproteins, whereas others with more serious hepatic disease are unable to manufacture these binding proteins.[22,24,25]

BINDING AFFINITY

The binding affinity of plasma protein for a drug can also alter the fraction of drug which is free (fu) (compare Fig. 5 with Fig. 3). For example, the plasma proteins in patients with uremia (severe end-stage renal failure) have less affinity for phenytoin than do proteins present in nonuremic individuals. As a result, the fu for phenytoin in uremic patients is estimated

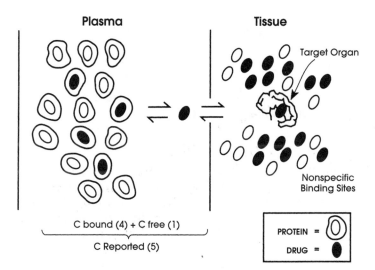

FIGURE 5.   The effect of decreased binding affinity on plasma drug concentration. Compare this figure with Figure 3. Although the protein concentration is normal, the decreased binding affinity of the drug for protein has decreased the reported drug concentration. The concentration of free, or active, drug remains the same because free drug that is released as a result of this decreased affinity is taken up by nonspecific binding sites in the tissue and/or cleared from the body. Thus, the pharmacologic effect that can be expected from the reported C of 5 will be the same as that produced by the reported C of 10 in Figure 3. In this illustration, fu (or the fraction of free drug to total drug concentration) is increased to 0.2.

to be in the range of 0.2 to 0.3 in contrast to the normal value of 0.1.[21,26] The "effective" or free drug concentration can be calculated by rearranging Equation 6:

$$fu = \frac{C\ free}{C\ bound + C\ free}$$

$$= \frac{C\ free}{C\ total}$$

C free = (fu)(C total)   [Eq. 9]

According to Equation 9, the concentration of free phenytoin in uremic patients is comparable to that in nonuremic patients—despite lower phenytoin plasma concentrations (C total)—because the fu for phenytoin is increased in uremic patients. The uremic patient with an fu of 0.2 and a reported phenytoin concentration of 5 mg/L would have the same free drug concentration (and same pharmacologic effect) as a patient with normal renal function who has a reported phenytoin concentration of 10 mg/L (using Equation 9):

$$C\ free = (fu)(C\ total)$$

$$\frac{C\ free}{(in\ a\ Uremic\ Patient)} = (0.2)(5\ mg/L)$$

$$= 1\ mg/L$$

$$\frac{C\ free}{(in\ a\ patient\ with\ Normal\ Renal\ Function)} = (0.1)(10\ mg/L)$$

$$= 1\ mg/L$$

In summary, any factor that alters protein binding becomes clinically important when a drug is highly protein bound (i.e., if fu is < 0.1 or 10% unbound). For example, if fu is increased from 0.1 (10% free) to 0.2 (20% free), the concentration of free or active drug for any given value of C (bound + free) would be double the usual values, that is:

$$C\ free = (fu)(C\ total)$$

$$= (0.1)(10\ mg/L)$$

$$= 1\ mg/L$$

vs.

$$= (0.2)(10\ mg/L)$$

$$= 2\ mg/L$$

If, on the other hand, the fu for a drug is $\geq$ 0.5 (50% free), it is unlikely that changes in plasma protein binding will be of clinical consequence. As an illustration, if the fraction unbound for a drug is increased from a normal value 0.5 (50% free) to 0.6 (60% free) because of decreased protein concentrations, the concentration of free active drug (assuming the same total concentration) would actually be increased by only 20%.

$$C \text{ free} = (fu)(C \text{ total})$$

$$= (0.5)(10 \text{ mg/L})$$

$$= 5 \text{ mg/L}$$

vs.

$$= (0.6)(10 \text{ mg/L})$$

$$= 6 \text{ mg/L}$$

As a general rule, if fraction unbound is increased in any given situation, the clinician should reduce the desired C by the same proportion.[27] That is, if fu is increased twofold, the desired C or "therapeutic range" should be reduced to one-half the usual value.

What is often misunderstood is that for drugs with significant plasma protein binding, changes in plasma binding will have a profound effect on the plasma drug concentration, because the bound concentration has been altered. As a consequence, the free fraction (fu) of drug in plasma is altered. However, the unbound drug concentration is, in most cases, relatively unaffected.[28] When considering changes in binding, it should be kept in mind that the free fraction (fu) is the ratio of unbound drug concentration to total drug concentration as outlined in Equation 6.

$$fu = \frac{C \text{ free}}{C \text{ bound} + C \text{ free}}$$

As depicted in Equation 6, fu is dependent on the binding characteristics and is not the "cause" of the free or unbound drug concentration as might be suggested in Equation 9.

$$C \text{ free} = (fu)(C \text{ total})$$

As an example, let us consider four patients, the first two with phenytoin concentrations of 10 and 20 mg/L, respectively. If both these patients had normal plasma binding (fu = 0.1), their respective C free phenytoin concentrations would be 1 and 2 mg/L. The increased potential effect of the C total phenytoin concentration of 20 mg/L with a C free of 2 mg/L seems intuitively obvious. The fact that the drug concentration (C bound and C free) is higher in the second patient is probably the result of either higher-than-average doses or decreased elimination.

Now let us consider two other patients each with a phenytoin concentration of 10 mg/L. However, in this case the first patient has normal plasma binding and an fu of 0.1. The second patient has decreased plasma binding and as a result an fu of 0.2. In this situation the first patient with a normal binding fu of 0.1 and C total of 10 mg/L would have a C free of 1 mg/L. The second patient with an altered binding fu of 0.2 and a C total of 10 mg/L would have a C free of 2 mg/L. It is important to recognize that although both patients have a phenytoin concentration of 10 mg/L, the second patient would be expected to have an increased drug effect because of the higher C free or unbound drug concentration. The reason that the second patient has an increased C free is not because of altered binding, but probably because the patient has been given higher-than-average doses or their metabolism is less than average.

MONITORING FREE OR UNBOUND PLASMA CONCENTRATIONS

Although many clinicians believe that monitoring free or unbound plasma concentrations is desirable, it is not common in general clinical practice. The reasons are several and include the fact that assay procedures for free or unbound drug are not commercially available for many compounds. Furthermore, the assay procedures available for free drug concentrations are more expensive and increase the cost of providing patient care. Also, most patients exhibit reasonably normal binding characteristics; therefore, monitoring unbound drug concentrations would not add significantly to the evaluation of their clinical status. Whereas in theory monitoring unbound drug concentrations should be clinically superior, there is little evidence demonstrating that monitoring unbound drug levels improves the correlation between the plasma concentration and the pharmacologic effect or therapeutic outcome.

If unbound drug concentrations are to be used in clinical practice, the clinician must be aware of factors that can alter the relationship between in vitro to in vivo plasma binding characteristics. For example, the method used to determine the free drug level (equilibrium dialysis, ultrafiltration, saliva sampling, etc.) and the conditions under which the sample is obtained can alter the in vitro assay results. This in turn can result in an inaccurate estimate of the in vivo binding characteristics.[15,29-32] For these reasons, the use of unbound or free plasma level monitoring is not the standard of practice and is used in only a limited number of clinical settings. If unbound serum drug concentrations are used infrequently, the results should be carefully evaluated and compared to both the expected free drug level and the clinical response of the patient.

Volume of Distribution (V)

The volume of distribution for a drug or the "apparent volume of distribution" does not necessarily refer to any physiologic compartment in the body.[1,36] It is simply the size of a compartment necessary to account for the total amount of drug in the body if it were present throughout the body at the same concentration found in the plasma (Fig. 6A). The equation for the volume of distribution is expressed as follows:

$$V = \frac{Ab}{C}$$ [Eq. 10]

where V is the apparent volume of distribution, Ab is the total amount of drug in the body, and C is the plasma concentration of drug.

The plasma volume of the average adult is approximately 3 liters (L). Therefore, apparent volumes of distribution that are larger than the plasma compartment (> 3 L) only indicate that the drug is also present in

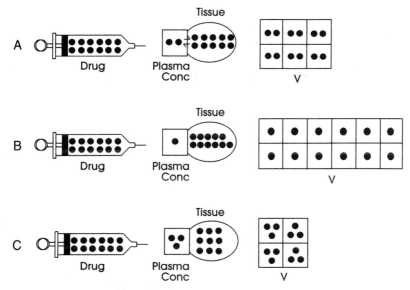

FIGURE 6. Volume of distribution. (A) The administration of a drug into the body produces a specific plasma concentration. The apparent volume of distribution (V) is the volume that accounts for the total dose administration based on the observed plasma concentration. **(B)** Any factor that decreases the drug plasma concentration (e.g., decreased plasma protein binding) will increase the apparent volume of distribution. **(C)** Conversely, any factor that increases the plasma concentration (e.g., decreased tissue binding) will decrease the apparent volume of distribution.

tissues or fluids outside the plasma compartment. The actual sites of distribution cannot be determined from the V value. For example, a drug with a volume of distribution similar to total body water (0.65 L/kg) does not indicate that the drug is equilibrated equally throughout the total body water. The drug may or may not be bound in certain tissues. However, the average binding results in an apparent volume of distribution that is approximately equal to that of total body water. Without additional specific information, the actual sites of a drug's distribution are only speculative.

The apparent volume of distribution is a function of the lipid versus water solubilities and of the plasma and tissue protein binding properties of the drug. Factors that tend to keep the drug in the plasma or increase C (such as low lipid solubility, increased plasma protein binding, or decreased tissue binding) reduce the apparent volume of distribution. It follows then that factors which decrease C (such as decreased plasma protein binding, increased tissue binding, and increased lipid solubility) increase the apparent volume of distribution.

LOADING DOSE

Because the volume of distribution is the factor that accounts for all of the drug in the body, it is an important variable in estimating the loading dose necessary to rapidly achieve a desired plasma concentration:

$$\text{Loading Dose} = \frac{(V)(C)}{(S)(F)} \qquad \text{[Eq. 11]}$$

where V is the volume of distribution, C is the desired plasma level, and (S)(F) represents the fraction of the dose administered that will reach the systemic circulation (Fig. 7).

For example, if one wishes to calculate an oral loading dose of digoxin (i.e., using digoxin tablets) for a 70 kg man that will produce a plasma concentration of 1.5 μg/L, Equation 11 can be used. If S is assumed to be 1.0, F to be 0.7, and V to be 7.3 L/kg,[1,3,37] the loading dose will be 1095 μg or 1.095 mg based on the following calculation:

$$\text{Loading Dose} = \frac{(V)(C)}{(S)(F)}$$

$$= \frac{(7.3 \text{ L/kg})(70 \text{ kg})(1.5 \text{ μg/L})}{(1)(0.7)}$$

$$= 1095 \text{ μg or } 1.095 \text{ mg}$$

A reasonable approximation of this dose would be 1 mg given orally as tablets. The usual clinical approach is to give the loading dose in divided doses (0.25 to 0.5 mg per dose every 6 hours). The patient is ob-

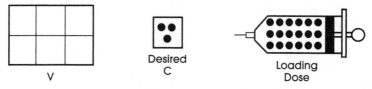

FIGURE 7. Loading dose. The volume of distribution is the major determinant of the loading dose. If the V for a drug is known, the loading dose that will produce a specific concentration can be calculated easily (see Equation 11).

served and evaluated for therapeutic response and digoxin toxicity before each successive dose is administered. In addition, some clinicians use a bioavailability factor > 0.7 (e.g., 0.75 or 0.8), which would further decrease the chance of exceeding the desired drug concentration.

Equation 11 can also be used to estimate the loading dose that will be required to achieve a higher plasma concentration than the present concentration (Fig. 8). This new formula is derived by replacing the C in Equation 11 with an expression that represents the increment in plasma concentration which is desired.

$$\text{Incremental Loading Dose} = \frac{(V)(C_{desired} - C_{initial})}{(S)(F)} \qquad \text{[Eq. 12]}$$

For example, if the previous patient had a digoxin level of 0.5 µg/L and the desired concentration was 1.5 µg/L, the loading dose would have been:

$$\text{Incremental Loading Dose} = \frac{(V)(C_{desired} - C_{initial})}{(S)(F)}$$

$$= \frac{(7.3 \text{ L/kg})(70 \text{ kg})(1.5 \text{ µg/L} - 0.5 \text{ µg/L})}{(1)(0.7)}$$

$$= 730 \text{ µg or } 0.73 \text{ mg}$$

A reasonable incremental loading dose in this case would be about 0.75 mg.

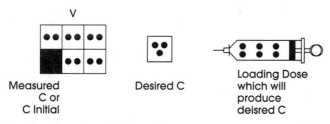

FIGURE 8. Loading dose to produce an increment in plasma level. If the V and initial plasma concentration for a drug are known, the incremental loading dose that will produce a higher desired plasma concentration can be calculated (see Equation 12).

FACTORS THAT ALTER VOLUME OF DISTRIBUTION (V) AND LOADING DOSE

In analyzing Equation 11, it becomes clear that any factor that alters the volume of distribution will theoretically influence the loading dose.

Decreased tissue binding of drugs in uremic patients is a common cause of a reduced apparent volume of distribution for several agents (Fig. 6C).[38,39] Decreased tissue binding will increase the C by allowing more of the drug to remain in the plasma. Therefore, if the desired plasma level remains unchanged, a smaller loading dose will be required. Digoxin is an example of a drug whose loading dose should be altered in uremic patients. This is discussed in Part Two: Digoxin.

Decreased plasma protein binding, on the other hand, tends to increase the apparent volume of distribution because more drug that would normally be in plasma is available to equilibrate with the tissue and the tissue binding sites (Fig. 6B). Decreased plasma protein binding, however, also increases the fraction of free or active drug so that the desired C that produces a given therapeutic response decreases. To summarize, diminished plasma protein binding increases V and decreases C in Equation 11, resulting in no net effect on the loading dose.

$$\overset{\leftrightarrow}{\text{Loading Dose}} = \frac{(\uparrow V)(C \downarrow)}{(S)(F)}$$

This is based on the assumption that the majority of drug in the body is actually outside the plasma compartment and that the amount of drug bound to plasma protein comprises only a small percentage of the total amount in the body.

This principle is illustrated by the pharmacokinetic behavior of phenytoin in uremic patients. Plasma phenytoin concentrations in uremic patients are frequently one half of those observed in normal patients given the same dose. The lower plasma levels, however, produce the same free or pharmacologically active phenytoin concentration as levels twice as high in non-uremic patients because the free fraction (fu) is increased from 0.1 to 0.2 in these individuals, indicating that the target plasma concentrations (bound + free) in uremics should be about half of the usual target concentration. Furthermore, a loading dose of phenytoin which produces a normal therapeutic effect is the same for both uremic and non-uremic patients because the volume of distribution increases by approximately twofold (0.65 L/kg to 1.44 L/kg) in uremic individuals.[26] Equation 11 indicates that there would be no change in the loading dose if the volume of distribution is increased by a factor of 2 and the desired drug concentration is decreased by a factor of ½.

$$\overset{\leftrightarrow}{\text{Loading Dose}} = \frac{(2 \times V)(1/2 \times C)}{(S)(F)}$$

TWO-COMPARTMENT MODELS

Pharmacokinetic Parameters

If one thinks of the body as a single compartment, pharmacokinetic calculations are relatively simple. However, there are some situations in which it is more appropriate to conceptualize the body as two, and occasionally, more than two compartments when thinking about drug distribution, elimination, and pharmacologic effect. The first compartment can be thought of as a smaller, rapidly equilibrating volume, usually made up of plasma or blood and those organs or tissues that have high blood flow and are in rapid equilibrium with the blood or plasma drug concentration. This first compartment has a volume referred to as Vi or initial volume of distribution. The second compartment equilibrates with the drug over a somewhat longer period. This volume is referred to as Vt or tissue volume of distribution.[36,40] The half-time for the distribution phase is referred to as the alpha (α) half-life, and the half-time for drug elimination from the body is referred to as the beta (β) half-life. The sum of Vi and Vt is the apparent volume of distribution (V). Drugs are assumed to enter into and be eliminated from Vi. That is, any drug that distributes into the tissue compartment (Vt) must re-equilibrate into Vi before it can be eliminated (Fig. 9).

Effects of a Two-Compartment Model on the Loading Dose and Plasma Concentration (C)

Because some time is required for a drug to distribute into Vt, a rapidly administered loading dose calculated on the basis of V (Vi + Vt) would result in an initial C that is higher than predicted because the initial volume of distribution (Vi) is always smaller than V. The consequences of such an inaccurate prediction depend on whether the target organ behaves as though it were located in Vi or Vt.

Drugs such as lidocaine, phenobarbital, procainamide, and theophylline exert therapeutic and toxic effects on target organs that behave as though they are located in Vi. In these instances, when loading doses are calculated based on the total volume of distribution, the concentration of drug delivered to the target organs could be much higher than expected and produce toxicity if the loading dose is not administered appropriately. This problem can be circumvented by first calculating the loading dose based on the total volume of distribution (V), then administering the loading dose at a rate slow enough to allow for drug distribution into Vt. This approach is common in clinical practice, and the guidelines for rates of drug administration are often based on the principle of two-compartment modeling with the receptors for clinical response (toxic or therapeutic) responding as though they were located in Vi. A second approach is to administer the loading dose in sufficiently small individual bolus doses such that the C in Vi does not exceed some predetermined critical concentration.[41,42]

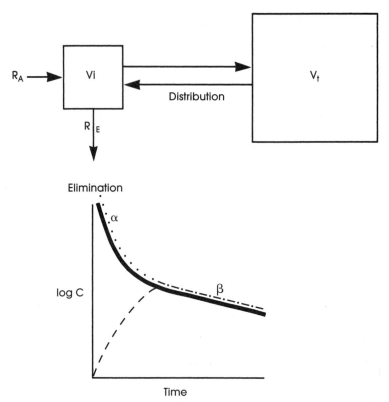

FIGURE 9. Two-compartment model. Volumes of distribution for a two-compartment model. Vi is the initial volume of distribution. Drug administration (R_A) and elimination (R_E) are assumed to occur in Vi. The lower graph shows that following rapid administration of drug into Vi, the plasma concentration (———) follows a biphasic decay pattern. The initial decay half-life ($\alpha t\frac{1}{2}$) is usually due to drug distribution into Vt. The second decay half-life ($\beta t\frac{1}{2}$) is usually due to drug elimination from the body. The dotted line (·····) represents the drug effect when the end-organ for effect is located in Vi. Note that drug effect parallels the plasma concentration at all times. The dashed line (-----) represents the drug effect when the end-organ for effect is located in Vt. Note that initially when all of the drug is in Vi there is no drug effect. However, as distribution takes place, the drug effect increases and begins to parallel the plasma concentration only in the elimination phase after distribution is complete.

Although not commonly discussed in pharmacokinetic terms, potassium is a good example of a drug that follows this principle of two-compartment modeling with the end-organ being located in Vi. Potassium is primarily an intracellular electrolyte but its cardiac effects parallel the plasma concentration. In addition, there is a slow equilibrium between plasma and tissue potassium concentrations. When potassium is given intravenously, the rate of administration must be carefully controlled as serious cardiac toxicity and death will occur if the patient experiences excessive plasma (Vi) concentrations.

This concept of two-compartment modeling is also important in evaluating the offset of drug effect. For drugs with the end-organ for clinical response located in Vi, rapid achievement of a therapeutic response followed quickly by a loss of the therapeutic response may be the result of drug being distributed into a larger volume of distribution rather than drug being eliminated from the body (see Part Two: Lidocaine).

When the drug's target organ is in the second or tissue compartment, Vt (e.g., digoxin, lithium), the rather high C, which may be observed before distribution occurs, is not dangerous. However, plasma concentrations that are obtained before distribution is complete will not reflect the tissue concentration at equilibrium. Therefore, these plasma samples cannot be used to predict the therapeutic or toxic potential of these drugs.[43,44] For example, clinicians usually wait 1 to 3 hours after an intravenous bolus dose of digoxin before evaluating the effect. This delay allows the digoxin to distribute to the site of action (myocardium) so that the full therapeutic or toxic effects of a dose can be observed (see Part Two: Digoxin and Fig. 4.1).

Slow drug distribution into the tissue compartment can pose problems in the accurate interpretation of a drug concentration when a drug is given by the intravenous route. It is not generally a problem when a drug is given orally, because the rate of absorption is usually slower than the rate of distribution from Vi into Vt. Nevertheless, digoxin and lithium are exceptions to this rule. Even when these drugs are given orally, several hours are required for complete absorption and distribution.

Plasma samples obtained less than 6 hours after an oral dose of digoxin or less than 12 hours after an oral dose of lithium are of questionable value. For these two drugs, the receptors in the end-organs behave as though they are located in the more slowly equilibrating tissue compartment or Vt. Plasma concentrations obtained during the distribution phase (before equilibrium with the deep tissue compartment is complete) will be increased, and the pharmacologic response will be much less than the plasma concentration would indicate.

Drugs With Significant and Nonsignificant Two-Compartment Modeling

As illustrated in Figure 9, the alpha phase for most drugs represents distribution of drug from Vi into Vt, and relatively little drug is eliminated during the distribution phase. Drugs that behave in this way are generally referred to as "nonsignificant" two-compartmental drugs. What this statement of "nonsignificant" means is that if the patient is not harmed by the initially elevated drug concentration in the alpha phase and no drug samples are taken in the alpha phase, then the drug can be successfully modeled as a one-compartment drug (i.e., only the elimination or beta phase is considered). It is important to recognize that for some drugs, increased drug plasma concentrations during the alpha phase can be clinically significant because the patient may experience serious toxicity if the end-organ behaves as though it lies within the initial volume of distribution (Vi). These drugs are considered to exhibit "nonsignificant" two-compartmental modeling only after the alpha phase or distribution has been completed. That is, plasma samples are obtained for pharmacokinetic modeling only during the beta or elimination phase.

Drugs with "significant" two-compartment modeling are those that are eliminated to a significant extent during the initial alpha phase. For these drugs (e.g., methotrexate), the alpha phase cannot be thought of simply as distribution, because significant elimination occurs as well. Two drugs that border on having significant two-compartment modeling are lithium and lidocaine. When a one-compartment model is used for drugs that exhibit significant drug elimination in the alpha phase, the actual trough concentrations will be lower than those predicted by the one-compartment model.

Some clinicians have suggested that these drugs could be more successfully monitored by use of two-compartmental model pharmacokinetics. The complexity of these models, however, as well as the number of plasma samples required for patient-specific dose adjustments, usually limits the use of two-compartmental modeling techniques.

Two-compartment computer models are available for therapeutic drug monitoring. Usually, the value of these two-compartment computer models is that they can compensate or adjust for drug samples that have been obtained in the distribution phase. If care is taken to avoid obtaining samples in the distribution phase, very similar pharmacokinetic interpretations are usually arrived at using the simpler one-compartment model.

Clearance (Cl)

Clearance can be thought of as the intrinsic ability of the body or its organs of elimination (usually the kidneys and the liver) to remove drug from the blood or plasma. Clearance is expressed as a volume per unit of time. It is important to emphasize that clearance is not an indicator of how much drug is being removed; it only represents the theoretical volume of blood or plasma which is completely cleared of drug in a given period. The amount of drug removed depends on the plasma concentration of drug and the clearance (Fig. 10).

At steady state, the rate of drug administration (R_A) and rate of drug elimination (R_E) must be equal [also see Elimination Rate Constant (K)].

$$R_A = R_E \qquad \text{[Eq. 13]}$$

STEADY STATE

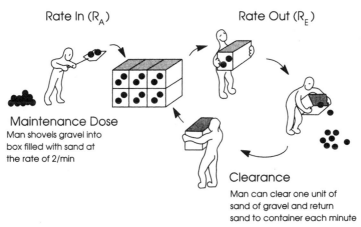

Rate In (R_A)

Rate Out (R_E)

Maintenance Dose
Man shovels gravel into
box filled with sand at
the rate of 2/min

Clearance
Man can clear one unit of
sand of gravel and return
sand to container each minute

FIGURE 10. Steady state, maintenance dose, clearance, elimination rate constant.
At steady state, the rate of drug administration (R_A) is equal to the rate of drug elimination (R_E), and the concentration of drug remains constant. In this example, the man on the left is able to shovel gravel or "drug" into a container of sand at the rate of 2/min. The man on the right is able to remove one unit of sand containing gravel or "drug" from the container, dump the gravel, and return the sand to the container each minute. The amount of gravel or "drug" removed per unit of time (rate of elimination) will be determined by the concentration of gravel per unit of sand as well as the clearance (volume of sand cleared of gravel). The elimination rate constant (K) can be thought of as the fraction of the total volume cleared per unit of time. In this case, K would be equal to $\frac{1}{6}$ or 0.17min^{-1}.

Clearance (Cl) can best be thought of as the proportionality constant that makes the average steady-state plasma drug level equal to the rate of drug administration (R_A):

$$R_A = (Cl)(Css\ ave) \qquad \text{[Eq. 14]}$$

where R_A is $(S)(F)(Dose)/\tau$ (see Equation 5), and Css ave is the average steady-state drug concentration.

If an average steady-state plasma concentration and the rate of drug administration are known, the clearance can be calculated by rearranging Equation 14:

$$Cl = \frac{(S)(F)(Dose/\tau)}{Css\ ave} \qquad \text{[Eq. 15]}$$

For example, if intravenous lidocaine is infused continuously at a rate of 2 mg/min and if the concentration of lidocaine at steady state is 3 mg/L, the calculated lidocaine clearance using Equation 15 would be 0.667 L/min:

$$Cl = \frac{(S)(F)(Dose/\tau)}{Css\ ave}$$
$$= \frac{(1)(1)(2\ mg/min)}{3\ mg/L}$$
$$= 0.667\ L/min$$

or a clearance of 40 L/hr if the administration rate of lidocaine were expressed as mg/hr.

$$Cl = \frac{(S)(F)(Dose/\tau)}{Css\ ave}$$
$$= \frac{(1)(1)(120\ mg/hr)}{3\ mg/L}$$
$$= 40\ L/hr$$

F is considered to be 1.0 because the drug is being administered intravenously. S is also assumed to be 1.0 because the hydrochloride salt represents only a small fraction of the total molecular weight for lidocaine and correction for the salt form is unnecessary.

MAINTENANCE DOSE

If an estimate for clearance is obtained from the literature, the clearance formula (Equation 15) can be rearranged slightly and used to calculate the rate of administration or maintenance dose which will produce a desired average plasma concentration at steady state:

$$\text{Maintenance Dose} = \frac{(Cl)(Css\ ave)(\tau)}{(S)(F)} \qquad \text{[Eq. 16]}$$

For example, using the literature estimate for theophylline clearance of 2.8 L/hr, the rate of intravenous administration for theophylline that will produce a steady-state plasma theophylline concentration of 10 mg/L is illustrated below:

$$\text{Maintenance Dose} = \frac{(Cl)(Css\ ave)(\tau)}{(S)(F)}$$
$$= \frac{(2.8\ L/hr)(10\ mg/L)(1\ hr)}{(1)(1)}$$
$$= 28\ mg\ given\ every\ hour$$

Since τ is 1 hour, the rate of administration is 28 mg/hr. If the theophylline were to be given every 12 hours, the dose would be 336 mg or 12 times the hourly administration rate to maintain the same average steady-state concentration.

$$\text{Maintenance Dose} = \frac{(Cl)(Css\ ave)(\tau)}{(S)(F)}$$
$$= \frac{(2.8\ L/hr)(10\ mg/L)(12\ hr)}{(1)(1)}$$
$$= 336\ mg\ to\ be\ given\ every\ 12\ hours$$

The units for volume and time in clearance are somewhat arbitrary but must be consistent with the units for the drug administration rate and drug concentration.

Administration rate	Mass/time
Drug concentration	Mass/volume
Clearance	Volume/time

As an example, if the drug administration rate is in mg/hr and concentration is in mg/L, then clearance would have to be in L/hr. Conversely, if the administration rate were mg/day and concentration in mg/L, then clearance would have to be in L/day. Again the units are somewhat arbitrary, but clinicians usually use values that are consistent with how the drug is used in clinical practice. In some cases conversions need to be made. Methotrexate is usually administered as grams or milligrams, but methotrexate concentrations are reported in units of micromolar or micromoles/L. Care should be taken to be sure the appropriate units are used (see Part Two: Methotrexate).

FACTORS THAT ALTER CLEARANCE (Cl)

Body Surface Area (BSA)

Most literature values for clearance are expressed as volume/kg/time or as volume/70 kg/time. There is some evidence, however, that drug clearance is best adjusted on the basis of body surface area rather than weight.[45-50] Body surface area can be calculated using Equation 17 or it can be obtained from various charts and nomograms[51-53] (see Appendix I).

$$\text{BSA in m}^2 = \left(\frac{\text{Patient's Weight in kg}}{70 \text{ kg}} \right)^{0.7} (1.73 \text{ m}^2) \qquad \text{[Eq. 17]}$$

The value of a patient's weight divided by 70 taken to the 0.7 power is an attempt to scale or size a patient as a fraction of the average 1.73 m^2 or 70 kg individual. Weight divided by 70 taken to the 0.7 power has no units and should be thought of as the fraction of the average-size person.

As an example, a 7-kg patient has a weight ratio relative to 70 kg of 0.1 and, therefore, may be thought of as having a size and thus a metabolic and renal capacity that is one tenth of the average 70-kg person.

$$\left(\frac{7 \text{ kg}}{70 \text{ kg}} \right) = 0.1$$

TABLE 2   Factors That Alter Clearance (Cl)

Body weight
Body surface area
Cardiac output
Drug-drug interactions
Extraction ratio
Genetics
Hepatic function
Plasma protein binding
Renal function

If the same weight individual was compared to the 70-kg standard using weight to the 0.7 power, the ratio becomes 0.2 or 20% the size and clearance capacity of the standard 70 kg or 1.73 m² individual.

$$\left(\frac{7 \text{ kg}}{70 \text{ kg}} \right)^{0.7} = 0.2$$

In the example above, the difference between 0.1 and 0.2 is large. However, when patients do not differ significantly from 70 kg, the difference between using weight versus weight to the power 0.7 or body surface area becomes less significant.

It is also important to remember that the 0.2 has no units and represents the fraction of the average-size (1.73 m² or 70 kg) individual. Occasionally, the value of 0.2 is mistaken for the surface area or size of the patient in m². This is not correct and can lead to dosing errors.

The following formulas can be used to adjust the clearance values reported in the literature for specific patients. There are other equations one can use depending on units used in the literature for clearance.

Patient's Cl = (Literature Cl per m²)(Patient's BSA) [Eq. 18]

Patient's Cl = (Literature Cl per 70 kg)$\left(\dfrac{\text{Patient's BSA}}{1.73 \text{ m}^2} \right)$ [Eq. 19]

Patient's Cl = (Literature Cl per 70 kg)$\left(\dfrac{\text{Patient's Weight in kg}}{70 \text{ kg}} \right)$ [Eq. 20]

Patient's Cl = (Literature Cl per kg)(Patient's Weight in Kg) [Eq. 21]

Equations 20 and 21 adjust clearance in proportion to weight, whereas Equations 18 and 19 adjust clearance in proportion to body surface area.

The underlying assumption in using weight or surface area to adjust clearance is that the patient's liver and kidney size (and hopefully function) vary in proportion to these physical measurements. This may not always be the case; therefore, clearance values derived from the patient populations having a similar age and size should be used whenever possible. If the patient's weight is reasonably close to 70 kg (BSA = 1.73 m²), the patient's calculated clearance will be similar whether weight or body surface area are used to calculate clearance. If, however, the patient's weight differs significantly from 70 kg, then the use of weight or surface area is likely to generate substantially different estimates of the patient's clearance. When a patient's size is substantially greater or less than the standard 70 kg, or 1.73 m², a careful assessment should be made to determine if the patient's body stature is normal, obese, or emaciated. In obese and emaciated patients, neither weight nor surface area is likely to be helpful in predicting clearance, since the patient's body size will not reflect the size or function of the liver and kidney.

Plasma Protein Binding

For highly protein-bound drugs, diminished plasma protein binding is associated with a decrease in reported steady-state plasma drug concentrations (total of unbound plus free drug) for any given dose that is administered [see Fig. 5 and Desired Plasma Concentration (C)]. According to Equation 15, a decrease in the denominator, Css ave, increases the calculated clearance.

$$Cl = \frac{(S)(F)(Dose/\tau)}{Css\ ave}$$

It would be misleading, however, to assume that because the calculated clearance is increased, the amount eliminated per unit of time has increased. Equation 15 assumes that when Css ave (total of bound plus free drug) changes, the free drug concentration, which is available for metabolism and renal elimination, changes proportionately. In actuality, the free or unbound fraction of drug in the plasma[13,54] generally increases (even though Css ave decreases) with diminished plasma protein binding. As a result, the amount of free drug eliminated per unit of time remains unchanged.[28] This should be apparent if one considers that at steady state, the amount of drug administered per unit of time (R_A) must equal the amount eliminated per unit of time (R_E). If R_A has not changed, R_E must remain the same.

In summary, when the same daily dose of a drug is given in the presence of diminished protein binding, an amount equal to that dose will be eliminated from the body each day at steady state despite a diminished steady-state plasma concentration and an increase in the calculated clearance. This lower plasma concentration (C bound + C free) is associated with a decreased C bound, no change in C free, and as a result there is an increase in the fraction of unbound drug (fu).

$$\uparrow fu = \frac{C\ free}{\downarrow C\ bound + C\ free} \qquad [Eq.\ 22]$$

Therefore, the pharmacologic effect achieved will be similar to that produced by the higher serum concentration observed under normal protein binding conditions. This example re-emphasizes the principle that clearance alone is not a good indicator of the amount of drug eliminated per unit of time (R_E) (Figs. 11 and 12).

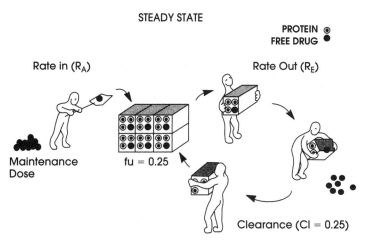

FIGURE 11. **Clearance (Cl) of a highly protein-bound drug with a low extraction ratio.** The free or unbound drug is available for clearance. Protein-bound drug is returned to the container so that the actual volume cleared of drug is ¼ of the total volume removed by the man and presented to the clearing organ (e.g., kidney or liver). (Compare with Figure 10.)

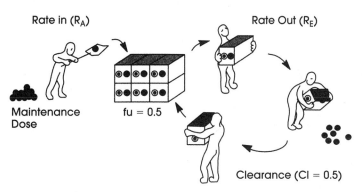

FIGURE 12. **Effect of diminished protein binding on clearance (Cl) of a highly protein-bound drug which has a low extraction ratio.** Compare this figure with Figure 11. The plasma concentration of drug has decreased, but the free concentration remains the same (fu is increased) (see Fig. 4). The volume cleared of drug has increased (½) compared to that cleared in Figure 11, even though the unbound concentration and amount of drug cleared per unit of time has remained unchanged. This illustrates the principle that the amount of a highly protein-bound drug cleared per unit of time or Rate of Elimination (R_E) remains the same if the increase in clearance is due to a decrease in plasma binding and the intrinsic metabolism or renal elimination remains unchanged.

This principle is illustrated by comparing phenytoin in an uremic and non-uremic patient at steady state. As noted previously in the discussion of desired plasma concentration, the steady-state unbound plasma phenytoin concentration (C free) will be the same in the uremic and non-uremic individual receiving the same daily dose and having the same metabolic capability. However, due to decreased protein binding, the concentration of bound (C bound) and therefore C total will be lower in the uremic than the non-uremic patient.

As an example, consider two patients with the same metabolic capability receiving phenytoin 300 mg/day. The first patient is non-uremic with a phenytoin concentration of 10 mg/L and normal plasma binding (fu = 0.1). The second patient is uremic with a phenytoin concentration of 5 mg/L and decreased plasma binding (fu = 0.2). If these two patients were to have their clearance calculated using Equation 15, it would appear as though the uremic patient has a higher clearance.

$$Cl = \frac{(S)(F)(Dose/\tau)}{Css\ ave}$$

Non-Uremic

$$Cl = \frac{(S)(F)(Dose/\tau)}{Css\ ave}$$

$$= \frac{(1)(1)(300\ mg/day)}{10\ mg/L}$$

$$= 30\ L/day$$

Uremic

$$Cl = \frac{(S)(F)(Dose/\tau)}{Css\ ave}$$

$$= \frac{(1)(1)(300\ mg/day)}{5\ mg/L}$$

$$= 60\ L/day$$

Although the calculated clearance for the uremic patient is higher than the non-uremic patient (60 L/day versus 30 L/day), the amount of drug cleared per day (300 mg) is the same, because at steady state the rate of drug administration (R_A) is equal to the rate of drug elimination (R_E) for both the uremic and non-uremic patient.

$$R_A = R_E$$

$$300\ mg/day = 300\ mg/day$$

When protein binding is decreased, the increase in calculated clearance is generally proportional to the change in fu. Although the calculated clearance may be used to estimate a maintenance dose, careful selection of the plasma level that will produce the desired unbound or free plasma level and pharmacologic effect is critical to the determination of a therapeutically correct maintenance dose.

Extraction Ratio

The direct proportionality between calculated clearance and fraction unbound (fu) does not apply to drugs that are so efficiently metabolized or excreted that some (perhaps all) of the drug bound to plasma protein is removed as it passes through the eliminating organ.[28,47,55] In this situation the plasma protein acts as a "transport system" for the drug, carrying it to the eliminating organs, and clearance becomes dependent on the blood or plasma flow to the eliminating organ. To determine whether the clearance for a drug with significant plasma binding will be influenced primarily by blood flow or plasma protein binding, its extraction ratio is estimated and compared to its fu value.

The extraction ratio is the fraction of the drug presented to the eliminating organ that is cleared after a single pass through that organ. It can be estimated by dividing the blood or plasma clearance of a drug by the blood or plasma flow to the eliminating organ. If the extraction ratio exceeds the free fraction (fu), then the plasma proteins are acting as a transport system and clearance will not change in proportion to fu. If, however, the extraction ratio is less than fu, clearance is likely to increase by the same proportion that fu changes. This approach does not take into account other factors that may affect clearance such as red blood cell binding, elimination from red blood cells, or changes in metabolic function.

Renal and Hepatic Function

Drugs can be eliminated or cleared as unchanged drug through the kidney (renal clearance) and by metabolism in the liver (metabolic clearance). These two routes of clearance are assumed to be independent of one another and additive.[36,40]

$$Cl_t = Cl_m + Cl_r \qquad \text{[Eq. 23]}$$

Where Cl_t is total clearance, Cl_m is metabolic clearance or the fraction cleared by metabolism, and Cl_r is renal clearance or the fraction cleared by the renal route. Because the kidneys and liver function independently, it is assumed that a change in one does not affect the other. Thus, Cl_t can be estimated in the presence of renal or hepatic failure or both. Because metabolic function is difficult to quantitate, Cl_t is most commonly adjusted when there is decreased renal function:

$$Cl\ Adjusted = (Cl_m) + \left[(Cl_r)\left(\frac{\text{Fraction of Normal Renal}}{\text{Function Remaining}}\right)\right] \qquad \text{[Eq. 24]}$$

A clearance that has been adjusted for renal function can be used to estimate the maintenance dose for a patient with diminished renal function (see Equation 16). This adjusted clearance equation, however, is only valid if the drug's metabolites are inactive and if the metabolic clearance is indeed unaffected by renal dysfunction as assumed. A decrease in the function of an organ of elimination is most significant when that organ serves as the primary route of drug elimination. However, as the major elimination pathway becomes increasingly compromised, the "minor" pathway becomes more significant because it assumes a greater proportion of the total clearance. For example, a drug that is usually 67% eliminated by the renal route and 33% by the metabolic route will be 100% metabolized in the event of complete renal failure; the total clearance, however, will only be one-third of the normal value.

As an alternative to adjusting Cl_t to calculate dosing rate, one can substitute fraction of the total clearance that is metabolic and renal for Cl_m and Cl_r. Using this technique the equation below can be derived.

Dosing Rate Adjustment Factor = [Eq. 25]

$$\left(\begin{array}{c}\text{Fraction Eliminated}\\\text{Metabolically}\end{array}\right) + \left[\left(\begin{array}{c}\text{Fraction Eliminated}\\\text{Renally}\end{array}\right)\left(\begin{array}{c}\text{Fraction of Normal Renal}\\\text{Function Remaining}\end{array}\right)\right]$$

The Dosing Rate Adjustment Factor can be used to adjust the maintenance dose for a patient with altered renal function.

As an example, take a drug that is 25% metabolized and 75% renally cleared and normally administered as 100 mg every 12 hours. If this drug were to be given to a patient who has only 33% of normal renal function, the Dosing Rate Adjustment Factor would be 0.5.

Dosing Rate Adjustment Factor =

$$\left(\begin{array}{c}\text{Fraction Eliminated}\\\text{Metabolically}\end{array}\right) + \left[\left(\begin{array}{c}\text{Fraction Eliminated}\\\text{Renally}\end{array}\right)\left(\begin{array}{c}\text{Fraction of Normal Renal}\\\text{Function Remaining}\end{array}\right)\right]$$

$$= (0.25) + [(0.75)(0.33)]$$

$$= (0.25) + [(0.25)]$$

$$= 0.5$$

The Dosing Rate Adjustment Factor of 0.5 suggests that the drug should be administered at half the usual rate. This could be accomplished by decreasing the dose and maintaining the same interval (e.g., 50 mg every 12 hours) or by maintaining the same dose and increasing the interval (e.g., 100 mg every 24 hours). Depending on the situation and therapeutic intent, either method (or a combination of dose and dosing interval adjustment) might be appropriate.

Most pharmacokinetic adjustments for drug elimination are based on renal function because hepatic function is usually more difficult to quantitate. Elevated liver enzymes do reflect liver damage but are not a good measure of function. Hepatic function is often evaluated using the prothrombin time, serum albumin concentration, and serum bilirubin concentration. Unfortunately, each of these laboratory tests is affected by variables other than altered hepatic function. For example, the serum albumin may be low due to decreased protein intake or increased renal or GI loss, as well as decreased hepatic function. Although liver function tests do not provide quantitative data, pharmacokinetic adjustments must still take into consideration liver function because this route of elimination is important for a significant number of drugs.

Cardiac Output

Cardiac output also affects drug metabolism. Hepatic or metabolic clearances for some drugs can be decreased by 25% to 50% in patients with congestive heart failure. For example, the metabolic clearances of theophylline[56] and digoxin[45] are reduced by approximately one-half in patients with congestive heart failure. Since the metabolic clearance for both of these drugs is much lower than the hepatic blood or plasma flow (low extraction ratio), it would not have been predicted that their clearances would have been influenced by cardiac output or hepatic blood flow to this extent. The decreased cardiac output and resultant hepatic congestion must, in some way, decrease the intrinsic metabolic capacity of the liver. The effect of diminished clearance on plasma drug concentrations is illustrated in Figure 13 (compare with Fig. 10).

NON STEADY STATE

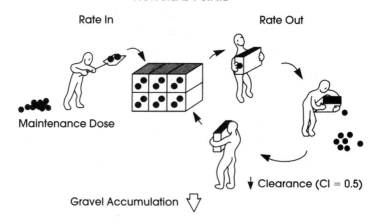

NEW STEADY STATE

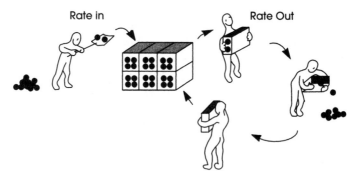

FIGURE 13. Effect of changes in clearance (Cl) on steady-state serum concentrations. Compare this figure with Figure 10. In the illustration above, the maintenance dose or amount of gravel added to the container per unit of time remains the same; however, the volume of sand cleared of gravel (clearance) has been halved. Initially, the amount of gravel or "drug" cleared per unit of time is less than the maintenance dose; the concentration of gravel in the container increases until a new steady state is reached. At this point, the rate at which gravel is added to the container again equals the rate at which gravels is eliminated from the container. If clearance had increased, the concentration of gravel would have decreased until the amount removed per unit of time (R_E) again equaled the rate of administration (R_A).

Elimination Rate Constant (K) and Half-Life (t½)

It is often desirable to predict how drug plasma levels will change with time. For drugs that are eliminated by first-order pharmacokinetics, these predictions are based on the elimination rate constant (K). The key characteristic of first-order elimination is that both clearance and volume of distribution do not vary with dose or concentration.

FIRST-ORDER PHARMACOKINETICS

First-order elimination pharmacokinetics refers to a process in which the amount or concentration of drug in the body diminishes logarithmically over time (Fig. 14).

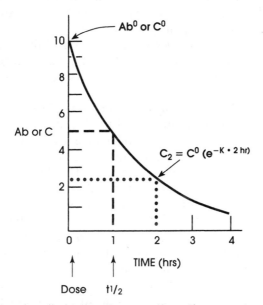

FIGURE 14. First-order elimination C versus time. The amount or concentration of drug diminishes logarithmically over time. The initial amount of plasma concentration produced by a loading dose is Ab^0 or C^0. The half-life (t½) is the time required to eliminate one-half of the drug. The concentration at the end of a given time interval (in this example, 2 hours) is equal to the initial concentration times the fraction of drug remaining at the end of that time interval ($e^{-K \cdot 2\,hr}$). The amount or concentration of drug lost in each 1-hour interval diminishes over time (5, 2.5, 1.25); however, the fraction of drug that is lost in each unit of time remains constant (0.5). For example, over the first hour (0–1 hr), of the total amount of drug in the body (10), one-half was lost (5). In the next time interval (1–2 hr), of the amount of drug that remained (5), one half was lost (2.5).

The rate of elimination (R_E) is proportional to the drug concentration; therefore, the amount of drug removed per unit of time (R_E) will vary in direct proportion to drug concentration. The fraction or percentage of the total amount of drug present in the body (Ab) that is removed at any instant in time, however, will remain constant and independent of dose or concentration. That fraction or percentage is expressed by the elimination rate constant, K. The equations that describe first-order elimination of a drug from the body are as follows:

$$Ab = (Ab°)(e^{-Kt}) \qquad \text{[Eq. 26]}$$

or

$$C = (C°)(e^{-Kt}) \qquad \text{[Eq. 27]}$$

where in Equation 26, Ab° and Ab represent the total amount of drug in the body at the beginning and end of the time interval, t, respectively; and e^{-Kt} is the fraction remaining at time t. In Equation 27, C° and C are the plasma concentrations at the beginning and end of the time interval, respectively. Because the drug concentration diminishes logarithmically, a graphic plot of the logarithm of the plasma level versus time yields a straight line (Fig. 15).

This type of graphical analysis of declining plasma drug concentrations is often used to determine if a drug is eliminated by a first-order process. The key element is that the drug concentration decay curve when plotted as C versus time is a concave curve (see Fig. 14) and when plotted as log C versus time is a straight line (see Fig. 15). One important assumption in this analysis is that there is no additional drug being absorbed or placed into the body during the decay process.

Because first-order drugs have a volume of distribution and clearance that are constant (assuming no change in a patient's clinical status), many but not all the dose to concentration relationships are proportional. As an example, the average steady-state concentration will be proportional to the dosing rate. Therefore, the steady-state concentration can be adjusted by altering the drug dosage rate in proportion to the desired change in concentration (Fig. 16).

Equation 27 can also be thought of as any initial drug concentration C_1 that is decayed over some time interval t_1 to calculate the subsequent drug concentration C_2.

$$C_2 = (C_1)(e^{-Kt_1}) \qquad \text{[Eq. 28]}$$

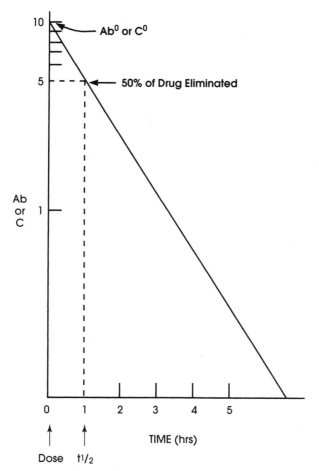

FIGURE 15. First-order elimination log C versus time. A graph of the log of Ab or C versus time yields a straight line. The half-life is the time required for Ab or C to decline to one-half the original value.

NON STEADY STATE

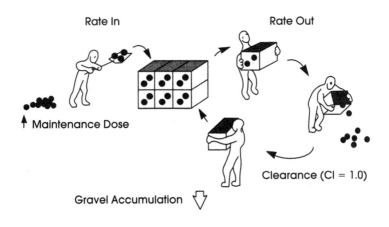

Rate In   Rate Out

↑ Maintenance Dose

Clearance (Cl = 1.0)

Gravel Accumulation ▽

NEW STEADY STATE

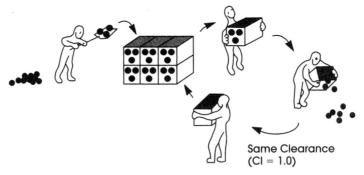

Same Clearance
(Cl = 1.0)

FIGURE 16. Effect of changes in maintenance dose on steady-state plasma concentrations. Compare this figure with Figure 10. In the illustration above, the clearance or volume of sand cleared of gravel remains the same; however, the maintenance dose or the amount of gravel added to the container per unit of time has been increased from 2/min to 3/min. Therefore, the concentration of gravel or "drug" increases until a new steady state is reached. At this point, the rate at which gravel is added to the container again equals the rate at which gravel is eliminated from the container. If the maintenance dose decreased, the concentration of gravel would have gradually decreased until a new steady state had been achieved.

ELIMINATION RATE CONSTANT (K)

The elimination rate constant, K, is the fraction or percentage of the total amount of drug in the body removed per unit of time and is a function of clearance and volume of distribution:

$$K = \frac{Cl}{V} \qquad \text{[Eq. 29]}$$

As the equation above illustrates, K can also be thought of as the fraction of the volume of distribution that will be cleared of drug per unit of time (see Fig. 10). For example, a drug with a clearance of 10 L/day and a V of 100 L would have an elimination rate constant of 0.1 days^{-1}.

$$K = \frac{10 \text{ L/day}}{100 \text{ L}}$$

$$= 0.1 \text{ days}^{-1}$$

The elimination rate constant of 0.1 days^{-1} indicates that in 1 day the volume cleared is 1/10th or 10% of the total volume of distribution. The value of K is based on the units used for clearance and volume of distribution and is somewhat arbitrary. As an example using the same clearance of 10 L/day expressed as 0.417 L/hr (10 L/day divided by 24 hours/day) and the V of 100 L, the corresponding K value would be 0.00417 hr^{-1} or 0.417% of the total volume of distribution cleared in 1 hour. As previously discussed, the units chosen for clearance and volume of distribution should be consistent with the units used to report the dose, concentration, and dosing interval [see Clearance (Cl) and Maintenance Dose].

Since the drug elimination rate constant is the slope of the natural log or ln C versus time plot, two plasma concentrations measured during the decay or elimination phase (i.e., between doses or following a single dose) can be used to calculate the K for a specific patient. The equation used to calculate K is a rearrangement of Equation 28:

$$C_2 = (C_1)(e^{-Kt})$$

$$\frac{C_2}{C_1} = e^{-Kt}$$

$$\ln\left(\frac{C_2}{C_1}\right) = -Kt$$

$$\ln\left(\frac{C_1}{C_2}\right) = Kt$$

$$\frac{\ln\left(\frac{C_1}{C_2}\right)}{t} = K$$

or

$$K = \frac{\ln\left(\frac{C_1}{C_2}\right)}{t} \qquad \text{[Eq. 30]}$$

where C_1 is the first or higher plasma concentration, C_2 is the second or lower plasma concentration, and t is the time interval between the plasma samples. For example, if C_1 is 5 mg/L and C_2 is 2 mg/L, and the time interval between the samples is 8 hours, the elimination rate constant (K) will be 0.115 hr^{-1}.

$$K = \frac{\ln\left(\dfrac{C_1}{C_2}\right)}{t}$$

$$= \frac{\ln\left(\dfrac{5\ \text{mg/L}}{2\ \text{mg/L}}\right)}{8\ \text{hr}}$$

$$= 0.115\ \text{hr}^{-1}$$

One of the key issues in using Equation 30 is that to estimate K accurately, the time between C_1 and C_2 should be at least one half-life [see Half-Life ($t\frac{1}{2}$)]. Said another way, C_2 should be equal to or less than half of C_1. This time interval of one half-life is a minimum, and an interval of longer than a half-life is desirable. Whereas K can be calculated from any two drug concentrations during a decay phase, when the interval is less than one half-life, assay error alone results in highly variable and inaccurate estimates of K.

HALF-LIFE (t½)

The elimination rate constant is often expressed in terms of a drug's half-life, a value that is more conveniently applied to the clinical setting. The half-life ($t\frac{1}{2}$) of a drug is the time required for the total amount of drug in the body or the plasma drug concentration to decrease by one-half (see Fig. 15). It sometimes is referred to as the β $t\frac{1}{2}$ to distinguish it from the half-life for distribution (α $t\frac{1}{2}$) in a two-compartment model, and it is a function of the elimination rate constant, K:

$$t\frac{1}{2} = \frac{0.693}{K} \qquad \text{[Eq. 31]}$$

If the K used in Equation 31 is derived from plasma concentrations obtained during the decay phase, then the time interval in which the samples are drawn should span at least one half-life as previously mentioned (see discussion of Equation 30).

Because the dosing interval is frequently equal to or shorter than the usual half-life for many drugs, it is often impractical to obtain peak and trough levels within a dosing interval to determine the half-life (e.g., theophylline, procainamide, digoxin, phenobarbital).

If the volume of distribution and clearance for a drug are known, the half-life can be estimated by using Equation 32 below. The half-life, like K, is dependent on and determined by Cl and V. This relationship is illustrated in Equation 32, which was obtained by substituting Equation 29 into Equation 31:

$$t\tfrac{1}{2} = \frac{0.693(V)}{Cl}$$
[Eq. 32]

The dependence of t½ or K on V and Cl is emphasized because the volume of distribution and clearance for a drug can change independently of one another and thus, affect the half-life or elimination constant in the same or opposite directions.

Another caution is appropriate at this point. It is a common misconception that because Equation 29 can be rearranged to:

$$Cl = (K)(V)$$
[Eq. 33]

that clearance is determined by K (or t½) and V; however, this is incorrect considering the physiologic model that is used in the application of pharmacokinetics to the clinical setting. Instead, K and t½ are dependent on clearance and the volume of distribution. Therefore, caution should be used when making any assumptions about the volume of distribution or clearance of a drug based solely on knowledge of its half-life. For example, if the half-life of a drug is prolonged, the clearance may be increased, decreased, or unchanged depending on corresponding changes in the volume of distribution. As a general principle, however, when the half-life of a drug is prolonged, it is more likely due to a decrease in clearance than an increase in volume of distribution. This is because the variability in both renal and hepatic function (i.e., clearance) is more likely to be altered than is the plasma and tissue distribution characteristics (volume of distribution) of a drug. However, there are situations when the volume of distribution is significantly altered and should be considered when using pharmacokinetics in the clinical setting (see Part Two: Aminoglycoside Antibiotics, Digoxin, Lidocaine, and Procainamide).

CLINICAL APPLICATION OF ELIMINATION RATE CONSTANT (K) AND HALF-LIFE (t½)

Time to Reach Steady State

Half-life is an important variable to consider when answering questions concerning time such as: "How long will it take a drug concentration to reach steady state on a constant dosage regimen?" or "How long will it

TABLE 3   Clinical Application of the Elimination Rate Constant (K) and Half-Life (t½)

1. Estimating the time to reach steady-state plasma concentrations after initiation or change in the maintenance dose
2. Estimating the time required to eliminate all or a portion of the drug from the body once it is discontinued
3. Predicting nonsteady-state plasma levels following the initiation of an infusion
4. Predicting a steady-state plasma level from a nonsteady-state plasma level obtained at a specific time following the initiation of an infusion
5. Given the degree of fluctuation in plasma concentration desired within a dosing interval, determine that interval; given the interval, determine the fluctuation in the plasma concentration

take for the drug concentration to reach steady state if the dosage regimen is changed?" When drugs are given chronically, they accumulate in the body until the amount administered in a given period (maintenance dose) is equal to the amount eliminated in that same period, that is, rate in equals rate out. When this occurs, drug concentrations in the plasma will plateau and will have reached "steady state" (see Figs. 10 and 16). The time required for a drug concentration to reach steady state is determined by the drug's half-life. It takes 1 half-life to reach 50%, 2 half-lives to reach 75%, 3 half-lives to reach 87.5%, 3.3 half-lives to reach 90%, and 4 half-lives to reach 93.75% of steady state. With each additional half-life, the residual fraction from steady state diminishes, and at some point (usually ≤10%) this residual is considered negligible, and steady state is assumed to have been achieved. In most clinical situations, the attainment of steady state can be assumed after 3 to 5 half-lives (Fig. 17).

Time for Drug Elimination

The half-life can also be used to determine how long it will take to effectively eliminate all the drug from the body after the drug has been discontinued. It takes 1 half-life to eliminate 50%, 2 half-lives to eliminate 75%, 3 half-lives to eliminate 87.5%, 3.3 half-lives to eliminate 90%, and 4 half-lives to eliminate 93.75% of the total amount of drug in the body. Again, in most clinical situations it can be assumed that all the drug has been effectively eliminated after 3 to 5 half-lives (Fig. 18).

Prediction of Plasma Levels Following Initiation of an Infusion

Often, when drugs are given by constant infusion, it is useful to predict the plasma concentrations that will be achieved at a specific period (Fig. 19). The rate at which a drug approaches steady state is also governed by the elimination rate constant; therefore, this parameter can be used to calcu-

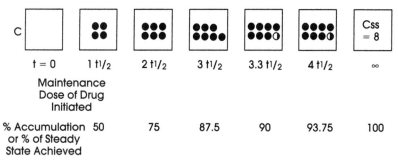

FIGURE 17. **First-order accumulation.** When a maintenance dose is initiated, it takes 3 to 5 half-lives to reach steady-state plasma levels; 3.3 half-lives represent 90% of steady-state. This example assumes that the maintenance dose administered will produce an average steady-state level (Css ave or Css) of 8.

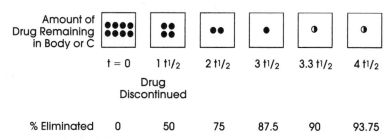

FIGURE 18. **First-order elimination: amount of drug remaining in the body after one to four half-lives have passed.** The amount of drug eliminated per unit of time diminishes over time, but the fraction eliminated in each time interval (in this case, 0.5 as the interval is one t½) remains the same; 3.3 t½ represents 90% eliminated or only 10% remaining.

late the fraction of steady state that is achieved at any time after the initiation of the infusion (t_1):

$$\text{Fraction of Steady State Achieved at time } t_1 = 1 - e^{-Kt_1} \qquad \text{[Eq. 34]}$$

The average plasma concentration at steady state (Css ave) can be calculated by rearranging the clearance formula (Equation 15):

$$Cl = \frac{(S)(F)(Dose/\tau)}{Css\ ave}$$

$$Css\ ave = \frac{(S)(F)(Dose/\tau)}{Cl} \qquad \text{[Eq. 35]}$$

The expected plasma concentration (C_1) at a specific time (t_1) after initiation of the infusion can be calculated by multiplying the average steady-state concentration (Css ave) by the fraction of steady state achieved at t_1.

$$C_1 = (Css\ ave)\left(\frac{\text{Fraction of Steady State}}{\text{Achieved at } t_1}\right) \qquad \text{[Eq. 36]}$$

If by substituting the appropriate parts of Equation 34 and Equation 35 into Equation 36 above, a new equation for plasma concentration C_1 at t_1 is derived:

$$C_1 = \frac{(S)(F)(Dose/\tau)}{Cl}(1 - e^{-Kt_1}) \qquad \text{[Eq. 37]}$$

All the units in Equation 37 must be consistent (e.g., time in τ, Cl, and t_1; volume in Cl, V, and C; mass in dose and C). According to Equation 37, as the duration of the infusion (t_1) approaches three to five half-lives, the fraction of steady state achieved approaches one, and for all practical purposes the patient is at steady state. Conversely, if a drug plasma concentration (C_1) was obtained before steady-state concentration was attained, the approximate steady-state concentration that should eventually be achieved can be estimated through rearrangement of Equation 37 and substituting Css ave for $(S)(F)(Dose/\tau)$:

$$Css\ ave = \frac{C_1}{1 - e^{-Kt_1}} \qquad \text{[Eq. 38]}$$

If the predicted steady-state concentration is unacceptably high, side effects or toxicities might be avoided by reducing the maintenance infusion before the achievement of steady state.

Prediction of Plasma Levels Following Discontinuation of an Infusion (Fig. 19)

The plasma concentration any time after an infusion is discontinued (C_2) can be estimated by multiplying the measured or predicted plasma concentration (C_1) at the time the infusion is discontinued by the fraction of drug remaining at t_2 hours from the end of the infusion.

$$\frac{\text{Fraction of Drug}}{\text{Remaining at } t_2} = (e^{-Kt_2}) \qquad \text{[Eq. 39]}$$

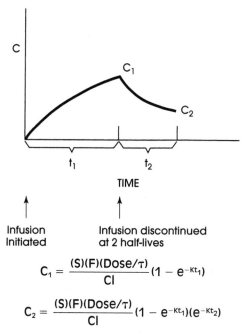

$$C_1 = \frac{(S)(F)(Dose/\tau)}{Cl}(1 - e^{-Kt_1})$$

$$C_2 = \frac{(S)(F)(Dose/\tau)}{Cl}(1 - e^{-Kt_1})(e^{-Kt_2})$$

FIGURE 19. Graphic representation of an infusion that is discontinued before steady state. C_1 is a concentration that is achieved any time (t_1) after the infusion is initiated, and C_2 is a concentration that results any interval of time (t_2) after the infusion has been discontinued.

$$C_2 = (C_1)(e^{-Kt_2}) \qquad \text{[Eq. 40]}$$

If the right side of Equation 37:

$$C_1 = \frac{(S)(F)(Dose/\tau)}{Cl}(1 - e^{-Kt_1})$$

is substituted for C_1 in Equation 40, the plasma concentration (C_2) at any time (t_2) after an infusion is discontinued is as follows:

$$C_2 = \frac{(S)(F)(Dose/\tau)}{Cl}(1 - e^{-Kt_1})(e^{-Kt_2}) \qquad \text{[Eq. 41]}$$

(see Figure 19).

Although Equation 41 may look complicated, it is really a series of simpler equations linked together to model the continuous infusion that was discontinued before steady state (Equation 37) followed by a first-order decay (Equation 39).

Calculation of a theophylline concentration, which will be expected 8 hours after a theophylline infusion of 80 mg/hr is discontinued, can be used to illustrate this principle. Assume that theophylline has been administered for 16 hours to a patient with a theophylline clearance of 2.8 L/hr and a half-life of 8 hours (K of 0.087 hr^{-1}). The calculations can be accomplished step by step as follows:

1. The expected steady-state theophylline concentration resulting from a theophylline infusion of 80 mg/hr to a patient with a theophylline clearance of 2.8 L/hr and an assumed S and F of 1 can be calculated using Equation 35:

$$\text{Css ave} = \frac{(S)(F)(Dose/\tau)}{Cl}$$

$$= \frac{(1)(1)(80 \text{ mg}/1 \text{ hr})}{2.8 \text{ L/hr}}$$

$$= 28.6 \text{ mg/L}$$

2. The expected concentration after 16 hours of infusion (t_1) can be calculated using Equation 37:

$$C_1 = \frac{(S)(F)(Dose/\tau)}{Cl}(1 - e^{-Kt_1})$$

$$C_1 = 28.6 \text{ mg/L } (1 - e^{-(0.087 \text{ hr}^{-1})(16 \text{ hr})})$$

$$= 28.6 \text{ mg/L } (1 - e^{-1.392})$$

$$= 28.6 \text{ mg/L } (1 - 0.25)$$

$$= 21.45 \text{ mg/L}$$

3. The expected concentration 8 hours after the end of the infusion can be calculated using Equation 40:

$$C_2 = (C_1)(e^{-Kt_2})$$

$$C_2 = 21.45 \text{ mg/L } (e^{-(0.087 \text{ hr}^{-1})(8 \text{ hr})})$$

$$= 21.45 \text{ mg/L } (e^{-0.696})$$

$$= 21.45 \text{ mg/L } (0.5)$$

$$= 10.7 \text{ mg/L}$$

Of course, these three steps could have been combined by using Equation 41 where t_1 would be 16 hours and t_2 would be 8 hours.

$$C_2 = \frac{(S)(F)(Dose/\tau)}{Cl}(1 - e^{-Kt_1})(e^{-Kt_2})$$

Whether the step-wise or single combined equation is used depends on how the sequence of events is visualized and therefore how the problem or equation is expressed (see Fig. 19).

Dosing Interval (τ)

The half-life can also be used to estimate the appropriate dosing interval or tau (τ) for maintenance therapy when a drug is administered intermittently and the absorption or input into the body is relatively rapid. For example, if the goal of therapy is to minimize plasma fluctuations to no more than 50% between doses, the dosing interval (τ) should be less than or equal to the half-life. The maintenance dose can be calculated using Equation 16:

$$\text{Maintenance Dose} = \frac{(Cl)(Css\ ave)(\tau)}{(S)(F)}$$

If tau is less than or equal to the half-life of a drug, the calculated maintenance dose will produce plasma concentrations that will fluctuate by ≤ 50% during that dosing interval. The plasma levels will be above the average steady-state plasma level for the first half of the dosing interval and below the average steady-state plasma level during the second half of the dosing interval (Fig. 20).

If the approximate half-life and dosing interval are known, the degree of change in plasma drug concentration that will occur over a dosing interval can be determined. Once the degree of fluctuation is known, one can then determine whether the primary determinant of plasma levels between dosing intervals is the volume of distribution or the clearance.

In certain situations, the dosing interval is much longer than the half-life and, for practical purposes, all the drug is eliminated before the next dose. Therefore, each new dose is essentially a new loading dose. In this situation, the peak concentration will be determined primarily by the volume of distribution because almost no drug remains from the previous dose.

Antibiotics are commonly dosed in this manner. The therapeutic index for antibiotics is usually so large that wide fluctuations in plasma levels are acceptable and perhaps even desirable.[57,58] Furthermore, the therapeutic effect may require a plasma level that is above the minimal bactericidal or inhibitory concentration for only a brief period relative to the dosing interval.[59]

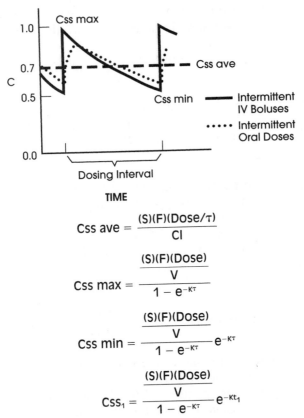

$$Css\ ave = \frac{(S)(F)(Dose/\tau)}{Cl}$$

$$Css\ max = \frac{\dfrac{(S)(F)(Dose)}{V}}{1 - e^{-K\tau}}$$

$$Css\ min = \frac{\dfrac{(S)(F)(Dose)}{V}}{1 - e^{-K\tau}}e^{-K\tau}$$

$$Css_1 = \frac{\dfrac{(S)(F)(Dose)}{V}}{1 - e^{-K\tau}}e^{-Kt_1}$$

FIGURE 20. **Plasma level-time curve for intermittent dosing at steady state.** When the dosing interval is equal to the half-life, plasma concentrations are above the average steady-state plasma concentration (Css ave) approximately 50% of the time. Oral administration dampens the curve considerably, and the maximum concentration at steady state (Css max) occurs later and is lower than that produced by IV bolus. The minimum concentration at steady state (Css min) is greater than that produced by IV bolus doses because of the effect of absorption. In the equations above, τ is the interval between doses and t_1 is the time from the theoretical peak concentration following a dose to the time of sampling.

When the dosing interval is much shorter than the half-life, the plasma concentration fluctuates very little throughout the dosing interval. In this case, the plasma concentration will be primarily determined by clearance. Digoxin and phenobarbital given orally and any drug administered by a constant infusion or as a sustained-release dosage form that releases the drug over the entire dosing interval are good examples of such a situation (also see Maximum and Minimum Plasma Concentrations).

Determining the parameter that primarily affects plasma concentration for any given dosage regimen (when τ is longer or shorter than $t\frac{1}{2}$) is important because one then knows which parameters can be calculated reliably from the reported steady-state plasma concentrations. For example, if a patient who has been taking a dose of 0.375 mg of digoxin daily has a reported steady-state trough plasma concentration of 3.8 µg/L, one can reliably calculate the digoxin clearance for this patient using Equation 15.

$$Cl = \frac{(S)(F)(Dose/\tau)}{Css\ ave}$$

Since the dosing interval is much shorter than the half-life, the trough concentration is a good approximation of the Css ave and therefore clearance is the major determinant of the patient's plasma concentration. One cannot reliably use the reported plasma concentration to calculate V because the average steady-state concentration is only a function of clearance (see Maximum and Minimum Plasma Concentrations).

With a new clearance value, one can estimate a new maintenance dose. Loading doses are based on volume of distribution and would require a literature estimate, as no patient-specific information about V can be determined from this drug level. In addition, using the value of V from the literature and our revised clearance, a new estimate of K (Equation 29) or t½ (Equation 32) can be obtained:

$$K = \frac{Cl_{revised}}{V_{assumed}}$$

$$t\tfrac{1}{2} = \frac{0.693(V_{assumed})}{Cl_{revised}}$$

Of course, the confidence in this new K or t½ would be dependent on the confidence in the assumed value of V derived from the literature.

Maximum and Minimum Plasma Concentrations

It is often important to estimate the maximum (Css max or peak) and minimum (Css min or trough) plasma drug concentrations produced by a given dose of drug within the dosing interval at steady state (see Fig. 20). For example, whereas it is critical in gentamicin therapy to achieve an acceptable peak concentration for efficacy, it is also important that the trough level be below a specified concentration to minimize concentration-related toxicity.

For drugs with a narrow therapeutic index (e.g., theophylline), it is useful to determine the degree of fluctuation in plasma drug concentration that will occur between doses. This can be particularly important if the dosing interval is longer than the half-life (i.e., fluctuations will be large) and Css min levels are being used to monitor therapy.

Most frequently, plasma samples for drug assays are drawn as a trough or just before a dose because Css min levels are the most reproducible. The reported plasma drug concentrations for these samples are often considered to be average steady-state concentrations (Css ave). However, when the dosing interval approaches or exceeds the drug's half-life, a patient's pharmacokinetic parameters can be more accurately estimated by using an equation that describes Css min rather than Css ave [see Minimum Plasma Drug Concentration (Css min)].

MAXIMUM PLASMA DRUG CONCENTRATION (Css MAX)

The maximum plasma drug concentration can be calculated from Equation 43 if the dose, salt form (S), bioavailability (F), volume of distribution (V), and elimination rate constant (K) are known:

$$\text{Css max} = \frac{\Delta C}{\text{Fraction of Drug Lost in } \tau} \qquad \text{[Eq. 42]}$$

or

$$\text{Css max} = \frac{\dfrac{(S)(F)(Dose)}{V}}{1 - e^{-K\tau}} \qquad \text{[Eq. 43]}$$

where ΔC and $(S)(F)(Dose)/V$ represent the change in drug concentration that occurs over the dosing interval, and $(1 - e^{-K\tau})$ represents the fraction of drug that is eliminated in the dosing interval.

Some pharmacokineticists have chosen to describe the fraction lost in a dosing interval $(1 - e^{-K\tau})$ as the "accumulation factor" and express it as:

$$\frac{1}{1 - e^{-K\tau}}$$

and the Css max equation as:

$$Css\ max = \left(\frac{(S)(F)(Dose)}{V}\right)\left(\frac{1}{1 - e^{-K\tau}}\right)$$

This equation is the same as Equation 43 expressed in a slightly different format.

Equation 43 assumes drug absorption and distribution rates are rapid in relation to the drug elimination half-life and the dosing interval. This assumption is valid as long as drug concentrations are not sampled during the absorption and distribution phase. Following intravenous injection, the absorption and distribution phases are relatively short compared to the dosing interval and half-life for most drugs. When drugs are administered orally, the primary concern is with the absorption phase because the distribution component associated with two-compartment modeling is usually negligible. Digoxin and lithium are two notable exceptions in that a distribution phase continues for several hours after oral administration.

For digoxin, the observed peak concentration following oral administration will be greater than that predicted by Equation 43 for Css max because drug distribution into tissue requires a minimum of 6 hours. When procainamide is dosed every 3 or 4 hours, as a nonsustained product, the observed peak concentration will be slightly lower than that predicted by Equation 43 because absorption is relatively slow compared to the dosing interval and the half-life of the drug. This tends to blunt or dampen the peak and trough level fluctuations of procainamide because elimination begins before all the drug enters the body. For most drugs, the time required to reach peak concentrations after oral administration is between 1 and 2 hours.

MINIMUM PLASMA DRUG CONCENTRATION (Css MIN)

The minimum plasma drug concentration can be estimated by subtracting ΔC or the change in plasma concentration in one dosing interval from the maximum plasma concentration:

$$Css\ min = Css\ max - \Delta C \qquad \text{[Eq. 44]}$$

or

$$\text{Css min} = \text{Css max} - \left(\frac{(S)(F)(Dose)}{V} \right) \qquad \text{[Eq. 45]}$$

Alternatively, Css min can be calculated by multiplying Css max by the fraction of drug which remains at the end of the dosing interval ($e^{-K\tau}$).

$$\text{Css min} = \text{Css max} \, (e^{-K\tau}) \qquad \text{[Eq. 46]}$$

Substituting Equation 43 for Css max into Equation 46 enables one to calculate Css min if the dose, elimination rate constant (K), volume of distribution (V), salt form (S), and bioavailability (F) are known:

$$\text{Css min} = \frac{\dfrac{(S)(F)(Dose)}{V}}{1 - e^{-K\tau}} \, e^{-K\tau} \qquad \text{[Eq. 47]}$$

If a steady-state sample is obtained at some time other than the peak or trough, the concentration can be calculated by the following equation:

$$\text{Css}_1 = \frac{\dfrac{(S)(F)(Dose)}{V}}{1 - e^{-K\tau}} \, e^{-Kt_1} \qquad \text{[Eq. 48]}$$

Where t_1 is the number of hours since the last dose, and Css_1 is the steady-state plasma concentration "t_1" hours after the last dose or Css max, which is "assumed" to occur at the time of dose administration (i.e., absorption or drug input is assumed to be instantaneous). Note that although steady state has been achieved, not all plasma concentrations within the dosing interval represent the average concentration or Css ave. If the dosing interval (τ) is short compared to the half-life, the plasma concentration changes very little within the dosing interval and all concentrations are a close approximation of Css ave (see Figs. 20 and 31).

One note of caution: When a slow absorption rate significantly dampens the plasma drug concentration-versus-time curve (e.g., sustained-release dosage forms), the Css min can usually be assumed to be a close approximation of the average steady-state concentration (Css ave) and Equation 15:

$$Cl = \frac{(S)(F)(Dose/\tau)}{Css\ ave}$$

is used to calculate the patient's pharmacokinetic parameter (i.e., clearance) (see Figs. 20 and 31). This assumption also is applicable when the dosing interval is short relative to the half-life. Although it would not be incorrect to use Equation 48:

$$Css_1 = \frac{\dfrac{(S)(F)(Dose)}{V}}{1 - e^{-K\tau}} e^{-Kt_1}$$

when the dosing interval is much shorter than the drug half-life, the complexity of the equation tends to obscure that fact that all drug concentrations within the dosing interval are essentially an approximation of Css ave. In addition, if pharmacokinetic revisions are made by manipulating K and/or V in Equation 48, it should be kept in mind that it is the product of K times V or clearance that has the most value or accuracy from the revision process. Again, when the dosing interval is much shorter than the half-life, peak and trough plasma levels are about equal to the average concentration and are, therefore, primarily determined by clearance. Although the product of the V and K obtained by manipulating Equation 48 may closely approximate clearance, there is less confidence in the V and K values.

Selecting the Appropriate Equation

It is often difficult to determine which of the many equations should be used to solve specific clinical problems. A technique used by this author to avoid the use of inappropriate equations is to draw a graphical representation of the plasma drug concentration-versus-time curve that would be expected on the basis of the dosage regimen the patient is receiving. Once the graph is drawn and the plasma concentration visualized, mathematical equations that describe the drug's pharmacokinetic behavior are selected. To facilitate this process, a series of typical plasma level-time curves and their corresponding formulas is presented in Figures 21 through 27.

LOADING DOSE OR BOLUS DOSE

When a loading dose or a bolus of drug has been administered (Figure 21), the initial plasma concentration (C) can be determined by rearranging the "loading dose" equation (See Equation 11):

$$C = \frac{(S)(F)(\text{Loading Dose})}{V} \qquad \text{[Eq. 49]}$$

A subsequent plasma level (C_1) any time (t_1) after the dose has been administered can be calculated by using a variation of the Equation 28 that describes first-order elimination:

$$C_2 = (C_1)(e^{-Kt_1})$$

where C_1 is replaced by $\dfrac{(S)(F)(\text{Loading Dose})}{V}$ and C_2 is replaced by C_1

$$C_1 = \frac{(S)(F)(\text{Loading Dose})}{V}(e^{-Kt_1}) \qquad \text{[Eq. 50]}$$

C_1 now represents the concentration remaining t_1 hours after the loading dose.

CONTINUOUS INFUSION TO STEADY STATE

The plasma concentration-versus-time curve produced by a continuous infusion which has been administered until steady state has been achieved is represented by Figure 22. The average steady-state concentration

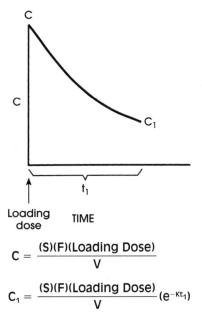

$$C = \frac{(S)(F)(\text{Loading Dose})}{V}$$

$$C_1 = \frac{(S)(F)(\text{Loading Dose})}{V} (e^{-Kt_1})$$

FIGURE 21. Graphic representation of the change in plasma level that occurs over time following a loading dose. C represents the initial concentration immediately following the administration of a loading dose, and C_1 represents the concentration at any interval of time (t_1) after the dose has been administered. Assume a one-compartment model and rapid absorption if the drug is given orally.

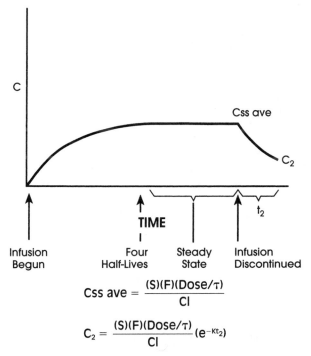

$$\text{Css ave} = \frac{(S)(F)(\text{Dose}/\tau)}{Cl}$$

$$C_2 = \frac{(S)(F)(\text{Dose}/\tau)}{Cl} (e^{-Kt_2})$$

FIGURE 22. Graphic representation of the plasma concentration-versus-time curve that results when an infusion is continued until steady state is reached and then discontinued. Css ave is the steady-state concentration, and C_2 is the concentration at any interval of time (t_2) after the infusion has been discontinued.

(Css ave) that will be produced by the infusion can be calculated using Equation 35:

$$\text{Css ave} = \frac{(S)(F)(\text{Dose}/\tau)}{Cl}$$

DISCONTINUATION OF INFUSION AFTER STEADY STATE

The curve representing a change in plasma concentration after the infusion has been discontinued is also represented in Figure 22. The concentration (C_2) produced any time (t_2) after the infusion has been discontinued can be calculated using a variation of the first-order elimination equation (Equation 28):

$$C_2 = (C_1)(e^{-Kt_1})$$

where C_1 is replaced by Css ave, and t_1 by t_2:

$$C_2 = (\text{Css ave})(e^{-Kt_2}) \qquad \text{[Eq. 51]}$$

or substituting $\dfrac{(S)(F)(\text{Dose}/\tau)}{Cl}$ for Css ave:

$$C_2 = \frac{(S)(F)(\text{Dose}/\tau)}{Cl}(e^{-Kt_2}) \qquad \text{[Eq. 52]}$$

INITIATION AND DISCONTINUATION OF INFUSION BEFORE STEADY STATE

When an infusion is initiated and discontinued before steady state is achieved (< 3 to $5\ t^{1/2}$) the plasma concentration time curve can be described as depicted in Figure 19. In this situation, the concentration (C_1) that occurs at any time (t_1) after the infusion has been initiated and the concentration (C_2) that occurs any time (t_2) after the infusion was discontinued can be approximated by Equation 37:

$$C_1 = \frac{(S)(F)(\text{Dose}/\tau)}{Cl}(1 - e^{-Kt_1})$$

and Equation 41:

$$C_2 = \frac{(S)(F)(\text{Dose}/\tau)}{Cl}(1 - e^{-Kt_1})(e^{-Kt_2})$$

The input model for Equations 37 and 41 is an infusion model. Whether a bolus or infusion model is used to represent the input or absorption of drug into the body depends on the relationship between the duration of drug input relative to the drug's half-life. For example, if a drug is administered rapidly as an intravenous bolus or if an orally administered drug is absorbed rapidly relative to the drug's half-life, very little drug will be cleared or eliminated during the administration or absorption process. Therefore, absorption can be thought of as instantaneous, and the bolus model $\left(\dfrac{(S)(F)(Dose)}{V} \right)$ can be used. If, however, a drug is absorbed over a long time relative to its half-life, a significant amount of drug will be eliminated during the input or absorption period and the plasma level concentrations resulting from oral administration would resemble those resulting from an infusion model. As a general rule, if the drug input time (t_{in}) is less than one-tenth its half-life, then it can be successfully modeled as a bolus dose; however, if the drug input time is greater than one-half its half-life, it is more appropriate to use an infusion model. When the duration of drug input falls between one-tenth and one-half of its half-life, an arbitrary choice can be made between a bolus dose and an infusion model.

As a clinical guideline, the author uses one-sixth of a drug half-life as an arbitrary break point. That is, for those drugs that are absorbed over a period equal to one-sixth of a half-life or less, the bolus model is used; for those drugs absorbed over a period that is greater than one-sixth of the half-life, the infusion model is used. Whereas the one-sixth of a half-life "rule" is arbitrary, it was selected because the difference in the calculated plasma concentrations when using the bolus or short infusion model is <10% (see Fig. 24).

If there is any uncertainty about which model is more appropriate, the infusion model should be used because it more closely approximates the actual absorption and plasma concentration curve during drug absorption and elimination. Figure 23 represents the plasma concentration obtained at the end of a short infusion, as calculated by Equation 53.

$$C_{t_{in}} = \frac{(S)(F)(Dose/t_{in})}{Cl}(1 - e^{-Kt_{in}}) \qquad \text{[Eq. 53]}$$

Note in the above equation that t_{in} represents the duration of drug input and that $(1 - e^{-Kt_{in}})$ represents the fraction of steady state that would be achieved during the infusion time. This concentration ($C_{t_{in}}$) therefore represents the peak level at the end of the infusion.

Conceptually, it is useful to compare Equation 53 above to Equation 37.

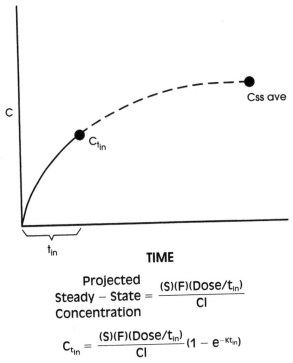

$$\text{Projected Steady - State Concentration} = \frac{(S)(F)(Dose/t_{in})}{Cl}$$

$$C_{t_{in}} = \frac{(S)(F)(Dose/t_{in})}{Cl}(1 - e^{-Kt_{in}})$$

FIGURE 23. Graphic representation of a short infusion. The plasma concentration at the end of a short infusion ($C_{t_{in}}$) can be calculated by multiplying the "projected steady-state concentration" (- - - -) by the fraction of steady state achieved ($1 - e^{-Kt_{in}}$) during the infusion period (t_{in}).

$$C_1 = \frac{(S)(F)(Dose/\tau)}{Cl}(1 - e^{-Kt_1})$$

Both equations represent the process of multiplying a steady-state average concentration by the fraction of steady state achieved. The dosing interval (τ) and duration of infusion (t_1) in Equation 37 are replaced in Equation 53 with the duration of drug input (t_{in}). Although both equations represent the same basic process, Equation 37 is most commonly used when a continuous infusion (e.g., theophylline, lidocaine, etc.) is discontinued before steady state is achieved, and Equation 53 is used when a dose is to be administered over a relatively short period (e.g., aminoglycoside antibiotics).

Once the infusion has been concluded, any subsequent drug concentration (C_2) can be calculated by multiplying the concentration at the end of the infusion ($C_{t_{in}}$) by the fraction remaining at any time interval since the end of the infusion (t_2).

$$C_2 = \frac{(S)(F)(Dose/t_{in})}{Cl}(1 - e^{-Kt_{in}})(e^{-Kt_2}) \qquad \text{[Eq. 54]}$$

The relationship between plasma concentrations predicted by the bolus dose equation (Equations 49 and 50) and the short infusion equation (Equations 53 and 54) is depicted in Figure 24. Note that the bolus

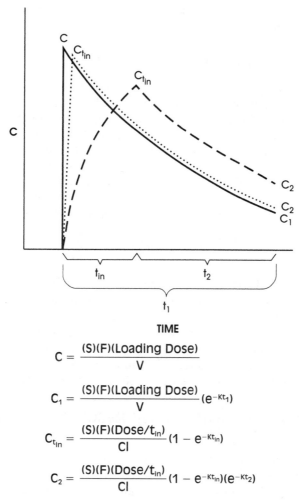

$$C = \frac{(S)(F)(Loading\ Dose)}{V}$$

$$C_1 = \frac{(S)(F)(Loading\ Dose)}{V}(e^{-Kt_1})$$

$$C_{t_{in}} = \frac{(S)(F)(Dose/t_{in})}{Cl}(1 - e^{-Kt_{in}})$$

$$C_2 = \frac{(S)(F)(Dose/t_{in})}{Cl}(1 - e^{-Kt_{in}})(e^{-Kt_2})$$

FIGURE 24. Graphic representation of a drug administered as a bolus (—) or as a short infusion (- - -) and (······). The bolus dose model assumes that drug input or absorption is instantaneous. The decay interval, t_1 (i.e., $t_{in} + t_2$), is therefore assumed to begin at the start of the infusion. In contrast, the infusion model assumes that the decay interval (t_2) begins at the conclusion of the infusion period (t_{in}). When t_{in} is $\leq 1/6^{th}$ of a $t\frac{1}{2}$ (······), the concentrations are approximately the same for the short infusion and bolus dose model. When t_{in} is $> 1/6^{th}$ of a $t\frac{1}{2}$ (- - -), the concentrations calculated by the short infusion and bolus dose model are substantially different.

dose is assumed to be instantaneously absorbed at the beginning of the infusion; therefore, the initial peak concentration is higher than would be predicted by the short infusion model. However, plasma concentrations corresponding to the conclusion of the short infusion model (t_{in} hours after starting the infusion) and all subsequent plasma levels are lower for the bolus-dose model than for the infusion model. If the infusion time t_{in} is less than one-sixth of a drug's half-life, then the difference between the plasma concentrations predicted by the bolus dose and the short infusion model will be minimal. Although either equation can be used, the bolus dose model is much simpler.

LOADING DOSE FOLLOWED BY INFUSION

When a patient is given a loading dose followed by an infusion, the plasma concentration (C_1) at any time (t_1) can be calculated by summing the equations that describe the concentration produced by the loading dose at t_1 (Equation 50) and the concentration produced by the infusion at t_1 (Equation 37). Refer to C_1 in Figure 21 and C_1 in Figure 19.

$$C_1 = \begin{matrix} \text{Concentration} \\ \text{Produced by the} \\ \text{Loading Dose at } t_1 \end{matrix} + \begin{matrix} \text{Concentration} \\ \text{Produced by the} \\ \text{Infusion at } t_1 \end{matrix}$$

$$C_1 = \left[\frac{(S)(F)(\text{Loading Dose})}{V}(e^{-Kt_1}) \right] + \left[\frac{(S)(F)(\text{Dose}/\tau)}{Cl}(1 - e^{-Kt_1}) \right]$$

Note that $(S)(F)(\text{Dose}/\tau)$ in the second portion of the above equation represents the infusion rate. It is important to recall in this situation that the loading dose is eliminated according to first-order pharmacokinetics as described in Figure 21 even when a maintenance infusion is initiated. This must be taken into account when predicting a plasma concentration. In other words, the maintenance infusion is accumulating while the concentration resulting from the loading dose is diminishing (Fig. 25).

INTERMITTENT ADMINISTRATION AT REGULAR INTERVALS TO STEADY STATE

When a drug is administered intermittently at regular dosing intervals until steady state is achieved (at least three to five half-lives), the average steady-state concentration can be calculated using Equation 35:

$$\text{Css ave} = \frac{(S)(F)(\text{Dose}/\tau)}{Cl}$$

Assuming absorption is rapid relative to $t\frac{1}{2}$, the steady-state maximum and minimum concentrations can be approximated using Equations 43 and 47, respectively.

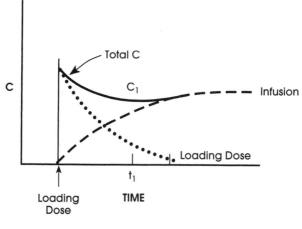

$$C_1 = \left[\frac{(S)(F)(\text{Loading Dose})}{V}(e^{-Kt_1}) \right] + \left[\frac{(S)(F)(\text{Dose}/\tau)}{Cl}(1 - e^{-Kt_1}) \right]$$

FIGURE 25. **Graphic representation of the plasma level-time curve that results from a loading dose followed by a maintenance infusion.** The curve represents a summation of a loading dose curve (⋯) and an infusion curve (- - - -). C_1 is the concentration any time (t_1) after the loading dose has been administered and after the maintenance infusion has been initiated.

$$\text{Css max} = \frac{\dfrac{(S)(F)(\text{Dose})}{V}}{1 - e^{-K\tau}}$$

$$\text{Css min} = \frac{\dfrac{(S)(F)(\text{Dose})}{V}}{1 - e^{-K\tau}}e^{-K\tau}$$

Prediction of a plasma concentration at any time (t_1) following the peak can be accomplished by using Equation 48. Figure 26 depicts the plasma concentration-versus-time curve that occurs with this type of dosing regimen (also see Maximum and Minimum Plasma Concentrations).

$$\text{Css}_1 = \frac{\dfrac{(S)(F)(\text{Dose})}{V}}{1 - e^{-K\tau}}e^{-Kt_1}$$

SERIES OF INDIVIDUAL DOSES

When a series of individual doses is administered and a concentration before steady state must be calculated, there are several approaches that can be taken. One approach is to sum the contributions of each individual dose. This is done by decaying the peak concentration of each dose to the time at which the plasma concentration needs to be predicted. Figure 27

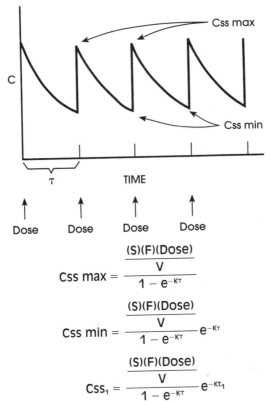

$$Css\ max = \dfrac{\dfrac{(S)(F)(Dose)}{V}}{1 - e^{-K\tau}}$$

$$Css\ min = \dfrac{\dfrac{(S)(F)(Dose)}{V}}{1 - e^{-K\tau}} e^{-K\tau}$$

$$Css_1 = \dfrac{\dfrac{(S)(F)(Dose)}{V}}{1 - e^{-K\tau}} e^{-Kt_1}$$

FIGURE 26. Graphic representation of the steady-state plasma concentration-versus-time curve which occurs when drugs are given intermittently at regular dosing intervals. Any maximum concentration (Css max) is interchangeable with any other maximum concentration, and any minimum concentration (Css min) is interchangeable with any other minimum concentration. In addition, any concentration (Css_1) at time t_1 within a dosing interval is interchangeable with a corresponding concentration at the same t_1 within any other interval.

represents a series of three doses whose individual contributions were calculated and then summed to estimate the total plasma concentration existing at some time point after the third dose. Note that this is simply the sum of three individual doses as modeled by Equation 50. This approach is most practical when the interval between doses or the amount of drug administered with each dose varies. Note that depending on where the brackets are placed, the Summation Equation may predict the concentration from one dose to the next or the contribution of each dose to the final concentration or C_{sum}. The approach of calculating the concentration from dose to dose is most useful when the pattern of drug accumulation and the potential of drug effect at each point in time is of interest. However, if the intent is to see how much each of the individual doses contribute or if an iterative solution for revision of a pharmacokinetic

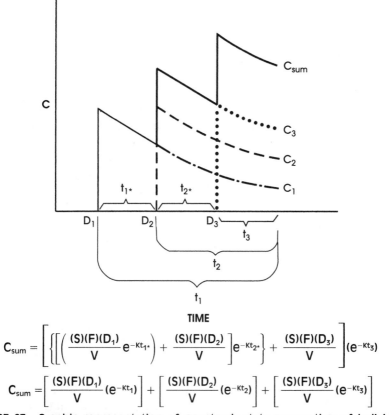

$$C_{sum} = \left[\left\{\left[\left(\frac{(S)(F)(D_1)}{V}e^{-Kt_{1*}}\right) + \frac{(S)(F)(D_2)}{V}\right]e^{-Kt_{2*}}\right\} + \frac{(S)(F)(D_3)}{V}\right](e^{-Kt_3})$$

$$C_{sum} = \left[\frac{(S)(F)(D_1)}{V}(e^{-Kt_1})\right] + \left[\frac{(S)(F)(D_2)}{V}(e^{-Kt_2})\right] + \left[\frac{(S)(F)(D_3)}{V}(e^{-Kt_3})\right]$$

FIGURE 27. Graphic representation of nonsteady-state summation of individual doses. The solid line represents the top Summation Equation and a plasma concentration as each dose is administered (D₁, D₂, D₃) as they accumulate. t₁* is the time from D₁ to D₂, t₂* is the time from D₂ to D₃, and t₃ is the time from D₃ to the time at which the plasma concentration (C_sum) is to be calculated. The dashed and dotted lines represent the bottom Summation Equation and the contribution of each of the individual doses to the total concentration or C_sum. The t₁, t₂, and t₃ represent the time from each administered dose to the time at which the plasma concentration (C_sum) is to be calculated.

parameter is to be performed, then the approach that allows one to see how much each dose is contributing to the final solution is preferred.

If each dose and the intervals between doses are the same, it may be simpler to multiply Css max or the peak concentration that would be achieved at steady state (Equation 43)

$$\text{Css max} = \frac{\dfrac{(S)(F)(Dose)}{V}}{1 - e^{-K\tau}}$$

by the fraction of steady state achieved after N doses:

$$\text{Fraction of Steady State Achieved After (N) Doses} = (1 - e^{-K(N)\tau})$$ [Eq. 55]

In Equation 55, τ is the interval between each dose and N represents the number of doses that have been administered. The peak concentration following N doses can be calculated by combining Equations 43 and 55. Any concentration (C_2) following the Nth dose can be calculated by multiplying the peak concentration following N doses by (e^{-Kt_2}), where t_2 is the number of hours since the last dose.

$$Css_2 = \frac{\frac{(S)(F)(Dose)}{V}}{1 - e^{-K\tau}}(1 - e^{-K(N)\tau})(e^{-Kt_2})$$ [Eq. 56]

Note that if the doses and dosing intervals were the same in Figure 27, the concentration (C_{sum}) could be calculated using Equation 56 where N would be 3 and t_2 would be the number of hours after the third dose. Equation 56 is most useful when a number of doses have been administered with a consistent τ but steady state has not yet been achieved. Equation 56 represents the concentration of drug produced by a series of consistently administered bolus doses that have not yet achieved steady state. This equation can be further expanded to represent a series of doses that are absorbed over a significant fraction of the drug's half-life (i.e., $t_{in} > \frac{1}{6}$th $t\frac{1}{2}$).

$$Css_2 = \frac{\frac{(S)(F)(Dose/t_{in})}{Cl}(1 - e^{-Kt_{in}})}{(1 - e^{-K\tau})}(1 - e^{-K(N)\tau})(e^{-Kt_2})$$ [Eq. 57]

Equation 57 is similar to Equation 56 except that the bolus dose input model is now replaced with the short infusion input model. Equation 57 is seldom used in clinical practice. This is because the half-life of the drug, which requires the use of a short infusion input model, is likely to be sufficiently brief such that steady state will be achieved after two to three doses have been administered.

SUSTAINED-RELEASE DOSAGE FORMS

Most sustained-release dosage forms are designed to produce concentrations that fluctuate little within the dosage interval. Therefore, in most cases concentrations produced by sustained-release products can be estimated by use of the equation that describes the average steady-state concentration (Equation 35):

$$\text{Css ave} = \frac{(S)(F)(Dose/\tau)}{Cl}$$

As illustrated below, the use of the Css ave formula for sustained-release products is based on the assumption that the time required for absorption (t_{in}) is approximately equal to the dosing interval (τ).

$$Css_2 = \frac{\dfrac{(S)(F)(Dose/t_{in})}{Cl}(1 - e^{-Kt_{in}})}{} (e^{-Kt_2}) \qquad \text{[Eq. 58]}$$

$$Css_2 = \frac{\dfrac{(S)(F)(Dose/\tau)}{Cl}(1 - e^{-K\tau})}{(1 - e^{-K\tau})} (e^{-Kt_2})$$

In the above equation, the $1 - e^{-K\tau}$ in the numerator and denominator cancel and assuming t_2 is zero, we have Equation 35.

$$\text{Css ave} = \frac{(S)(F)(Dose/\tau)}{Cl}$$

If the t_{in} is exactly equal to τ, the input from one dose stops at the same time the next dose begins its infusion process. As a result, an average steady-state concentration with no rise or fall within the dosing interval is achieved. This would be exactly the same as changing an IV bag for a constant infusion without interrupting the infusion process. In practice, absorption times are not exactly equal to the dosing interval, but for most sustained-release drug products, they are reasonably close and, therefore, plasma concentrations can be considered as an average steady-state value. It should be emphasized, however, that the use of Equation 35 is not universal and depends on not only the absorption of the drug product, but also the dosing interval selected and half-life of the drug in the specific patient. As a general rule, absorption times that exceed the dosing interval are not a problem. However, if the duration of absorption (t_{in}) is substantially less than the dosing interval, then there will be some fluctuation of the plasma concentrations. A useful approach is to consider the duration over which the plasma concentrations will decay following the end of absorption. This can be approximated by subtracting the absorption time from the dosing interval.

$$\tau - t_{in} = \frac{\text{Time Within the Dosing}}{\text{Interval With No Drug Absorption}} \qquad \text{[Eq. 59]}$$

If this time within the dosing interval when there is no drug input is short compared to the drug's half-life, it suggests that there will be little fluctuation of the plasma concentration within the dosing interval. As a clinical guideline, if $\tau - t_{in}$ is $\leq \frac{1}{3}$ $t\frac{1}{2}$, the average steady-state equation (Equation 35) can be used. Note that this guideline is very similar to the guidelines used for substituting the average steady-state equation (Equation 35) for the intermittent bolus dose equation (Equation 48) (see Fig. 31 and Interpretation of Plasma Drug Concentrations: Choosing a Model to Revise or Estimate a Patient's Clearance at Steady State). Note, however, in Figure 31 the time of decay is considered to be the entire dosing interval as the absorption is assumed to be instantaneous and t_{in} is zero.

ALGORITHM FOR CHOOSING THE APPROPRIATE EQUATION

Selecting the appropriate equation to use in a specific clinical situation can be a complex process. The algorithm in Figure 28 offers a step-wise approach to this process. The rules follow those outlined in the text. First, one must consider whether steady state has been achieved; then, the appropriate model is chosen to predict or calculate drug concentrations.

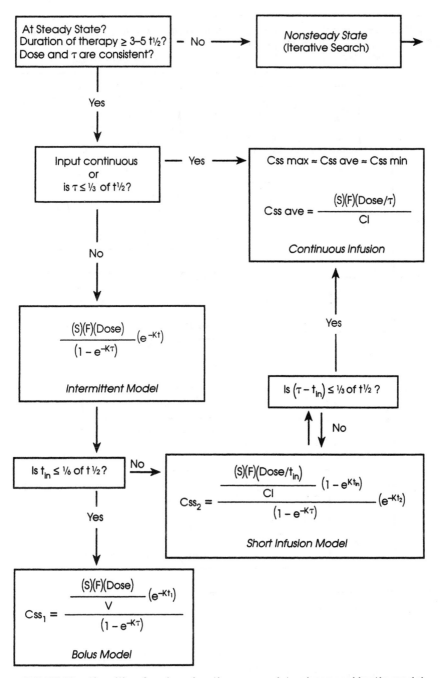

FIGURE 28. Algorithm for choosing the appropriate pharmacokinetic model.

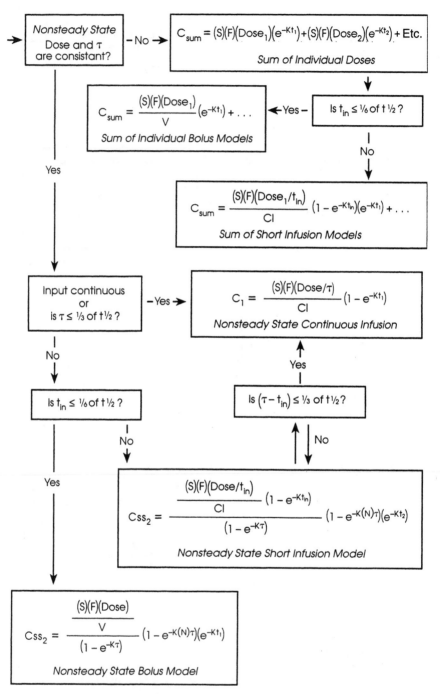

FIGURE 28—continued. Algorithm for choosing the appropriate pharmacokinetic model.

Interpretation of Plasma Drug Concentrations

Plasma drug concentrations are measured in the clinical setting to determine whether a therapeutic or toxic concentration has been produced by a given dosage regimen. This process is based on the assumption that plasma drug concentrations reflect drug concentrations at the receptor and, therefore, can be correlated with pharmacologic response. This assumption is not always valid. When plasma samples are obtained at inappropriate times or when other factors (such as delayed absorption or altered plasma binding) confound the usual pharmacokinetic behavior of a drug, the interpretation of serum drug concentrations can lead to erroneous pharmacokinetic and pharmacodynamic conclusions and ultimately inappropriate patient care decisions. These factors are discussed below.

PLASMA SAMPLING TIME

To properly interpret a plasma concentration, it is essential to know when a plasma sample was obtained in relation to the last dose administered and when the drug regimen was initiated. If a plasma sample is obtained before distribution of the drug into tissue is complete (e.g., digoxin), the plasma concentration will be higher than predicted on the basis of dose and response. Peak (Css max) plasma levels are helpful in evaluating the dose of antibiotics used to treat severe, life-threatening infections. Although serum concentrations for many drugs peak 1 to 2 hours after an oral dose is administered, factors such as slow or delayed absorption can significantly delay the time at which peak serum concentrations are attained. Large errors in the estimation of Css max can occur if the plasma sample is obtained at the wrong time (Fig. 29). Therefore, with few exceptions, plasma samples should be drawn as trough or just before the next dose (Css min) when determining routine drug concentrations in plasma. These trough levels are less likely to be influenced by absorption and distribution problems.

    When the full therapeutic response of a given drug dosage regimen is to be assessed, plasma samples should not be obtained until steady-state concentrations of the drug have been achieved. If drug doses are increased or decreased on the basis of drug concentrations that have been measured while the drug is still accumulating, disastrous consequences can occur. Nevertheless, in some clinical situations it is appropriate to measure drug levels before steady state. For example, pharmacokinetic parameters for a drug administered to a severely ill patient may change so rapidly that extrapolations from a reported plasma concentration may not be valid from

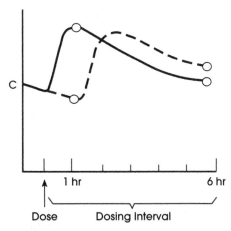

FIGURE 29. Schematic representation of the effect of delayed absorption (- - - -) on plasma level measurements. Note the magnitude of error at 1 hour (theoretical time to reach Css max) as compared to 6 hours (Css min).

one day to the next. Similarly, if there is reason to suspect that the pharmacokinetic parameters in a given patient are likely to differ substantially from those reported in the literature (e.g., lidocaine in a patient with congestive heart failure),[60] or the accumulation process is prolonged because of a long $t\frac{1}{2}$ (e.g., phenobarbital),[33,61] it may be reasonable to obtain plasma samples before steady state to avoid excessive accumulation or unnecessarily prolonged subtherapeutic concentrations from the current dose. If possible, plasma samples should be drawn after a minimum of two half-lives because clearance values calculated from drug levels obtained less than one half-life after a regimen has been initiated are very sensitive to small differences in the volume of distribution and minor assay errors (Fig. 30).

REVISING PHARMACOKINETIC PARAMETERS

The process of using a patient's plasma drug concentrations and dosing history to determine patient-specific pharmacokinetic parameters can be complex and difficult. If the relationship between pharmacokinetic equations, the specific parameters, and the resultant plasma levels is understood, however, this process can be simplified. A single plasma sample obtained at the appropriate time can yield information to revise either the volume of distribution or clearance, but not both. Drug concentrations measured from poorly timed samples may prove to be useless in estimating a patient's V or Cl values. Thus, the goal is to obtain plasma samples at times that are likely to yield data that can be used with confidence to estimate pharmacokinetic parameters. In addition, it is important to evaluate available plasma concentration data to determine whether they can

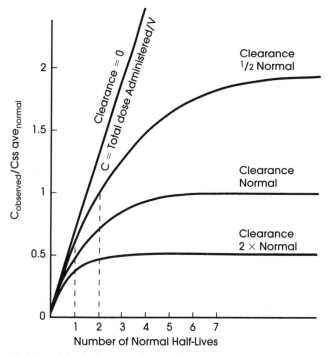

FIGURE 30. Relationship between observed plasma concentrations ($C_{observed}$) and the normal steady-state concentration (Css ave$_{normal}$) following initiation of a maintenance regimen at various clearance values. At steady state, the plasma concentrations are inversely proportional to clearance. Plasma concentrations obtained at or before one normal half-life are all very similar regardless of clearance. After two half-lives, alterations in a patient's clearance and ultimately steady-state concentrations can be detected by unexpectedly high or low plasma drug concentrations. After three half-lives, more confident predictions of steady-state concentrations can be made.

be used to estimate, with some degree of confidence, V and/or Cl. Which pharmacokinetic parameter is revised has much to do with the timing of the sample and the drug's pharmacokinetic profile. The goal in pharmacokinetic revisions is not only to recognize which pharmacokinetic parameter can be revised, but also the accuracy or confidence one has in the revised or patient-specific pharmacokinetic parameter.

Volume of Distribution

A plasma concentration that has been obtained soon after administration of an initial bolus is primarily determined by the dose administered and the volume of distribution. This assumes that both the absorption and distribution phases have been avoided. This is illustrated by Equation 50 (also see Figs. 21 and 32):

$$C_1 = \frac{(S)(F)(\text{Loading Dose})}{V}(e^{-Kt_1})$$

When e^{-Kt_1} approaches 1 (i.e., when t_1 is much less than $t\frac{1}{2}$), the plasma concentration (C_1) is primarily a function of the administered dose and the apparent volume of distribution. At this point, very little drug has been eliminated from the body. As a clinical guideline, a patient's volume of distribution can be estimated when t_1, or the interval between the administration and sampling time, is less than or equal to one-third of the drug's half-life. As t_1 exceeds one-third of a half-life, the measured concentration is increasingly influenced by clearance. As more of the drug is eliminated (i.e., t_1 increases), it is difficult to estimate the patient's V with any certainty. The specific application of this clinical guideline depends on the confidence with which one knows clearance. If clearance is extremely variable and uncertain, a time interval of less than one-third of a half-life might be appropriate. On the other hand, if a patient-specific value for clearance has already been determined, then t_1 could exceed one-third of a half-life and a reasonably accurate estimate of volume of distribution could be obtained. It is important to recognize that the pharmacokinetic parameter that most influences the drug concentration is not determined by the model chosen to represent the drug level. For example, even if the dose is modeled as a short infusion (Equation 54), the volume of distribution can still be the important parameter controlling the plasma concentration. V is not clearly defined in the equation; nevertheless, it is incorporated into the elimination rate constant (K):

$$C_2 = \frac{(S)(F)(Dose/t_{in})}{Cl}(1 - e^{-Kt_{in}})(e^{-Kt_2})$$

Although one would not usually select Equation 54 to demonstrate that the drug concentration is primarily a function of volume of distribution, it is important to recognize that the relationship between the observed drug concentration and volume is not altered as long as the total elapsed time $[t_{in} + t_2]$ does not exceed one-third of a half-life.

Our assumption in evaluating the volume of distribution is that although we have not sampled beyond one-third of a $t^1/_2$, we have waited until the drug absorption and distribution process is complete.

Clearance

A plasma drug concentration that has been obtained at steady state from a patient who is receiving a constant drug infusion is determined by clearance. This is illustrated by Equation 35:

$$Css\ ave = \frac{(S)(F)(Dose/\tau)}{Cl}$$

Note that the average steady-state plasma concentration is not influenced by volume of distribution. Therefore, plasma concentrations that represent the average steady-state level can be used to estimate a patient's clearance value, but they cannot be used to estimate a patient's volume of distribution. As illustrated in Figure 31, all steady-state plasma concentrations within a dosing interval that is short relative to a drug's half-life ($\tau \le \frac{1}{3}$ t½) approximate the average concentration. Therefore, these concentrations are also primarily a function of clearance and only minimally influenced by V. If the average drug concentration is assumed to occur approximately in the middle of the dosing interval, the trough concentration will have decayed from the average for only half of the dosing interval or by one-sixth of a drug half-life (assuming the dosing interval is one-third of a half-life or less). Under these conditions, the trough concentration is approximately 90% of the average drug level, an error that is usually acceptable in clinical practice. Thus, in this circumstance, the equation for Css ave (Equation 35) or the equation which represents a steady-state

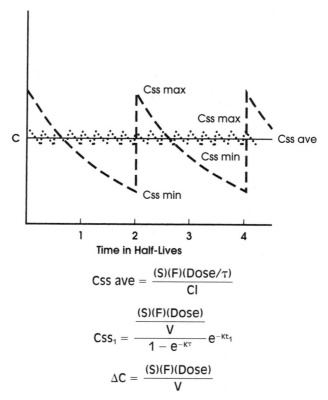

$$Css\ ave = \frac{(S)(F)(Dose/\tau)}{Cl}$$

$$Css_1 = \frac{\dfrac{(S)(F)(Dose)}{V}}{1 - e^{-K\tau}}\, e^{-Kt_1}$$

$$\Delta C = \frac{(S)(F)(Dose)}{V}$$

FIGURE 31. Plasma concentrations relative to Css ave (——) when τ is much less than (· · ·) and greater than (- - - -) the half-life. When τ is much less than t½ (· · ·), all plasma concentrations approximate the average concentration (Css ave) and are, therefore, primarily a function of clearance. When τ is much greater than t½ (- - - -), the plasma concentrations fluctuate significantly. The degree to which plasma concentrations are determined by clearance and/or volume of distribution is a function of when the plasma level is obtained within the dosing interval. Also note that with the bolus model, the difference between Css max and Css min (ΔC) is a function of the dose and volume of distribution.

plasma concentration sampled any time within the dosing interval (Equation 48) can be used to estimate a patient-specific clearance.

$$Css_1 = \frac{\dfrac{(S)(F)(Dose)}{V}}{1 - e^{-K\tau}} e^{-Kt_1}$$

If Equation 48 is used, the expected volume of distribution should be retained and the elimination rate constant adjusted such that Css_1 at t_1 equals the observed drug plasma concentration. Clearance could then be calculated using Equation 33:

$$Cl = (K)(V)$$

Sensitivity Analysis

Whether a measured drug concentration is a function of clearance or volume of distribution is not always apparent. When this is difficult to ascertain, one can examine the sensitivity or responsiveness of the predicted plasma concentration to a parameter by changing one parameter while holding the other constant. For example, Equation 37 represents a plasma concentration (C_1) at some time interval (t_1) after a maintenance infusion has been started.

$$C_1 = \frac{(S)(F)(Dose/\tau)}{Cl}(1 - e^{-Kt_1})$$

When the fraction of steady state that has been reached $(1 - e^{-Kt_1})$ is small, large changes in clearance are frequently required to adjust a predicted plasma concentration to the appropriate value. If a large percentage change in the clearance value results in a disproportionately small change in the predicted drug level, then the volume of distribution and the amount of drug administered are the primary determinants of the observed concentration. This concept is illustrated graphically in Figure 30. Note that plasma concentrations within the first two half-lives are all very similar, while the steady-state concentrations are quite different. Within the first two half-lives of initiating a maintenance regimen, very large changes in clearance are required to account for small changes in plasma levels.

This type of sensitivity analysis is useful to reinforce the concept that the most reliable revisions in pharmacokinetic parameters are made when the predicted drug concentration changes by approximately the same percentage as the pharmacokinetic parameter undergoing revision. To illustrate this principle, let us examine the relationship between a theophylline drug concentration obtained 6.93 hours after starting a theophylline infusion of 30 mg/hr in a patient with the following expected parameters for theophylline: Cl 3 L/hr, V 30 L, K 0.1 hr^{-1}, t½ 6.93 hr. Because the drug being administered is theophylline, S and F are assumed to be 1.0. Using Equation 37, the expected plasma concentration $[C_1]$ is calculated to be 5 mg/L:

$$C_1 = \frac{(S)(F)(Dose/\tau)}{Cl}(1 - e^{-Kt_1})$$

$$= \frac{(1)(1)(30 \text{ mg/hr})}{3 \text{ L/hr}}(1 - e^{-(0.1 \text{ hr}^{-1})(6.93 \text{ hr})})$$

$$= 10 \text{ mg/L} (1 - 0.5)$$

$$= 5 \text{ mg/L}$$

As can be seen from the calculations, the expected steady-state concentration is 10 mg/L and the fraction of steady state achieved $(1 - e^{-Kt_1})$ is 0.5 since the time of sampling is at one drug half-life and 50% of the steady-state plasma concentration has been achieved. If the observed plasma concentration was 6 mg/L, only slightly higher than the calculated or expected value of 5 mg/L, one might expect the patient's clearance on revision to be only slightly less than the expected 3 L/hr. This relationship, however, is deceiving because, in order to calculate a plasma concentration of 6 mg/L at 6.93 hr with a volume of 30 L, a clearance of approximately 1.32 L/hr with a corresponding K and t½ of 0.044 hr^{-1} and 15.7 hr, respectively, is required.

$$C_1 = \frac{(S)(F)(Dose/\tau)}{Cl}(1 - e^{-Kt_1})$$

$$= \frac{(1)(1)(30 \text{ mg/hr})}{1.32 \text{ L/hr}}(1 - e^{-(0.044 \text{ hr}^{-1})(6.93 \text{ hr})})$$

$$= 22.7 \text{ mg/L} (1 - 0.737)$$

$$= 22.7 \text{ mg/L} (0.263)$$

$$= 5.97 \text{ mg/L}$$

As can be seen from this illustration, the clearance value of 3 L/hr had to be reduced by more than one-half (1.32 L/hr) to increase the predicted drug concentration by ≈20%. This poor response of the calculated drug concentration to a change in clearance suggests that clearance is not the primary pharmacokinetic parameter responsible for the drug concentration. Therefore, any estimates of clearance and future dosing regimen based on these calculations would be tenuous at best.

When a predicted drug concentration changes in direct proportion to an alteration in only one of the pharmacokinetic parameters, it is likely that a measured drug concentration can be used to estimate that patient-specific parameter. When both clearance and volume of distribution have a significant influence on the prediction of a measured drug concentration, revision of a patient's pharmacokinetic parameters will be less certain, because there is an infinite number of combinations for clearance and volume of distribution values that could be used to predict the observed drug concentration. When this occurs, the patient's specific pharmacokinetic characteristics can be estimated by adjusting one or both of the pharmacokinetic parameters. Nevertheless, in most cases such as this, additional plasma level sampling will be needed to accurately predict the patient's clearance or volume of distribution so that subsequent dosing regimens can be adjusted.

If a plasma drug concentration calculated from a specific equation is similar to the reported value, the pharmacokinetic parameters used in that equation may not necessarily be the most important determinants of the drug concentration. Equation 48 and Figure 31 can be used to demonstrate this principle.

$$Css_1 = \frac{\frac{(S)(F)(Dose)}{V}}{1 - e^{-K\tau}} e^{-Kt_1}$$

When the dosing interval is much shorter than the drug's half-life, the changes in concentration within a dosing interval are relatively small, and any drug concentration obtained within a dosing interval can be used as an approximation of the average steady-state concentration. Even though Equations 43 and 47:

$$Css\ max = \frac{\frac{(S)(F)(Dose)}{V}}{1 - e^{-K\tau}}$$

$$Css\ min = \frac{\frac{(S)(F)(Dose)}{V}}{1 - e^{-K\tau}} e^{-K\tau}$$

could be used to predict peak and trough concentrations, a reasonable approximation could also be achieved by using Equation 35 for Css ave:

$$Css\ ave = \frac{(S)(F)(Dose/\tau)}{Cl}$$

This suggests that even though Equations 43 and 47 do not contain the parameter clearance per se, the elimination rate constant functions in such a way that the clearance derived from Equations 43 or 47 and 35 would all essentially be the same.

In the situation in which the dosing interval is greater than one-third of a half-life, the use of Equations 43 and 47 are appropriate as not all drug concentrations within the dosing interval can be considered as the Css ave. However, as long as the dosing interval has not been extended beyond one half-life, clearance is still the primary pharmacokinetic parameter that is responsible for the drug concentrations within the dosing interval. Although the elimination rate constant and volume of distribution might be manipulated in Equations 43 and 47, it is only the product of those two numbers (i.e., clearance) that can be known with any certainty:

$$Cl = (K)(V)$$

If a drug is administered at a dosing interval that is much longer than the apparent half-life (see Fig. 31), peak concentrations may be primarily a function of volume of distribution. Since most of the dose is eliminated within a dosing interval, each dose can be treated like a new loading dose. Of course for steady-state conditions, at some point within the dosing interval, the plasma concentration (Css ave) will be determined by clearance. Trough plasma concentrations in this situation are a function of both clearance and volume of distribution. Since clearance and volume of distribution are critical to the prediction of peak and trough concentrations when the dosing interval is much longer than the drug t½, a minimum of two plasma concentrations is needed to accurately establish patient-specific pharmacokinetic parameters and a dosing regimen that will achieve desired peak and trough concentrations. Aminoglycoside antibiotics are examples of drugs that are administered at dosing intervals that exceed their apparent half-life; therefore, if it is important to achieve targeted peak and trough concentrations, at least two plasma concentrations would be needed (see Part Two: Aminoglycoside Antibiotics).

When an observed drug concentration correlates with the level that was predicted based on pharmacokinetic parameters from the literature, the particular pharmacokinetic parameter that is the primary determinant of the observed drug concentration should be determined before making future predictions. Successful prediction of an appropriate loading dose to achieve specific plasma levels, for example, does not guarantee that the maintenance dose is correct. Therefore, critical evaluation of the parameters affecting a patient's measured drug concentration will minimize incorrect assumptions about the applicability of literature-based pharmacokinetic parameters to a specific patient's situation or about the predictability of future plasma concentrations.

CHOOSING A MODEL TO REVISE OR ESTIMATE A PATIENT'S CLEARANCE AT STEADY STATE

As previously discussed, a drug's half-life often determines the pharmacokinetic model that should be used to estimate a pharmacokinetic parameter that is specific for the patient receiving treatment. A common problem encountered clinically, however, is that the half-life observed in the patient often differs from the expected value. Since a change in either clearance or volume of distribution or both may account for this unexpected value, the pharmacokinetic model is often unclear. One way to approach this dilemma is to first calculate the expected change in plasma drug concentration associated with each dose:

$$\Delta C = \frac{(S)(F)(Dose)}{V} \qquad \text{[Eq. 60]}$$

where ΔC is the change in concentration following the administration of each dose [(S)(F)(Dose)] into the patient's volume of distribution (V). This change in concentration can then be compared to the steady-state trough concentration measured in the patient.

$$\frac{(S)(F)(Dose)}{V} \quad \text{versus} \quad Css \ min$$

or

$$\Delta C \quad \text{versus} \quad Css \ min$$

Note in Figure 31 that when the dosing interval (τ) is much less than the drug half-life, ΔC will be small when compared to Css min. As the dosing interval increases relative to τ, ΔC will increase relative to Css min. Therefore, a comparison of ΔC or (S)(F)(Dose)/V to Css min can serve as a guide to estimating the drug $t\frac{1}{2}$ and the most appropriate pharmacokinetic model or technique to use for revision. With few exceptions, drugs are most often dosed at intervals less than or equal to their half-lives. Therefore, clearance is the pharmacokinetic parameter most often revised or calculated for the patient in question. The following guidelines can be used to select the pharmacokinetic model that is the least complex and therefore the most appropriate to estimate a patient-specific pharmacokinetic parameter.

Condition 1

- When:

$$\frac{(S)(F)(Dose)}{V} \leq \frac{1}{4} \ Css \ min$$

- Then:

$$\tau \leq \frac{1}{3} \ t\frac{1}{2}$$

- Under these conditions:

$$\text{Css min} \approx \text{Css ave}$$

- And Cl can be estimated by Equation 15:

$$Cl = \frac{(S)(F)(Dose/\tau)}{\text{Css ave}}$$

- Rules/Conditions: Must be at steady state.

Condition 2

- When:

$$\frac{(S)(F)(Dose)}{V} \leq \text{Css min}$$

- Then:

$$\tau \leq t\frac{1}{2}$$

- Under these conditions:

$$\text{Css min} + (\tfrac{1}{2})\frac{(S)(F)(Dose)}{V} \approx \text{Css ave} \qquad \text{[Eq. 61]}$$

- And Cl can be estimated by Equation 15:

$$Cl = \frac{(S)(F)(Dose/\tau)}{\text{Css ave}}$$

- Rules/Conditions:
  Must be at steady state
  C is Css min
  Bolus model for absorption is acceptable
    That is, dosage form is not sustained release
    Short infusion model does not apply $t_{in} \leq \frac{1}{6} t$

Condition 3

- When:

$$\frac{(S)(F)(Dose)}{V} > \text{Css min}$$

- Then:

$$\tau > t\tfrac{1}{2}$$

- Under these conditions:

$$Css\ min + \frac{(S)(F)(Dose)}{V} = Css\ max \qquad \text{[Eq. 62]}$$

where V is an assumed value from the literature.

- K is revised (K Revised):

$$K\ Revised = \left(\frac{Css\ min + \dfrac{(S)(F)(Dose)}{V}}{\dfrac{Css\ min}{\tau}} \right) = \frac{\ln\left(\dfrac{Css\ max}{Css\ min}\right)}{\tau} \qquad \text{[Eq. 63]}$$

- Clearance is revised (Cl Revised) using K Revised in Equation 33:

Cl Revised = (K Revised) (V)

- Rules/Conditions:
  Must be at steady state
  C is Css min
  Bolus model for absorption is acceptable
    That is, dosage form is not sustained release
    Short infusion model does not apply $t_{in} \leq \tfrac{1}{6}\ t\tfrac{1}{2}$

Note that the approaches used become more complex as the dosing interval increases relative to the drug half-life. If a drug is administered at a dosing interval less than or equal to one-third of its half-life and the technique in Condition 3 is used to revise clearance, the revised clearance would be correct. The calculation is not wrong, just unnecessarily complex. However, if a drug is administered at a dosing interval that exceeds one half-life and the technique in Condition 1 is used to revise clearance, the revised clearance value would be inaccurate because Css min cannot be assumed to be equal to Css ave. While it could be argued that the technique used in Condition 3 would suffice for all the previous conditions, it is more cumbersome and tends to focus on the intermediate parameters, K and V rather than Cl. One should also be aware that as the dosing interval increases, the confidence in a revised clearance diminishes because the volume of distribution, which is an assumed value from the literature, begins to influence the revised clearance to a greater degree. As a general rule, the confidence in Cl is usually good when the dosing interval is $< t\tfrac{1}{2}$, steady-state has been achieved, and drug concentrations are obtained properly.

NONSTEADY-STATE REVISION OF CLEARANCE (ITERATIVE SEARCH)

The techniques described in the previous section allow one to calculate a revised clearance directly. However, there are a number of situations in which revision of the clearance value is possible, but there are no explicit solutions. These situations require an iterative search technique. The first situation is when the parameter being revised appears in both the exponential and nonexponential portions of the equations, as illustrated by Equation 37.

$$C_1 = \frac{(S)(F)(Dose/\tau)}{Cl}(1 - e^{-Kt_1})$$

Although it may not be obvious that clearance appears in both the exponential and nonexponential portions of the equation, the elimination rate constant consists of both clearance and V.

$$C_1 = \frac{(S)(F)(Dose/\tau)}{Cl}\left(1 - e^{-\left(\frac{Cl}{V}\right)t_1}\right)$$

Therefore, if V is held constant, the revision process would be associated with a changing clearance (and the corresponding elimination rate constant) to match the observed plasma concentration [C_1]. The clearance that "fits" or calculates a value for C_1 that is the same as the assayed concentration would be the revised clearance. As stated earlier, there is no direct solution and the clearance value (which when placed in Equation 37 calculates the specific C1) can only be found by trial and error. The second situation that requires an iterative search is any time there are multiple exponential terms (e^{-Kt}) where t differs. This might occur when there are multiple bolus doses being administered and the plasma concentration is the sum of the residual of each of these doses (see Fig. 27). Another example is the short infusion model at steady state or Equation 58.

$$C_2 = \frac{\dfrac{(S)(F)(Dose/t_{in})}{Cl}(1 - e^{-Kt_{in}})\,(e^{-Kt_2})}{(1 - e^{-K\tau})}$$

In Equation 58, clearance is expressed in both the exponential (i.e., $K = Cl/V$) and nonexponential portions. In addition, each of the exponential terms has a different value for t, which in itself is a condition that would require an iterative search to find a unique solution for Cl.

Although an iterative search process can be cumbersome, in most cases approximate values for the revised clearance can be arrived at within one to three attempts. One technique is to adjust the Cl by the ratio that the predicted C_1 and the assayed drug concentration are different. If, for example, the predicted drug concentration is 10 mg/L and the assayed drug concentration is 12 mg/L, the Cl in Equation 58 would be decreased by about 20% in the hope that a 20% decrease in Cl would increase the calculated C_1 by 20%. However, this may not be the case because in Equation 58 there is not a proportional relationship between Cl and C_1. If the required change in Cl is significantly out of proportion to the ratio of C_1 to the assayed drug concentration, it is a strong indication that Cl is not the only pharmacokinetic parameter responsible for C_1. Therefore, any estimates of Cl under conditions where a large change in Cl is required to make small changes in C_1 would be tenuous at best. Many pharmacokineticists use programmed calculators or computers to facilitate these repetitive trial and error calculations. While use of computers is to be encouraged as a labor-saving device, the user must understand the fundamental process and the limits of the method (see Interpretation of Plasma Drug Concentrations: Sensitivity Analysis and Bayesian Analysis).

NONSTEADY-STATE REVISION OF CLEARANCE (MASS BALANCE)

The mass balance technique has been suggested as a more direct alternative to the iterative approach.[62,63] The mass balance technique is relatively simple and can be best visualized by examining the relationship between the rate of drug administration and the rate of drug elimination. At steady state, the rate of drug elimination (R_E) is equal to the rate of administration (R_A) and the change in the amount of the drug in the body with time is zero.

$$R_A - R_E = \frac{\text{Change in the Amount of Drug in the Body with Time}}{} = 0$$

Under nonsteady-state conditions, however, there will be a change in the amount of drug in the body with time. This change can be estimated by multiplying the difference in the plasma concentration (ΔC) by the volume of distribution and dividing by the time interval between the two drug concentrations.

$$R_A - R_E = \frac{(\Delta C)(V)}{t} \qquad \text{[Eq. 64]}$$

By substituting the appropriate values in the above equation, an estimate of clearance can be derived as follows:

$$R_A - R_E = \frac{(\Delta C)(V)}{t}$$

$$(S)(F)(Dose/\tau) - R_E = \frac{(C_2 - C_1)(V)}{t}$$

$$(S)(F)(Dose/\tau) - \frac{(C_2 - C_1)(V)}{t} = R_E$$

$$(S)(F)(Dose/\tau) - \frac{(C_2 - C_1)(V)}{t} = (Cl)(C\ ave)$$

$$\frac{(S)(F)(Dose/\tau) - \dfrac{(C_2 - C_1)(V)}{t}}{C\ ave} = Cl \qquad \text{[Eq. 65]}$$

Note that the average plasma concentration (C ave) is generally assumed to be the average of C_1 and C_2.

$$C\ ave = \frac{C_1 + C_2}{2} \qquad \text{[Eq. 66]}$$

While this C ave is not the steady-state average, it is assumed to be the average concentration that results in the elimination of drug as the concentration proceeds toward steady state. Equation 65 is an accurate method for estimating clearance if the following conditions are met:

1. t, or time interval between C_1 and C_2, should be equal to at least one but no longer than two of the revised drug half-lives. This rule helps to ensure that the time interval is not so short as to be unable to detect any change in concentration and yet not so long that the second concentration (C_2) is at steady state.
2. The plasma concentration values should be reasonably close to one another. If the drug concentrations are increasing, C_2 should be less than two times C_1; if the plasma concentrations are declining, C_2 should be more than one-half of C_1 (i.e., $0.5 < C_2/C_1 < 2.0$). This rule limits the change in concentration so that the assumed value for V will not be a major determinant for the value of Cl calculated from Equation 65.
3. The rate of drug administration $[(S)(F)(Dose/\tau)]$ should be regular and consistent. This rule helps to ensure a reasonably smooth progression from C_1 to C_2 such that the value of C ave $((C_1 + C_2)/2)$ is approximately equal to the true average drug concentration between C_1 and C_2.

The mass balance approach is a useful technique if the above conditions are met. It is relatively simple and allows for the calculation of clearance under nonsteady-state conditions by a direct solution process. There are certain situations in which the above conditions are not met but the mass balance technique still works relatively well. For example, if the time interval between C_1 and C_2 is substantially greater than two half-lives but the value of C_2 is very close to C_1, then Equation 65 approximates Equation 15 because the average plasma concentration approximates the average steady-state value.

$$\frac{(S)(F)(Dose/\tau) - \dfrac{(C_2 - C_1)(V)}{t}}{C\ ave} = Cl$$

$$\frac{(S)(F)(Dose/\tau) - (\approx 0)}{C\ ave} = Cl$$

$$\frac{(S)(F)(Dose/\tau)}{C\ ave} = Cl$$

The mass balance approach is most commonly applicable for drugs that are given as a continuous intravenous infusion, as a sustained-release product, or at a dosing interval that is much less than the half-life.

As an example, let's look at a patient who has a phenobarbital level of 10 mg/L on day 1 and is given 100 mg daily for 10 days. At the end of the 10th day the phenobarbital level is reported to be 18 mg/L. Given that the usual $t\frac{1}{2}$ of phenobarbital is approximately 4 or 5 days, it seems unlikely that the phenobarbital level of 18 mg/L represents steady state (i.e., less than 3 to 5 $t\frac{1}{2}$'s on this regimen). One of several approaches could be taken to resolve this problem. One approach would be to write an equation that was the sum of the initial concentration decayed to the time of the second sample plus each of the 10 doses decayed individually to the time of the second sample. To solve the equation, values of S, F, and V would have to be assumed and then in an iterative fashion values of K would be substituted until the equation equaled the observed phenobarbital level of 18 mg/L:

$$C_{sum} = C(e^{-Kt}) + \left[\frac{(S)(F)(D_1)}{V}(e^{-Kt_1})\right] + \left[\frac{(S)(F)(D_2)}{V}(e^{-Kt_2})\right] + \cdots$$

The K value could then be used in combination with the assumed V in Equation 33 to calculate a clearance value.

$$Cl = (K)(V)$$

A second approach might be to again start with the initial concentration decayed to the time of the second sample and add to that concentration the contribution of a continuous infusion model that was accumulating toward steady-state. The continuous infusion model could be used because the interval of 1 day between the phenobarbital doses is sufficiently short compared to the $t\frac{1}{2}$ so that the accumulation is a relatively smooth process (see Part Two: Phenobarbital and Fig. 9.1).

$$C_1 = [C(e^{-Kt_1})] + \left[\frac{(S)(F)(Dose/\tau)}{Cl} (1 - e^{-Kt_1}) \right]$$

In the above equation, Cl/V would be substituted for K or (K)(V) for Cl so there is only one unknown to be resolved in the equation.

Lastly, the mass balance approach could be used.

$$\frac{(S)(F)(Dose/\tau) - \dfrac{(C_2 - C_1)(V)}{t}}{Css \text{ ave}} = Cl$$

Where t would be the 10-day interval between the initial phenobarbital level and the second level. This last approach using mass balance is a direct solution and does not require an iterative search. The solution for clearance should be reasonably good as long as the three rules previously mentioned are met. If there are concerns that the value of Cl is incorrect, this value of Cl could be used in one of the previous equations to see if the more complex equation will predict the observed second phenobarbital concentration. A word of caution: If the clearance value predicts the phenobarbital concentration well (calculated value is close to the observed value), it does not necessarily mean the clearance is correct—only that regardless of which equation is used, you will calculate the same answer.

Single-Point Determination of Clearance

A drug concentration obtained approximately 1.44 half-lives after a single bolus dose is primarily a function of clearance. This concept is represented in Figure 32. The ability to predict clearance using this principle is based on a complex relationship between volume of distribution, clearance, and half-life. As can be seen from Equation 49 for C and Equation 32 for $t\frac{1}{2}$:

$$C = \frac{(S)(F)(Loading\ Dose)}{V} \qquad\qquad t\frac{1}{2} = \frac{(0.693)(V)}{Cl}$$

if clearance is held constant, and volume of distribution is decreased, the initial plasma levels will be higher and the elimination half-life will be decreased. However, if volume of distribution is increased, the initial plasma concentrations will be lower and the elimination half-life will be longer.

By examining Figure 32, it can be seen that over a range of volume of distribution values, there is a locus or point about which the decaying plasma concentration-versus-time curves appears to pivot. This pivot point is at 1.44 half-lives. For this reason, a single plasma concentration

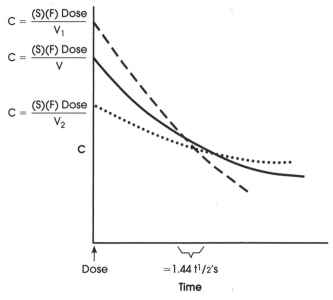

$$C = \frac{(S)(F)\,Dose}{V_1}$$

$$C = \frac{(S)(F)\,Dose}{V}$$

$$C = \frac{(S)(F)\,Dose}{V_2}$$

C

Dose $\approx 1.44\ t^1/2's$

Time

FIGURE 32. Single-point determination of clearance. The plasma concentrations following a single bolus dose when clearance is held constant and volume of distribution is altered tend to pivot around a single point that occurs at approximately 1.44 half-lives after the dose. When the volume of distribution is small (- - - V_1), the concentrations before the 1.44 half-life points are elevated, relative to the concentrations found in patients with larger volumes of distribution (· · · V_2). The opposite is true after the 1.44 half-life point.

obtained at 1.44 half-lives following an initial bolus dose[64-66] can be used to estimate a clearance. This approach is essentially a rearrangement of Equation 30:

$$K = \frac{\ln\left(\dfrac{C_1}{C_2}\right)}{t}$$

where (S)(F)(Dose)/V is substituted for C_1, and C_2 is the measured plasma concentration at time t after the loading dose.

$$K = \frac{\ln\left(\dfrac{(S)(F)(Loading\ Dose)/V}{C_2}\right)}{t} \qquad \text{[Eq. 67]}$$

Equation 33 below can then be used with the assumed value for V to calculate the patient's clearance.

$$Cl = (K)(V)$$

It is important to recognize that if the patient's clearance or volume of distribution values differ substantially from those assumed, a sampling time based on a literature-derived half-life may not represent 1.44 half-lives for the patient. In this instance, accurate patient-specific clearance would not be derived from this method outlined using Equations 67 and 33. For example, if a patient has a very low clearance and a longer-than-expected elimination half-life, plasma samples obtained at 1.44 times the drug's reported half-life will represent a sampling time that is sooner than 1.44 times the patient's actual half-life. Plasma samples obtained at this time are primarily a function of volume of distribution and would be influenced much less by clearance. Conversely, if the patient's clearance is much greater than the literature value, a sample obtained at 1.44 of the usual $t\frac{1}{2}$'s may represent several of the patient's true half-lives. Under these conditions, the observed plasma concentration is influenced to a large degree by both volume of distribution and clearance. As a result, the ability to extract (with any level of confidence) revised values for clearance or volume of distribution is extremely limited.

It is often difficult to accurately plan a sampling time that can be used for the single-point method. However, if sensitivity testing reveals that clearance is the primary determinant of a concentration obtained approximately 1.44 half-lives after a bolus dose, this concentration may be used to ascertain a patient-specific clearance.

BAYESIAN ANALYSIS

As previously discussed, the usual approach when using pharmacokinetics in the clinical setting is to solve our kinetic problem by using simple manipulations of an equation and then solving the equation by revising or changing one or sometimes two variables, usually volume of distribution and/or clearance. This technique works well if the clinician has a good understanding of pharmacokinetics and good clinical judgment. One of the potential dangers is that a clinical decision might be made using pharmacokinetic data that have a very low level of reliability. To help guard against this type of error, many pharmacokinetic computer programs use Bayesian analysis.

The mathematics in this approach is complicated and requires significant computational capacity. However, the concept is relatively simple. The basic approach used in this analysis technique is to adjust each element in the equation to the degree that it helps solve the equation and to the degree that it is likely that the initial estimates are wrong. Depending on the way the program is designed, everything from adherence to bioavailability, concentration measurement variability, and our usual parameters of clearance and volume of distribution can be considered in the revision process. There are three key issues with the Bayesian approach. One is that the average population value is a good and a reasonable estimate for the patient. Second is that the uncertainty or variability in the individual parameters is known. Third is that the pharmacokinetic model is appropriate.

As an example, we can consider Equation 50 below:

$$C_1 = \frac{(S)(F)(\text{Loading Dose})}{V}(e^{-Kt_1})$$

If we take a situation in which we obtain two drug samples relatively soon after a loading dose of 100 mg is administered, both of the drug concentrations would have information about V but very little information about clearance. In this problem, we will start by assuming that S and F are 1, V is 10 L, Cl is 1 L/hr, K = 0.1 hr^1 (t$\frac{1}{2}$ = 6.93 hr), and the two sampling times are at 0.5 and 1 hours after the dose.

$$C_1 = \frac{(S)(F)(\text{Loading Dose})}{V}(e^{-(K)(t_1)})$$

$$= \frac{(1)(1)(100 \text{ mg})}{10 \text{ L}}(e^{-(0.1 \text{ hr}^{-1})(0.5 \text{ hr})})$$

$$= 10 \text{ mg/L } (0.951)$$

$$= 9.51 \text{ mg/L}$$

and the second concentration would be:

$$= \frac{(1)(1)(100 \text{ mg})}{10 \text{ L}}(e^{-(0.1 \text{ hr}^{-1})(1 \text{ hr})})$$

$$= 10 \text{ mg/L } (0.905)$$

$$= 9.05 \text{ mg/L}$$

If the laboratory reported the drug concentration at 0.5 and 1 hour to be 9.8 and 8.7 mg/L, respectively, we would, from a clinical point of view, simply look at the expected values of 9.51 and 9.05 and consider the predictions to be excellent. We would assume that the less than 10% differences in the predicted and observed drug concentrations were due to assay error. Knowing that the two drug levels were obtained very soon after the initial loading dose suggests that our volume of distribution is approximately correct. However, very little information about clearance is "contained" in the two drug samples. This would mean that our maintenance dosing regimen should be based on our original estimate of 1 L/hr for clearance. We would use the expected clearance value not because we know it is correct, but rather because we do not have any additional information that would suggest changing our original expectation.

There are computer programs (and clinicians with calculators) that would use what is commonly thought of as an "exact fit" method of analysis.

This method tries to make everything fit the drug concentrations as closely as possible. In our example, S, F, t_1, and C_1, would be assumed to be exact values, and any differences between the observed values in C and the expected value are due to differences in our expected V and Cl. Following this line of reasoning, Equation 30 and the two drug concentrations can be used to calculate a new elimination rate constant of 0.238 hr^{-1}:

$$K = \frac{\ln\left(\dfrac{C_1}{C_2}\right)}{t}$$

where C_1 is 9.8 mg/L, C_2 is 8.7 mg/L, and t is the 0.5 hour time interval between the first and second sample. (Note: these two samples were obtained less than one $t\frac{1}{2}$ apart, indicating that the calculated K will be suspect.)

$$K = \frac{\ln\left(\dfrac{9.8\ \text{mg/L}}{8.7\ \text{mg/L}}\right)}{0.5\ \text{hr}}$$

$$= 0.238\ \text{hr}^{-1}$$

Now using Equation 28 and rearranging to solve for C_1, just after the bolus dose or one-half hour before the first sample, we calculate a drug level of 11.04 mg/L.

$$C_2 = C_1(e^{-(K)(t)})$$

$$9.8\ \text{mg/L} = C_1(e^{-(0.238\ \text{hr}^{-1})(0.5\ \text{hr})})$$

$$9.8\ \text{mg/L} = C_1(0.888)$$

$$\frac{9.8\ \text{mg/L}}{(0.888)} = C_1$$

$$11.04\ \text{mg/L} = C_1$$

Now using this concentration of 11.04 mg/L that would correspond to the C in Equation 49, we can calculate a revised volume of distribution of 9.1 L.

$$C = \frac{(S)(F)(\text{Loading Dose})}{V}$$

$$11.04\ \text{mg/L} = \frac{(1)(1)(100\ \text{mg})}{V}$$

$$V = \frac{(1)(1)(100\ \text{mg})}{11.04\ \text{mg/L}}$$

$$V = 9.1\ \text{L}$$

Note that the revised V of 9.1 L is reasonably close to the initial estimate of 10 L. This is as we would expect considering that the timing of the samples is close to the loading dose.

However, if we use the revised K of 0.238 hr^{-1} and V of 9.1 L in Equation 33 to calculate a revised value for Cl, we would calculate 2.17 L/hr.

$$Cl = (K)(V)$$

$$Cl = (0.238hr^{-1})(9.1\ L)$$

$$Cl = 2.17\ L/hr$$

This revised clearance is more than twice our initial estimate of 1 L/hr and would have a major impact on the maintenance regimen.

This revision is an example of making too much out of too little information. A Bayesian pharmacokinetics program would try to balance the change in the calculated drug concentrations as a result of a change in clearance, and attempt to come up with a reasonable estimate or compromise considering that there is an expected assay error as well as some error in V and Cl. The end result would probably be a slightly higher clearance, a slightly smaller volume of distribution, and some slight differences in the observed and predicted drug concentrations. This approach would help to avoid the huge change in clearance that occurred using the "exact fit" type of analysis. This Bayesian analysis would be similar to our initial conclusion that the observed and predicted drug concentrations are a close fit and confirm V but do not contain much information on Cl.

When drug levels are obtained at an "optimal" time, and the appropriate pharmacokinetic parameter is being analyzed, both the "exact fit" and Bayesian approaches usually give essentially the same answer. It should also be pointed out that while the Bayesian approach will help to prevent the error of making too much of too little, it cannot correct or account for large real errors. Bayesian computer programs cannot adjust for gross errors. For example, errors in dose (200 mg administered vs. 100 mg recorded as given), sample labeling (sample labeled with incorrect patient name), model (linear vs. nonlinear elimination), etc. cannot be successfully corrected by Bayesian or any other type of computer program. Another potential problem with Bayesian programs occurs when the patient is truly different from the expected patient population. In this situation, the computer will tend to place less emphasis on the drug concentrations from the patient and try to revise toward parameters that are more like the average patient. This problem should be taken in the context that in most clinical situations, data that are very unusual are often errors. Regardless of what type of approach is taken, it is important for the clinician to evaluate the drug concentration in the context of the patient and use rational judgment as to how pharmacokinetics is used in designing drug regimens.

ASSAY SPECIFICITY

The accuracy and specificity of assays used by the clinical laboratory to measure serum drug concentrations are critical. Historically, laboratories developed their assay procedures using a variety of analytical methods ranging from radioimmunoassays to high-performance liquid chromatography (HPLC) assay procedures. Currently, however, the vast majority of drug assays performed in the clinical setting are some variant of commercially available immunobinding assay procedures. The most commonly used procedures are fluorescence polarization immunoassay (FPIA) and enzyme immunoassay [enzyme multiplied immunoassay technique (EMIT) and enzyme-linked immunosorbent assay (ELISA)].[67,68]

These assays are generally specific; however, in isolated instances, metabolites or other drug-like substances are also recognized by the antibody.[69–73] Most assay interferences are the result of cross-reactivity with the drug's metabolites, but in some cases endogenous compounds or drugs with similar structures can cross-react, resulting in either a falsely elevated or decreased assayed drug concentraton.[72–77]

Pharmacokinetic parameters derived from nonspecific assays or plasma concentrations that are in error may influence clinicians to make decisions that are not optimal for patient care.[74–77] Whereas the current literature is usually associated with relatively specific drug assays, caution should always be exercised when using serum drug concentrations as part of the clinical decision-making process. This is especially true when the older literature is used, because pharmacokinetic parameters that have been derived from assays with differing specificities are not interchangeable. The usual therapeutic range will also be altered when more specific assays are used.

For assays that measure the parent compound only, it is important to determine the pharmacologic activity and pharmacokinetic behavior of the metabolites. Many drugs have active metabolites that may affect a patient's pharmacologic response (Table 4); the pharmacokinetic behavior of these metabolites cannot be predicted by assaying only the parent compound. One example of this is the active metabolite of procainamide, N-acetyl-procainamide (NAPA), which accumulates to rather high concentrations in patients with renal failure.[79] For this drug, therefore, an assay that measures only procainamide could underestimate the pharmacologic response of the patient.

Whenever possible, one should evaluate the patient's clinical response directly. If drug levels and clinical response do not correlate as predicted, it may be due to a laboratory error. Similarly, factors unique to the patient, such as concurrent disease states or antagonist drug therapy, may alter one's interpretation of the plasma drug concentration. For example, it is a common clinical observation that higher-than-usual plasma concentrations of digoxin are required to achieve a clinical response in patients with atrial fibrillation. Furthermore, for drugs that have high plasma

TABLE 4 Examples of Drugs with Active Metabolites[33,78]

Amitriptyline
Carbamazepine
Chlordiazepoxide
Chlorpromazine
Chlorpropamide
Diazepam
Lidocaine
Meperidine
Metronidazole
Primidone
Procainamide
Propranolol
Warfarin

protein binding, the same therapeutic effect will be achieved with a lower plasma concentration when plasma protein binding is decreased. This is because for most clinical assays both bound and free drug levels are measured, and decreased binding lowers the bound concentration but not the free, pharmacologically active concentration [see Desired Plasma Concentration (C)]. The formation of aberrant metabolites and tachyphylaxis are other reasons why plasma drug concentrations fail to correlate with an expected therapeutic response.

Creatinine Clearance (Cl$_{Cr}$)

Because many drugs are partially or totally eliminated by the kidney, an accurate estimation of renal function is an important component in the application of pharmacokinetics to designing drug therapy regimens. Creatinine clearance as determined by a urine collection and corresponding plasma sample is considered by many clinicians to be the most accurate test of renal function. In the clinical setting, the time delay and the difficulty in obtaining the 24-hour creatinine collection limit the utility of the 24-hour urine collection. In addition, all too often, the urine collection is inaccurate because a portion is accidentally discarded or the time of collection is shorter or longer than requested.[80,81] Perhaps the most common error is an incomplete collection, which will result in an underestimation of renal function. Because decisions with regard to drug dosing must often be made quickly, several authors have suggested a variety of methods by which Cl$_{Cr}$ can be estimated using a serum creatinine value. The most accurate of these equations include serum creatinine, body weight or size, age, and gender.[81,82]

CREATININE PHARMACOKINETICS

The pharmacokinetics of creatinine are presented in far more detail elsewhere,[80,83–86] but a brief overview is necessary. Creatinine is a metabolic byproduct of muscle, and its rate of formation (R$_A$) is primarily determined by an individual's muscle mass or lean body weight. It varies, therefore, with age (lower in the elderly) and gender (lower in females).[87–89] For any given individual, the rate of creatinine production is assumed to be constant. Once creatinine is released from muscle into plasma, it is eliminated almost exclusively by renal glomerular filtration. Any decrease in the glomerular filtration rate ultimately results in a rise in the serum creatinine level until a new steady state is reached and the amount of creatinine cleared per day equals the rate of production. In other words, at steady state, the rate in must equal the rate out. Since the rate of creatinine production remains constant even when renal clearance diminishes, the serum creatinine must rise until the product of the clearance and the serum creatinine again equals the rate of production. This concept is represented by Equation 14 and has been discussed earlier in the section on clearance:

$$\leftrightarrow R_A = (\downarrow Cl)(\uparrow Css\ ave)$$

where $\leftrightarrow R_A$ is a constant rate of creatinine production, $\downarrow Cl$ is the decreased creatinine clearance, and $\uparrow Css\ ave$ is the increased steady-state serum creatinine level or SCr$_{ss}$ such that when steady state is achieved the product of (Cl)(Css ave) will be equal to the R_A or production rate of creatinine.

ESTIMATING CREATININE CLEARANCE FROM STEADY-STATE SERUM CREATININE CONCENTRATIONS

The degree to which a steady-state serum creatinine rises is inversely proportional to the fall in creatinine clearance. Therefore, the new creatinine clearance can be estimated by multiplying a normal Cl_{Cr} value by the fractional change in the serum creatinine: Normal SCr/Patient's SCr_{ss}. For the 70 kg man, it can be assumed that the normal SCr is 1.0 mg/dL and that the corresponding Cl_{Cr} is 120 mL/min:

$$\text{New } Cl_{cr} = (120 \text{ mL/min})\left[\frac{1 \text{ mg/dL}}{SCr_{ss}}\right] \qquad \text{[Eq. 68]}$$

On the basis of this concept, one can see that each time the serum creatinine doubles, the creatinine clearance falls by half and that small changes in the serum creatinine at low concentrations are of much greater consequence than equal changes in the serum creatinine at high concentrations. To illustrate, if a patient with a normal serum creatinine of 1.0 mg/dL is reported to have a new steady-state serum creatinine of 2 mg/dL, the creatinine clearance has decreased from 120 mL/min to 60 mL/min. However, if a patient with chronic renal dysfunction has a usual serum creatinine of 4 mg/dL (Cl_{Cr} = 30 mL/min), a similar 1.0 mg/dL increase in the serum creatinine to 6 mg/dL would result in a small drop in the Cl_{Cr} (5 mL/min) and a new clearance value of 24 mL/min. However, at some point even small changes in Cl_{Cr} can be physiologically significant to the patient. As an example, for a patient with a creatinine clearance of 100 mL/min to have their renal function decline by 10 mL/min is of very little consequence, but for a patient with a creatinine clearance of 15 mL/min, a 10 mL/min decrease would probably change their clinical status from a patient with very poor renal function to a patient who would require dialysis.

The estimation of Cl_{Cr} from SCr_{ss} alone is reasonably satisfactory as long as the patient's daily creatinine production is average (i.e., 20 mg/kg/day); the patient weighs approximately 70 kg and the serum creatinine is at steady state (i.e., not rising or falling). These conditions are usually present in the young healthy adult, but young healthy adults are not the typical patient for whom pharmacokinetics manipulations are most useful.

Adjusting to Body Size: Weight or Body Surface Area

To account for any changes in creatinine production and clearance that may result from a difference in body size, Equation 68 can be modified to compensate for any deviation in body surface area (BSA) from the 70 kg patient (1.73 m²):

The patient's BSA can be obtained from a nomogram (see Appendix I), estimated from Equation 17:

$$\text{BSA in m}^2 = \left(\frac{\text{Patient's Weight in kg}}{70 \text{ kg}} \right)^{0.7} (1.73 \text{ m}^2)$$

or calculated from the following equation[90]:

$$\text{BSA in m}^2 = (W^{0.425})(H^{0.725})0.007184 \qquad \text{[Eq. 69]}$$

where the Body Surface Area (BSA) is in meters squared (m²), W is weight in kilograms, and H is the patient's height in centimeters.

A disadvantage of using only weight or body surface area is that the elderly or emaciated patients who have a reduced muscle mass do not have a "normal" creatinine clearance of 120 mL/min/1.73 m² with a serum creatinine value of 1.0 mg/dL. For this reason, it may be erroneous to assume that an SCr of 1.0 mg/dL is indicative of a creatinine clearance of 120 mL/min/1.73 m² in these individuals.

On average, as patients age, their muscle mass represents a smaller proportion of their total weight and creatinine production is decreased (Table 5). There are a number of equations that consider age, gender, body size, and serum creatinine when calculating or estimating creatinine clearance for adults.[88,91,92] Although all these methods are similar and equivalent in clinical practice, the most common method used by clinicians is probably the one proposed by Cockcroft and Gault.[91]

TABLE 5   Expected Daily Creatinine Production for Males[89]

Age (yr)	Daily Creatinine Production (mg/kg/day)
20–29	24[a]
30–39	22
40–49	20
50–59	19
60–69	17
70–79	14
80–89	12
90–99	9

[a]Daily creatinine production for females would be expected to be 85% of the above values.

$$\text{Cl}_{cr} \text{ for males (mL/min)} = \frac{(140 - \text{Age})(\text{Weight})}{(72)(\text{SCr}_{ss})} \qquad \text{[Eq. 70]}$$

$$\text{Cl}_{cr} \text{ for females (mL/min)} = (0.85)\frac{(140 - \text{Age})(\text{Weight})}{(72)(\text{SCr}_{ss})} \qquad \text{[Eq. 71]}$$

where age is in years, weight is in kg, and serum creatinine is in mg/dL. Equations 70 and 71 calculate creatinine clearance as mL/min for the patient's characteristics entered into the equation.

The two most critical factors to consider when using the above equations are the assumptions that 1) the serum creatinine is at steady state and 2) the weight, age, and gender of the individual reflect normal muscle mass. For example, when estimating a creatinine clearance for an obese patient, the nonobese or ideal body weight should be used in Equations 70 and 71. This estimate can be based on ideal body weight tables or the following equations.[93]

$$\frac{\text{Ideal Body Weight}}{\text{for males in kg}} = 50 + (2.3)(\text{Height in Inches} > 60) \qquad \text{[Eq. 72]}$$

$$\frac{\text{Ideal Body Weight}}{\text{for females in kg}} = 45 + (2.3)(\text{Height in Inches} > 60) \qquad \text{[Eq. 73]}$$

It should be pointed out, however, that an ideal body weight derived from a patient's height, as in Equations 72 and 73, may not represent the actual nonobese weight of a patient. Although there are some potential flaws in estimating the nonobese weight from height, the ideal body weight (IBW) is usually preferable to using the actual weight (total body weight) when a patient is markedly obese. As a clinical guideline, one approach is to make an adjustment for ideal body weight if the patient's actual weight is >120% of their ideal body weight.

$$\text{"Clinically Obese" if: } \left[\left(\frac{\text{TBW}}{\text{IBW}}\right) \times 100\right] > 120 \qquad \text{[Eq. 74]}$$

Some clinicians use a value of >130% of ideal body weight as their definition of clinically obese. In any case, an adjustment of a patient's weight that is close to their ideal body weight is not warranted given the inherent errors in the assumptions and literature estimates required when applying pharmacokinetic principles to patient care situations.

There are studies indicating that total body weight overestimates and ideal body weight underestimates renal function in the morbidly obese patient. It has been suggested that an adjusted body weight between ideal and total body weight be used to estimate renal function in obese individuals. While this adjustment factor is variable, 40% of the excess weight is commonly used:[94,95]

$$\text{Adjusted Body Weight} = \text{IBW} + 0.4(\text{TBW} - \text{IBW}) \qquad \text{[Eq. 75]}$$

where IBW is the patient's ideal body weight in kg as calculated from Equation 72 or 73, and TBW is the patient's total body weight in kg.

There are other factors not considered in these equations for IBW and Adjusted Body Weight. As an example, in patients with extensive third spacing of fluid (i.e., edema or ascites), the liters (kilograms) of excess third space fluid should probably not be included in the patient's estimate of total body weight. As an example, consider a 5 foot 4 inch male patient weighing 75 kg and having an estimated 15 kg of edema and ascitic fluid. Using the patient height (64 inches) and weight (75 kg) might suggest that the patient is more than 120% over his ideal body weight and therefore "clinically obese" for the purposes of doing pharmacokinetic calculations.

$$\frac{\text{Ideal Body Weight}}{\text{for males in kg}} = 50 + (2.3)(\text{Height in inches} > 60)$$

$$= 50 + (2.3)(4)$$

$$= 59.2$$

$$\text{"Clinically Obese" if: } \left[\left(\frac{\text{TBW}}{\text{IBW}} \right) \times 100 \right] > 120$$

$$: \left[\left(\frac{75}{59.2} \right) \times 100 \right] = 127$$

However, the patient is not obese but rather has a significant amount of interstitial fluid accumulated. This is obvious if we subtract the excessive third space fluid weight of 15 kg from his total weight of 75 kg, resulting in a weight of 60 kg. Clearly, the difference between the "nonexcess third space fluid weight" of 60 kg and the estimated IBW of 59.2 kg is so small that the patient would not be considered clinically obese.

Likewise, when calculating an Adjusted Body Weight, it would be the patient's weight minus any significant third space fluid weight that would be used in Equation 75. The excessive third space fluid weight may or may not be important to consider in making pharmacokinetic calculations. As an example, significant third space fluid does contribute to the apparent volume of distribution for some drugs (see Part Two: Aminoglycoside Antibiotics) but is unlikely to be an important contributor to volume of distribution if the apparent volume of distribution is large (e.g., digoxin) or if there is significant plasma protein binding (e.g., phenytoin, cyclosporine, lidocaine).

Third space fluid weight is unlikely to contribute to and should not be used when initial estimates of clearance are made. However, while not directly influencing clearance, it is possible that the presence of ascites or edema may indicate the presence of a disease process that is known to alter clearance.

Patients who weigh significantly less than their ideal body weight or are emaciated also require special consideration when estimating renal function. While it may seem counterintuitive, a creatinine clearance calculated for an emaciated subject using the patient's weight also tends to overpredict the patient's creatinine clearance. This is because patients who are emaciated tend to have a disproportionally greater loss in muscle mass than total body weight. Consequently, serum creatinine in the denominator of Equations 70 and 71 decreases more than the weight in the numerator, resulting in an overestimate of creatinine clearance. For this reason, the actual rather than ideal body weight should be used when calculating creatinine clearance in emaciated subjects. Even then, creatinine clearance is likely to be overestimated.

In addition, it has been suggested that when serum creatinine values are < 1.0 mg/dL, more accurate predictions of creatinine clearance can be obtained if these levels are upwardly adjusted or normalized to a value of 1.0 mg/dL. This suggestion is based on the assumption that low serum creatinine values are related to small muscle mass and a decreased creatinine production rather than to an unusually large creatinine clearance. It is a common practice for clinicians to normalize serum creatinine values < 1 mg/dL to 1 mg/dL.[96,97] However, there is evidence suggesting that using the actual serum creatinine values of < 1 mg/dL results in more accurate estimates of creatinine clearance.[98,99] Because of this continuing controversy and the difficulty in estimating creatinine clearance accurately, it is important to use clinical judgment in evaluating the risk versus the benefit of drug therapy. When a serum creatinine of < 1 mg/dL is used in Equations 70 or 71, most clinicians would recommend setting an upper limit for creatinine clearance. As an example, a 50-year-old man weighing 60 kg with a serum creatinine of 0.5 mg/dL would have a calculated creatinine clearance of 150 mL/min if the serum creatinine of 0.5 mg/dL is used:

$$\text{Cl}_{cr} \text{ for males (mL/min)} = \frac{(140 - \text{Age})(\text{Weight})}{(72)(\text{SCr}_{ss})}$$

$$= \frac{(140 - 50)(60)}{(72)(0.5)}$$

$$= 150 \text{ mL/min}$$

and a value of 75 mL/min if the serum creatinine is normalized to 1 mg/dL:

$$\text{Cl}_{cr} \text{ for males (mL/min)} = \frac{(140 - \text{Age})(\text{Weight})}{(72)(\text{SCr}_{ss})}$$

$$= \frac{(140 - 50)(60)}{(72)(1)}$$

$$= 75 \text{ mL/min}$$

Even if the first method is used, many clinicians would suggest that an upper limit for a calculated creatinine clearance should be set at somewhere near 120 mL/min. Of course in specific situations (e.g., very large, nonobese, young healthy male patient), a creatinine clearance of more than 120 mL/min might be appropriate to consider. Therefore, whether to normalize a patient's serum creatinine and whether there should be some upper limit for the calculated value of creatinine clearance should be dictated by clinical judgment rather than a specific rule.

Pediatric Patients

Estimation of creatinine clearance in children is difficult. There are several approaches,[100–102] and the fact that muscle mass and renal function continue to mature for the first year of life makes the infant especially challenging. One of the more commonly used equations for children from ages 1 to 18 years is as follows:[100]

$$\text{Cl}_{cr} \text{ for Children (mL/min/1.73m}^2\text{)} = \frac{(0.48)(\text{Height in cm})}{\text{SCr}_{ss}} \qquad \text{[Eq. 76]}$$

The above equation calculates the creatinine clearance that would exist if the child were the size of the standard 1.73 m^2 or 70 kg patient. Although Equation 76 does not calculate the creatinine clearance for the child, it is useful as a guide to the child's relative renal function; values near 100 mL/min per 1.73 m^2 would be considered relatively normal, and many dosing guides express creatinine clearance in this way. To calculate the actual creatinine clearance for the child, the creatinine clearance value calculated in Equation 76 should be adjusted for the patient's body size:

$$\text{Cl}_{cr} \text{ for Children (mL/min)} = (\text{Cl}_{cr} \text{ mL/min/1.73 m}^2)\left(\frac{\text{BSA}}{1.73 \text{ m}^2}\right) \qquad \text{[Eq. 77]}$$

where the body surface area is in m^2 as calculated from the nomogram in Appendix I,

or

$$\frac{Cl_{cr} \text{ for Children}}{(mL/min)} = (Cl_{cr} \text{ mL/min/1.73 m}^2)\left(\frac{\text{Weight in kg}}{70 \text{ kg}}\right)^{0.7} \quad \text{[Eq. 78]}$$

Although Equation 76 was designed to be used for children between the ages of 1 and 18 years, it appears to be less accurate in children < 100 cm tall.[92]

While use of Equation 76 does not require the child's weight to calculate creatinine clearance, it is assumed that the muscle mass for the child is normal for the child's height. For example, a child with an unusually low muscle mass for his height would produce less creatinine than a child of the same height with a normal amount of muscle mass. In this case, the creatinine clearance would be overestimated. Similarly, caution needs to be exercised in obese children. Equation 76 does not require the child's weight, and assuming the obese child has a normal amount of muscle mass for their height, the calculated creatinine clearance as mL/min/1.73 m² should be reasonably accurate. However, if the creatinine clearance as mL/min/1.73 m² is to be converted into a creatinine clearance for the child using Equations 77 or 78, caution is warranted. Whether calculating BSA or weight in kg, it is the child's estimated nonobese weight that would be most logical to use.

The principles and cautions to be exercised when calculating creatinine clearance in children are the same as in adults. The serum creatinine should be at steady state, and the muscle mass should be reasonably average for the child's size.

ESTIMATING TIME TO REACH A STEADY-STATE SERUM CREATININE LEVEL

All the above methods for estimating Cl_{cr} require a steady-state serum creatinine concentration. When a patient's renal function suddenly changes, some period of time will be required to achieve a new steady-state serum creatinine concentration. In this situation, it is important to be able to estimate how long it will take for the SCr to reach steady state. If a rising serum creatinine is used in any of the previous equations, the patient's creatinine clearance will be overestimated.

As presented earlier, half-life is a function of both the volume of distribution and clearance. If the volume of distribution of creatinine (0.5 to 0.7 L/kg)[103,104] is assumed to remain constant, the time required to reach 95% of steady state in patients with normal renal function is less than 1 day.[103,105] As an example, the average 70 kg patient with a creatinine clearance of 120 mL/min (7.2 L/hr) with a volume of distribution for creatinine of 45.5 L (0.65 L/kg) would be expected to have a creatinine t½ of 4.4 hours as calculated by Equation 32:

$$t\frac{1}{2} = \frac{0.693(V)}{Cl}$$

$$= \frac{0.693(45.5\ L)}{7.2\ L/hr}$$

$$= 4.4\ hr$$

Under these conditions, 90% of steady state should be achieved in approximately 15 hours (3.3 t½'s). However, if the same patient had a creatinine clearance of 10 mL/min (0.6 L/hr) the creatinine t½ would be 52.5 hours and many days would be required to ensure that steady state had been achieved. One useful approach is to remember that as a drug (in this case creatinine) concentration is accumulating toward steady state, half of the total change will occur in the first half-life. Therefore, two serum creatinine concentrations obtained several hours apart (8 to 12 hours) that appear to be similar (i.e., not increasing or declining) and that represent reasonably normal renal function probably represent steady-state conditions. As renal function declines, proportionately longer intervals between creatinine measurements are required to assure that steady-state conditions exist.

In clinical practice, patients occasionally have a slowly increasing serum creatinine. As an example, a patient might have the following serum creatinine concentrations on four consecutive days: 1 mg/dL, 1.2 mg/dL, 1.6 mg/dL, and 1.8 mg/dL. First it should be recognized that the increase in serum creatinine from day 1 to day 2 could be due to assay error alone as the absolute error for most creatinine assays is ± 0.1 to 0.2 mg/dL. Also, given that the t½ of creatinine at concentrations in the range of 1 to 2 mg/dL is approximately 4 to 8 hours, steady state should have been achieved in the first day. Therefore, the continued increase in serum creatinine probably reflects ongoing changes in creatinine clearance over the 4 days. The difficult clinical issue is not what the creatinine clearance is on each of the 4 days, but rather what it will be tomorrow, what the cause is, and how to prevent or minimize the ongoing renal damage.

ESTIMATING CREATININE CLEARANCE FROM NONSTEADY-STATE SERUM CREATININE CONCENTRATIONS

Using nonsteady-state serum creatinine values to estimate creatinine clearance is difficult, and a number of approaches have been proposed.[83,84] The author uses Equation 79 below to estimate creatinine clearance when steady-state conditions have not been achieved.

$$Cl_{cr} \text{ mL/min} = \cfrac{\left(\dfrac{\text{Production of Creatinine}}{\text{in mg/day}}\right) - \left[\left(\dfrac{(SCr_2 - SCr_1)(V_{cr})}{t}\right)(10 \text{ dL/L})\right]}{(SCr_2)(10 \text{ dL/L})}$$

$$\left(\dfrac{1000 \text{ mL/L}}{1440 \text{ min/day}}\right)$$

[Eq. 79]

The daily production of creatinine in mg is calculated by multiplying the daily production value in mg/kg/day from Table 5 by the patient's weight in kg. The serum creatinine values in Equation 79 are expressed in units of mg/dL; t is the number (or fraction) of days between the first serum creatinine measurement (SCr_1) and the second (SCr_2). The volume of distribution of creatinine (V_{cr}) is calculated by multiplying the patient's weight in kg times 0.65 L/kg. Equation 79 is essentially a modification of the mass balance Equation 65:

$$\cfrac{(S)(F)(\text{Dose}/\tau) - \dfrac{(C_2 - C_1)(V)}{t}}{Css \text{ ave}} = Cl$$

where the daily production of creatinine in mg has replaced the infusion rate of the drug and the second serum creatinine value replaced Css ave. The second serum creatinine is used primarily because Equation 79 is most commonly applied when creatinine clearance is decreasing (serum creatinine rising), and using the higher of the two serum creatinine values results in a lower, more conservative estimate of renal function. Some have suggested that the iterative search process, as represented by the combination of Equations 28 and 37, be used:

$$C_2 = (C)(e^{-Kt}) + \frac{(S)(F)(\text{Dose}/\tau)}{Cl}(1 - e^{-Kt_1})$$

where C_2 represents SCr_2, and C represents SCr_1. (S)(F)(Dose/τ) represents the daily production of creatinine, and t represents the time interval between the first and second serum creatinine concentrations. Cl represents the creatinine clearance with the corresponding elimination rate constant K being the creatinine clearance divided by the creatinine volume of distribution. As discussed previously [see Interpretation of Plasma Drug Concentrations: Nonsteady-State Revision of Clearance (Iterative Search)], the solution would require an iterative search, and the inherent errors in the calculation process probably do not warrant this type of calculation.

The use of Equation 79 can be illustrated by considering a 45-year-old, 70 kg man who has a serum creatinine concentration of 1.0 mg/dL on day 1 and a concentration of 2.0 mg/dL 24 hours later on day 2. Using

Table 5, the expected daily production of creatinine for this patient would be 1400 mg/day (20 mg/kg/day × 70 kg). The volume of distribution for creatinine is 45.5 L (0.65 L/kg × 70 kg), and the time between samples (t) is 1 day. Using these values, Equation 79 estimates a creatinine clearance of 32.8 mL/min.

$$Cl_{cr}\ mL/min = \frac{\left(\begin{array}{c}\text{Production of}\\ \text{Creatinine in mg/day}\end{array}\right) - \left[\left(\dfrac{(SCr_2 - SCr_1)(V_{cr})}{t}\right)(10\ dL/L)\right]}{(SCr_2)(10\ dL/L)}$$

$$\left(\frac{1000\ mL/L}{1440\ min/day}\right)$$

$$= \frac{(1400\ mg/day) - \left[\left(\dfrac{(2\ mg/dL - 1\ mg/dL)(45.5\ L)}{1\ day}\right)(10\ dL/L)\right]}{(2\ mg/dL)(10\ dL/L)}$$

$$\left(\frac{1000\ mL/L}{1440\ min/day}\right)$$

$$= \frac{(1400\ mg/day) - [455\ mg/day]}{(2\ mg/L)(10)}\left(0.694\ \frac{mL/L}{min/day}\right)$$

$$= 47.25\ L/day\left(0.694\ \frac{mL/L}{min/day}\right)$$

$$= 32.8\ mL/min$$

Although Equation 79 can be used to estimate a patient's creatinine clearance when a patient's serum creatinine is rising or falling, there are potential problems associated with this and all other approaches using nonsteady-state serum creatinine values. First, a rising serum creatinine concentration may represent a continually declining renal function. To help compensate for the latter possibility, the second creatinine (SCr$_2$) rather than the average is used in the denominator of Equation 79. Furthermore, there are nonrenal routes of creatinine elimination that become significant in patients with significantly diminished renal function.[103] Because as much as 30% of a patient's daily creatinine excretion is the result of dietary intake, the ability to predict a patient's daily creatinine production in the clinical setting is limited.[105] One should also consider the potential errors in estimating creatinine production for the critically ill patient, the errors in serum creatinine measurements, and the uncertainty in the volume of distribution estimate for creatinine. Estimating creatinine clearance in a patient with a rising or falling serum creatinine should be viewed as a best guess under difficult conditions, and ongoing reassessment of the patient's renal function is warranted.

EVALUATING CREATININE CLEARANCE: URINE COLLECTIONS

The accuracy of a reported creatinine clearance is dependent on the complete and accurate collection of urine over a 12- or 24-hour period. Errors in the collection process should always be considered. The predicted amount of creatinine produced or excreted for the patient (considering age, gender, weight, and body stature) should be compared with the amount of creatinine actually collected in the urine sample. At steady state, rate in (creatinine production) equals rate out (creatinine excretion). If the amount collected differs significantly from the patient's predicted production, the reported creatinine clearance is likely to be inaccurate. The patient's age, gender, and muscle mass should be considered when estimating the amount of creatinine produced. Increasing age and smaller muscle mass will reduce the expected amount of creatinine produced (see Table 5).

This principle will be illustrated using the following example. The data below were reported for a 55-year-old, 50 kg male patient for whom a 24-hour urine collection for Cl_{Cr} was ordered.

Total Collection Time:	24 hours
Urine Volume:	1200 mL
Urine Creatinine Concentration:	42 mg/dL
Serum Creatinine:	1.5 mg/dL
Creatinine Clearance:	23 mL/min (Uncorrected)
	30 mL/min (Corrected)

The creatinine clearance of 23 mL/min (uncorrected) represents the patient's creatinine clearance as calculated from the urine collection. The creatinine clearance of 30 mL/min (corrected) represents what the patient's creatinine clearance would have been if the patient were 70 kg or 1.73 m². This "corrected" value is most useful as a relative estimate of renal function when the patient is substantially smaller or larger than our average 70 kg, 1.73 m² patient.

The uncorrected Cl_{Cr} was calculated using the following equation:

$$Cl_{cr} = \frac{(U)(V)}{P} \qquad \text{[Eq. 80]}$$

Where U is the urine creatinine concentration in mg/dL, V the volume of urine per time of collection in mL/min, and P the plasma creatinine concentration in mg/dL. Equation 80 results in a Cl_{Cr} in the units of mL/min:

$$Cl_{cr} = \frac{(U)(V)}{P}$$

$$= \frac{(42 \text{ mg/dL})(1200 \text{ mL}/1440 \text{ min})}{1.5 \text{ mg/dL}}$$

$$= 23 \text{ mL/min}$$

The laboratory computer performs these calculations of the uncorrected or corrected creatinine clearance. By performing the above calculation, all we have checked is the math skill of the computer and not the validity of the collection.

To determine whether the collection was complete, the total amount of creatinine collected in the 24-hour period should be calculated.

Since the patient weighs 50 kg, the apparent creatinine production per day can be calculated using the urine collection data and the appropriate conversion factors as follows:

Apparent Rate of Creatinine Production mg/kg/day	=	Amount of Creatinine Excreted per Day in mg Patient's Weight in kg	=	(U)(V) Patient's Weight in kg	[Eq. 81]

$$= \frac{(42 \text{ mg/dL})(1200 \text{ mL/day})(1 \text{ dL}/100 \text{ mL})}{50 \text{ kg}}$$

$$= 10.08 \text{ mg/kg/day}$$

This apparent production rate of creatinine of 10 mg/kg/day is considerably less than the normal production rate of 19 mg/kg/day as estimated from Table 5 for our 55-year-old man. Therefore, one possibility is that the urine collection was incomplete, and the reported value for creatinine clearance is much less than the patient's actual Cl$_{cr}$. However, if the patient has a smaller than average muscle mass, the urine collection may be considered adequate and the reported creatinine clearance of 23 mL/min is the best estimate of the patient's renal function. In clinical practice it is important to evaluate the patient for their "body composition." Patients who have a muscle mass that is less than average usually appear emaciated or very thin and/or have been physically inactive for a prolonged period (e.g., patients who are bedridden secondary to chronic illness or a spinal cord injury). Whether to accept the 24-hour urine collection as complete would depend on our assessment of the patient's physical stature.

An alternative approach to evaluating the 24-hour urine collection could be to compare the Cl_{cr} as calculated from Cockcroft and Gault, Equation 70, to the uncorrected creatinine clearance from the 24-hour urine collection:

$$\frac{Cl_{cr} \text{ for males}}{(mL/min)} = \frac{(140 - Age)(Weight)}{(72)(SCr_{ss})}$$

$$= \frac{(140 - 55)(50)}{(72)(1.5 \text{ mg/dL})}$$

$$= 39.4 \text{ mL/min}$$

In this case, Equation 70 calculated a Cl_{cr} of approximately 40 mL/min and the 24-hour urine collection as a value of 23 mL/min. Clearly they both cannot be correct. Because Equation 70 and the 24-hour collection both used the SCr of 1.5 mg/dL, the difference must be the rate of creatinine production. Equation 70 assumes the average creatinine production for our 55-year-man is about 19 mg/kg/day (see Table 5). This is in contrast to the creatinine in the 24-hour collection, suggesting a production rate of about 10 mg/kg/day. Which is correct? As previously stated, if the patient has an unusually small muscle mass for their size, age, and gender, one might conclude that Equation 70 overestimated the production rate and the creatinine clearance. In this case, the 24-hour urine collection would be the most reasonable estimate of the patient's creatinine clearance. However, if the patient appears to have a normal amount of muscle mass (i.e., average physical stature for a 55-year-old man), then one might conclude that the 24-hour collection was inadequate and has underestimated the patient's creatinine production rate and therefore the creatinine clearance. In this case, the creatinine clearance of 40 mL/min from Equation 70 might be considered the better estimate of the patient's renal function.

Dialysis of Drugs

PHARMACOKINETIC MODELING—STANDARD HEMODIALYSIS

The pharmacokinetic model for drugs in patients undergoing standard intermittent hemodialysis generally follows one of two patterns. In Figure 33, a maintenance drug dose produces plasma concentrations that are relatively constant between dialysis periods. This plasma concentration of drug represents the steady-state condition with very little fluctuation of the drug concentration between doses. This pattern occurs when the input is continuous (intravenous or oral sustained-release) or the dosing interval is much less than the drug half-life (i.e., $\tau < \frac{1}{3}\ t\frac{1}{2}$). The rapid decline in the drug concentration corresponds to periods of hemodialysis when drug is being rapidly removed, and the rapid return of the plasma drug concen-

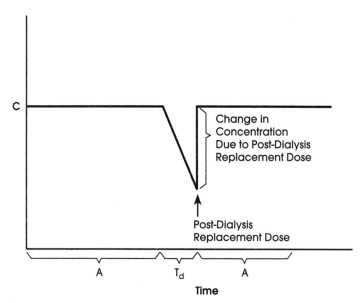

FIGURE 33. Plasma concentration curve between dialysis procedures. This figure represents a plasma concentration curve for a patient receiving a maintenance dose of a drug between dialysis procedures at intervals that result in small fluctuations in plasma concentration. The dosing interval during the interdialysis period (A) is arbitrary but should be less than the half-life of the drug. During the intradialysis period (T_d), the drug is rapidly removed by the dialysis procedure. The subsequent increase in the plasma concentration of drug is due to the postdialysis replacement dose. This model assumes that the drug is significantly removed during dialysis and does not include the distribution phase following the postdialysis replacement dose.

tration to steady state reflects the administration of a postdialysis replacement dose. This pattern can be represented by the following equations:

$$Cl_{pat} = Cl_m + Cl_r \qquad \text{[Eq. 82]}$$

$$Css\ ave = \frac{(S)(F)(Dose/\tau)}{Cl_{pat}} \qquad \text{[Eq. 83]}$$

$$Dose = \frac{(Css\ ave)(Cl_{pat})(\tau)}{(S)(F)} \qquad \text{[Eq. 84]}$$

where Cl_{pat} is the patient's drug clearance during nondialysis periods and is the sum of the patient's metabolic clearance (Cl_m) and residual renal clearance (Cl_r). S and F are the salt form and bioavailability of the drug, and τ is the dosing interval. Equation 83 may be used to predict the average steady-state plasma concentration, and Equation 84 may be used to calculate the maintenance dose based on the estimated Cl_{pat} and the desired Css ave. In addition to the maintenance dose, the patient may also require additional doses following dialysis to replace the drug lost during the dialysis period.

$$\begin{matrix} \text{Postdialysis} \\ \text{Replacement} \\ \text{Dose} \end{matrix} = \begin{bmatrix} \text{Amount of Drug} \\ \text{in the Body} \\ \text{Prior to Dialysis} \end{bmatrix} \begin{bmatrix} \text{Fraction of Drug} \\ \text{Lost During Dialysis} \end{bmatrix}$$

$$\begin{matrix} \text{Postdialysis} \\ \text{Replacement} \\ \text{Dose} \end{matrix} = (V)(Css\ ave)\left(1 - e^{-\left(\frac{Cl_{pat} + Cl_{dial}}{V}\right)(T_d)}\right) \qquad \text{[Eq. 85]}$$

$$\begin{matrix} \text{Postdialysis} \\ \text{Replacement} \\ \text{Dose} \end{matrix} = (V)(Css\ ave)(1 - e^{-K_{dial}(T_d)}) \qquad \text{[Eq. 86]}$$

In the above equations (V)(Css ave) is the amount of drug in the body at the beginning of dialysis, and the elimination rate constant during the dialysis (K_{dial}) represents the sum of the patient's clearance and the clearance by dialysis divided by the volume of distribution ((Cl_{pat} + Cl_{dial})/V). T_d is the duration of dialysis. If the patient's maintenance dose is given once daily, then the patient's dose would be calculated using Equation 84 on nondialysis days. On dialysis days, the patient would receive, in addition to the maintenance dose, a postdialysis replacement dose as calculated by Equation 85 or 86.

The second pharmacokinetic model for drug dosing in patients undergoing hemodialysis is depicted in Figure 34. In this model, a single dose

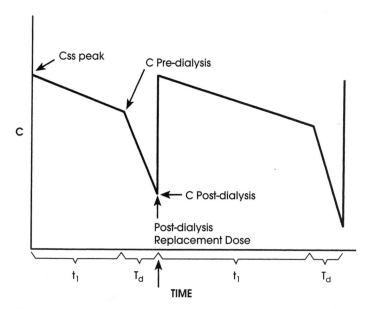

FIGURE 34. Plasma profile for a drug administered only at the postdialysis period for a patient receiving intermittent hemodialysis. The interdialysis period (t_1) represents the time from the steady-state peak concentration to the beginning of dialysis and may vary according to the number of days between each hemodialysis period. The intradialysis period is represented by T_d. The postdialysis dose represents the amount of drug that is lost from the body due to the patient's clearance during the interdialysis period and the dialysis clearance during the intradialysis period.

is given at the conclusion of each dialysis period. Significant amounts of drug are lost between dialysis periods, and additional drug is lost during dialysis. In this model, the dose administered at the end of dialysis replaces all of the drug lost by the patient's own clearance, as well as by dialysis clearance, and returns the drug level to a targeted "peak" concentration. This replacement dose can be calculated by use of Equations 87 or 88:

$$\text{Postdialysis Replacement Dose} = (V)(\text{Css peak})\left(1 - \left[\left(e^{-\left(\frac{Cl_{pat}}{V}\right)(t_1)}\right)\left(e^{-\left(\frac{Cl_{pat} + Cl_{dial}}{V}\right)(T_d)}\right)\right]\right)$$

[Eq. 87]

$$\text{Postdialysis Replacement Dose} = (V)(\text{Css peak})\left(1 - \left[\left(e^{-(K_{pat})(t_1)}\right)\left(e^{-(K_{dial})(T_d)}\right)\right]\right)$$

[Eq. 88]

where t_1 is the interdialysis period or the period from the peak concentration to the beginning of dialysis, and T_d is the dialysis period or the time interval from the beginning to the end of the dialysis procedure. K_{pat} and

K_{dial} are the elimination rate constants during the interdialysis period where drug loss is due to Cl_{pat} alone and the dialysis period where drug loss is the result of both Cl_{pat} and Cl_{dial}.

In some cases it may be appropriate to calculate the drug concentrations at the beginning and end of the dialysis period. This can be accomplished by use of Equations 89 and 90.

$$\text{Predialysis Concentration} = (\text{Css peak})\left(e^{-\left(\frac{Cl_{pat}}{V}\right)(t_1')}\right) \qquad \text{[Eq. 89]}$$

$$\text{Postdialysis Concentration} = \left(\frac{\text{Predialysis}}{\text{Concentration}}\right)\left(e^{-\left(\frac{Cl_{pat} + Cl_{dial}}{V}\right)(T_{d'})}\right) \qquad \text{[Eq. 90]}$$

These equations are used when there are specifically targeted peak and/or trough concentrations or when transient declines in the plasma concentrations might result in therapeutic failures, as with antiarrhythmics or anticonvulsant agents. Depending on the therapeutic intent, the specific drug concentrations may be of more or less interest. As an example, in the case of aminoglycoside antibiotics, the predialysis and not the postdialysis concentration should be thought of as the "trough" in assessing the risk of aminoglycoside toxicity. This is because the pattern of decay is more rapid during the intradialysis period and as a result, the postdialysis aminoglycoside "trough" concentration is transient and does not easily translate into drug exposure and risk of toxicity (Fig. 34). Given that the interval between dialysis runs is often about 48 hours, it is not possible to achieve the usually targeted high peak and low trough aminoglycoside concentrations in the dialysis patient. For these patients the usual gentamicin/tobramycin steady-state peak and predialysis trough concentration are approximately 5 and 2 mg/L. Because of this, the risk of aminoglycoside toxicity may be greater in dialysis patients.

ESTIMATING DRUG DIALYZABILITY

To calculate dosing requirements for patients undergoing intermittent hemodialysis, the dialysis clearance must be known. Although a number of general references are available,[85,86,106–110] it is frequently difficult to find information on specific drugs, especially for drugs that are poorly dialyzable. To determine the dialyzability of a drug, the apparent volume of distribution, plasma protein binding, the patient's clearance, and the drug's half-life should be considered as follows:

1. Divide the volume of distribution by fu or the usual free fraction to calculate the apparent unbound volume of distribution. This is the volume against which the drug will be dialyzed. If the unbound vol-

ume of distribution exceeds 3.5 L/kg or approximately 250 L/70 kg, it is unlikely that the drug will be dialyzable.

$$\text{Unbound Volume of Distribution} = \frac{V}{fu} \qquad \text{[Eq. 91]}$$

2. Estimate the patient's clearance. If this value is > 10 mL/min/kg or 700 mL/min/70kg, it is unlikely that hemodialysis will add significantly to the patient's intrinsic drug elimination process. This is because most drugs have a hemodialysis clearance less than 150 mL/min.
3. If the usual dosing interval is much less than the drug's $t\frac{1}{2}$, it is unlikely that hemodialysis will significantly alter the dosing regimen. The key here is to schedule the drug administration shortly after rather than shortly before dialysis, so that even if the drug is dialyzable, very little is remaining to be removed by dialysis.
4. Drugs with a low molecular weight are more likely to be removed significantly by dialysis. Drugs with a molecular weight > 1000 daltons are unlikely to be removed by standard hemodialysis. High-flux hemodialysis can remove molecules with molecular weight > 1000 daltons (see High-Flux Hemodialysis below).

For almost all drugs, if any one of the above criteria is met, it is unlikely that the drug in question will be significantly removed by standard hemodialysis. However, if a drug has an unbound volume < 3.5 L/kg, a clearance of < 10 mL/min/kg, a τ that is not greater than the drug's $t\frac{1}{2}$, and a molecular weight < 1000 daltons, it is possible, but not a certainty, that hemodialysis will significantly alter the drug elimination pattern. In these cases it is necessary to review the literature to establish whether the drug is significantly removed by hemodialysis. If Cl_{dial} adds significantly to the patient's clearance, then additional drug replacement following hemodialysis may be appropriate.

As an additional check, the drug half-life during the dialysis period can be calculated:

$$t\frac{1}{2} \text{ during Hemodialysis} = \frac{(0.693)(V)}{(Cl_{pat} + Cl_{dial})} \qquad \text{[Eq. 92]}$$

If the $t\frac{1}{2}$ during hemodialysis greatly exceeds the duration of dialysis, very little drug will be removed during any individual period of dialysis.

Whereas the techniques outlined above can be used to estimate the dialyzability of drugs and thereby model their pharmacokinetic behavior during dialysis, there are a number of potential limitations. For many drugs relatively little is known about either the activity or dialyzability of their metabolites. In addition, these guidelines must be used cautiously in acute overdose situations, because saturation of plasma and tissue binding as well as possible alterations in the pathways for elimination may occur when drug concentrations are very high. Considerable differences in dialysis equipment, the types of membranes used in hemodialysis, and the duration of dialysis can result in data that may not be applicable to all dialysis situations.

Although it would be ideal to have data derived from the specific dialysis equipment used for the patient in question, this will not be the case in most instances. Instead, one must rely on the data in the literature to estimate the average amount of drug that most likely would be removed during the patient's hemodialysis.

Dialysis procedures also vary in duration and effectiveness, but most standard hemodialysis runs are approximately 3 hours. The duration of dialysis can usually be found on the hemodialysis record sheets and should be checked to be certain that the initial plans for dialysis were successfully completed. Also, if the patient's blood flow through the artificial kidney (dialysis membrane) during the dialysis period is less than the usual 200 to 350 mL/min, the estimated drug loss during dialysis should probably be reduced.

The uncertainties and potential problems associated with predictions of drug levels during hemodialysis suggest that plasma drug concentrations guide the approach to therapy when possible. When plasma samples are obtained, the distribution phase associated with IV drug administration, as well as the transient period of disequilibrium between the plasma and tissue compartments associated with the hemodialysis process, should be avoided. Although this disequilibrium between the plasma and tissue during dialysis is not documented for most drugs, it would seem reasonable to wait at least 60 minutes following the end of hemodialysis if postdialysis trough plasma samples are to be obtained.

HIGH-FLUX HEMODIALYSIS

High-flux or high-efficiency hemodialysis refers to a dialysis process that utilizes a dialysis membrane that has larger pores through which both solvent (water) and solute (electrolytes, drugs, etc.) can pass.[85,86] Because the pore size is larger, high-flux hemodialysis is more capable of removing smaller compounds more efficiently and some larger compounds that standard hemodialysis cannot remove. This process is more efficient than the standard dialysis procedure, making the above techniques to estimate dialyzability less reliable as a predictor but not invalid. To illustrate, vancomycin with its large molecular weight (approximately 1500 daltons) is relatively unaffected by standard hemodialysis. This is because the pore size associated with standard hemodialysis membranes only allows passage of compounds with a molecular weight of less than 1000 daltons and has a limited ability to remove drugs with a molecular weight between 500 and 1000 daltons. However, when a high-flux dialysis membrane is used, the large pore size allows compounds of greater than 1000 daltons to pass through and be eliminated. As a result, during a usual 3-hour high-flux hemodialysis run, there is a rapid drop in the vancomycin drug concentrations followed by a postdialysis rebound in concentration indicating that approximately 17% of the body stores of vancomycin is removed.[111-113]

For those compounds that are eliminated to a significant extent during standard dialysis, even more drug is eliminated during high-flux hemodialysis. However, the differences in elimination are usually one of degree and not in most cases as significant as seen with vancomycin.

CONTINUOUS RENAL REPLACEMENT THERAPY (CRRT)

Continuous renal replacement therapy utilizes an ultrafiltration process with a large pore membrane similar to those in high-flux hemodialysis to filter free water and solute, including unbound drug. The rate of plasma filtration varies but ranges from 0.5 to 2 L/hr. Of course, patients could not tolerate this rate of fluid removal unless the vast majority of fluid being removed was continuously being replaced. Dialysate is sometimes added to the ultrafiltration process, which can further increase solute and drug elimination through a passive diffusion process. Total CRRT output (ultrafiltration + dialysate) is usually in the range of 1 to 2 L/hr. The advantage of CRRT is that it is more hemodynamically forgiving than standard or high-flux hemodialysis and is used in critically ill patients who cannot tolerate intermittent hemodialysis, usually because of hypotension.[85,86,114,115]

CRRT is also referred to as continuous arteriovenous hemofiltration (CAVH) or continuous venovenous hemofiltration (CVVH); when dialysate is added to the process, it is referred to as CAVHD or CVVHD. CRRT with or without dialysate is well documented to remove vancomycin and other drugs.[116-120] Although the absolute clearance of CRRT is not high, it is continuous and can add significantly to the elimination of some drugs.

One approach to identifying which drugs might be significantly influenced by CRRT is to calculate the maximum CRRT dialysis clearance (Cl_{CRRT}). Because the CRRT membranes, like standard and high-flux membranes, do not allow plasma proteins to pass through, only the unbound drug (Cu) can be removed by CRRT. One method of estimating the maximum Cl_{CRRT} is to multiply the total CRRT flow rate (volume of ultrafiltrate + volume of dialysate per interval of time) by the fraction of unbound drug in plasma (fu). This process assumes that both the ultrafiltrate and the dialysate will have a concentration of drug that is equal to the concentration of unbound drug in plasma. This assumption is probably true for the ultrafiltrate but may not be true if the drug is a large molecule and equilibrates slowly with the dialysate.

$$\text{Cl}_{\text{CRRT}} \text{ Maximum} = (\text{fu})(\text{CRRT Flow Rate}) \qquad \text{[Eq. 93]}$$

In Equation 93, fu is the fraction of drug unbound in plasma, and CRRT flow rate is the average volume output of ultrafiltration + dialysate per unit of time. Units for CRRT flow rate are usually expressed as mL/min or L/hr depending on the preference of the clinician. If the Cl_{CRRT} Maximum is $\leq 25\%$ of the patient's residual clearance (Cl_{pat}), then CRRT will not add significantly to the patient's drug elimination process and no dose adjustment would be necessary relative to the presence or absence of CRRT. If Cl_{CRRT} Maximum adds significantly to the patient's clearance, then the literature will have to be reviewed to identify either CL_{CRRT} values or recommended replacement doses for patients undergoing CRRT.[117–122]

Dose calculations are similar to the usual methods because the CRRT process is intended to be continuous. In many cases, the $t\frac{1}{2}$ is extended, even when the patient is receiving CRRT, and doses can be calculated using a variation of Equation 16:

$$\text{Maintenance Dose} = \frac{(\text{Cl}_{\text{pat}} + \text{Cl}_{\text{CRRT}})(\text{Css ave})(\tau)}{(\text{S})(\text{F})} \qquad \text{[Eq. 94]}$$

where Css ave is the average targeted steady-state concentration, Cl_{pat} the metabolic clearance (Cl_{m}) plus an estimate of the patient's residual renal clearance (Cl_{r}), and CL_{CRRT} is an estimate of the CRRT clearance from one of the literature sources or Equation 93 above. When there is likely to be significant fluctuation in drug concentration between doses (i.e., $\tau > \frac{1}{3}$ $t\frac{1}{2}$), the following equation can be used:

$$\text{Dose} = \frac{(\text{Css}_1)(\text{V})(1 - e^{-\text{K}_{\text{CRRT}}\tau})}{(\text{S})(\text{F})(e^{-\text{K}_{\text{CRRT}}t_1})} \qquad \text{[Eq. 95]}$$

This equation solving for dose is a rearrangement of Equation 48, where Css_1 is the desired drug concentration, usually Css max or Css min, t_1 is the time interval from the dose to Css_1, and K_{CRRT} represents the elimination rate constant consisting of Cl_{pat} ($\text{Cl}_{\text{m}} + \text{Cl}_{\text{r}}$) plus CL_{CRRT} divided by the drug's volume of distribution.

As with hemodialysis, patients undergoing CRRT need to be monitored to ensure that the CRRT process is proceeding as planned. Because patients receiving CRRT are critically ill and the process is complex, CRRT therapy is often adjusted on an hour-by-hour and day-by-day basis. The two most important issues to consider are whether the CRRT process has been interrupted and/or whether the CRRT flow rate has been significantly altered. Small changes in CRRT flow rates are normal, but if the patient's CRRT vascular access fails or for some other reason the process is discontinued or the flow rates changed, then many of the drug dosing recommendations will also have to be altered.

PERITONEAL DIALYSIS

Peritoneal dialysis, and especially continuous ambulatory peritoneal dialysis (CAPD), is occasionally used as an alternative to intermittent hemodialysis. This technique takes advantage of the large semipermeable surface area of the intraperitoneal space and is performed by instilling dialysate fluid via a catheter into the peritoneal space. The dialysate is allowed to equilibrate with the surrounding tissue vasculature and then is removed. This creates a clearance mechanism for solutes including body waste products and drugs. The usual volume instilled into the peritoneal space for an adult is ≈ 2 L, although this can vary somewhat depending on the size of the patient and the intent of dialysis. The efficiency of peritoneal dialysis in removing both drugs and body waste products depends on a number of factors. Assuming that the solute in plasma comes to equilibrium with the dialysate fluid, one would expect the concentration of drug in the dialysate to equal the unbound plasma drug concentration. Therefore, the maximum expected CAPD clearance (Cl_{CAPD}) would be approximately equal to the following:

$$Cl_{CAPD} \text{ Maximum} = (fu)(\text{Volume of Dialysate}/T_D) \qquad \text{[Eq. 96]}$$

where fu is the fraction of unbound drug in plasma, Volume of Dialysate is the peritoneal exchange volume, and T_D is the dwell time or the time the dialysate is allowed to remain in the peritoneal space before removal.

Using the usual volume of dialysate instilled into the peritoneal space of ≈ 2000 mL, the usual exchange or dwell time (T_D) of ≈ 6 hours and if fu is assumed to be 1 (no plasma binding), the expected Cl_{CAPD} Maximum for solute and drugs would be approximately 5.5 mL/min.

$$Cl_{CAPD} \text{ Maximum} = (fu)(\text{Volume of Dialysate}/T_D)$$

$$= (1)(2 \text{ L}/6 \text{ hr})$$

$$= 0.333 \text{ L/hr}$$

or

$$= (0.333 \text{ L/hr})(1000 \text{ mL/L})(1\text{hr}/60\text{min})$$

$$= 5.5 \text{ mL/min}$$

Drugs with a residual Cl_{pat} substantially greater than 5.5 mL/min or 0.333 L/hr will not be significantly influenced by peritoneal dialysis. As a general guideline, if the Cl_{CAPD} Maximum is $< 25\%$ of the patient's residual clearance (Cl_{pat}), one would not anticipate a need to adjust a drug's dose if peritoneal dialysis is initiated or discontinued. One of the assumptions in Equation 96 is that equilibrium is achieved between the unbound plasma drug concentration (Cu) and the dialysate fluid. This assumption is probably true for drugs of relatively low molecular weight (i.e., < 500 daltons). Larger compounds may not come to equilibrium within the usual 6-hour dwell time, and very large molecules (e.g., proteins) cannot diffuse across the peritoneal cell walls.

In theory, the Cl_{CAPD} for these larger compounds could be calculated by taking into account the fraction of steady-state equilibrium achieved in the dialysate dwell time as follows:

$$Cl_{CAPD} \approx (fu)\left(\frac{\text{Volume Dialysate}}{T_D}\right)(1 - e^{-(Keq)(T_D)}) \qquad \text{[Eq. 97]}$$

Where, again, fu is the free fraction in plasma of the compound or drug in question, T_D is the dwell time of the dialysate, Keq the equilibrium rate constant for the equilibrium between the unbound drug in plasma and the dialysate, and $[1 - e^{(-Keq)(T_D)}]$ is the fraction of equilibrium achieved during the dialysate dwell time (T_D). Whereas the free fraction or fu is available for many drugs, it should be recognized that in renal disease the free fraction is often increased. Also, the equilibrium rate constant (Keq) is not generally available for most drugs. The fraction of equilibrium achieved can be estimated, however, based on a drug's molecular weight. For example, urea and creatinine, with molecular weights of approximately 60 and 113 daltons, respectively, appear to come to equilibrium relatively rapidly. The average equilibrium half-time for urea and creatinine appears to be approximately 0.66 hr and 2 hr, respectively. Therefore, in the usual 6-hour exchange, urea has essentially reached equilibrium and creatinine approximately 85% of equilibrium.[85,123] Interestingly, the aminoglycoside antibiotics with fu ≈ 1 and molecular weight ≈ 500 daltons have a CAPD clearance that approaches the dialysis exchange rate when the dwell time (T_D) is ≈ 6 hours.[123–125] If equilibrium is approached in 6 hours, this suggests that the equilibrium half-time is probably in the range of 2 hours. Vancomycin, on the other hand, has a peritoneal dialysis clearance of only 1 to 3 mL/min. Given that vancomycin has a fu approaching 1,[33,116,126] this low Cl_{CAPD} suggests that equilibrium between plasma and dialysate is not achieved within the usual 6-hour dwell time. This observation is consistent with the fact that vancomycin is a large molecule with a molecular weight of ≈ 1500 daltons.

The significance of high plasma protein binding on drug clearance is fairly obvious. Compounds that are extensively bound to plasma proteins and have low free concentrations are not likely to be significantly cleared by peritoneal dialysis unless their residual clearance is exceedingly low. The influence of molecular weight and time to reach equilibrium on a drug's dialyzability is less well understood because relatively few data are available. However, the clearance of compounds that appear to come to equilibrium rapidly is likely to be altered if the dwell time is changed. For example, if a patient is taking a drug that has low molecular weight, more drug will be removed if the peritoneal dialysate fluid is exchanged more frequently as predicted by Equation 96. As a result, replacement doses of a drug that are necessitated by dialysis are likely to be influenced by the dialysate exchange rate. In contrast, replacement doses of drugs with high molecular weights are not likely to be significantly influenced by the exchange rate. This is because an increase in the exchange rate is offset by the decrease in dwell time and the fraction of equilibrium achieved. Consequently, the total calculated clearance by Equation 96 would tend to overestimate Cl_{CAPD} and if possible Equation 97 should be used for these larger, more slowly equilibrating compounds.

Because the surface area of the peritoneal membrane is large and peritoneal infections are frequent, it has become a common practice to administer antibiotics directly into the peritoneal space.[127-130] When administered by the peritoneal route, the drug does not remain in the peritoneal space but diffuses from the high concentration in the dialysate fluid to the plasma and the systemic circulation. The most common antibiotics administered intraperitoneally are the cephalosporins, aminoglycosides, and vancomycin. Techniques used to administer these drugs vary from intermittently adding large doses of drug to a single dialysate exchange on a daily or weekly basis, to the addition of smaller amounts of drug in each individual exchange. When drugs are placed in the peritoneal dialysate fluid either intermittently or with each exchange, the ability to achieve peak and trough concentrations is limited (see Part Two: Aminoglycoside Antibiotics and Vancomycin for usual dosing recommendations).

REFERENCES

1. Huffman DH, et al. Absorption of digoxin from different oral preparations in normal subjects during steady state. Clin Pharmacol Ther 1974;16:310.
2. Lisalo E. Clinical pharmacokinetics of digoxin. Clin Pharmacokinet 1977;2:1.
3. Mooradian AD. Digitalis. An update of clinical pharmacokinetics: therapeutic monitoring techniques and treatment recommendations. Clin Pharmacokinet 1988; 15:165–179.
4. Weinberger M, et al. The relation of product formulation to absorption of oral theophylline. N Engl J Med 1978;299:852.
5. Hendeles L, et al. Food-induced dose dumping from a once-a-day theophylline product as a cause of theophylline toxicity. Chest 1985;87:758.
6. Mallis GI, et al. Superior bioavailability of digoxin solution in capsules. Clin Pharmacol Ther 1975;18;761.
7. Marcus FI, et al. Digoxin bioavailability: formulations and rates of infusions. Clin Pharmacol Ther 1976;20:253.

8. Nahata MC, Powell DA. Bioavailability and clearance of chloramphenicol after intravenous chloramphenicol succinate. Clin Pharmacol Ther 1981;30:368.

9. Niles AS, Shand DG. Clinical pharmacology of propranolol. Circulation 1975;52:6.

10. Boyer RW, et al. Pharmacokinetics of lidocaine in man. Clin Pharmacol Ther 1971; 12:105.

11. Fahr A. Cyclosporin clinical pharmacokinetics. Clin Pharmacokinet 1993;24:472–495.

12. Koch-Weser J, Sellers EM. Binding of drugs to serum albumin. N Engl J Med 1976;294:311.

13. Levy RH, Shand D, ed. Clinical implications of drug-protein binding. Clin Pharmacokinet 1984;9(Suppl):1.

14. Levine M, Chang T. Therapeutic drug monitoring of phenytoin. Rationale and current status. Clin Pharmacokinet 1990;19:341–358.

15. Barre J, Didey F, Delion F, Tillement JP. Problems in therapeutic drug monitoring: free drug level monitoring. Ther Drug Monit 1988;10:133–143.

16. Perucca E. Pharmacological and therapeutic properties of valproate: a summary after 35 years of clinical experience. CNS Drugs 2002;10:695–714.

17. Furst DE, Tozer TN, Melmon KL. Salicylate clearance, the resultant of protein binding and metabolism. Clin Pharmacol Ther 1979;3:380–389.

18. Fremstad D, et al. Increased plasma binding of quinidine after surgery. A preliminary report. Eur J Clin Pharmacol 1976;10:441.

19. Tucker GT, et al. Binding of anilide-type local anaesthetics in human plasma. Anesthesiology 1970;33:287.

20. Borga O, et al. Plasma protein binding of basic drugs. Clin Pharmacol Ther 1977;22:539.

21. Adler DS, et al. Hemodialysis of phenytoin in a uremic patient. Clin Pharmacol Ther 1975;18:65.

22. Piafsky KM. Disease-induced changes in the plasma binding of basic drugs. Clin Pharmacokinet 1980;5:246.

23. Pike E, et al. Binding and displacement of basic drugs, acidic and neutral drugs in normal and orosomucoid deficient plasma. Clin Pharmacokinet 1981;6:367.

24. Edwards DJ, et al. Alpha-1-acid glycoprotein concentration and protein binding in trauma. Clin Pharmacol Ther 1982;31:62.

25. Routledge PA, et al. Relationship between alpha-1-acid glycoprotein and lidocaine disposition in myocardial infarction. Clin Pharmacol Ther 1981;30:154.

26. Odar-Cederlof I, et al. Kinetics of diphenylhydantoin in uremic patients: consequence of decreased protein binding. Eur J Clin Pharmacol 1974;7:31.

27. Koch-Weser J, Sellers EM. Binding of drugs to serum albumin. N Engl J Med 1976;294:311.

28. Benet LZ, Hoener BA. Changes in plasma protein binding have little clinical relevance. Clin Pharmacol Ther 2002;3:115–121.

29. Svensson CK, Woodruff MN, Baxter JG, Lalka D. Free drug concentration monitoring in clinical practice. Rationale and current status. Clin Pharmacokinet 1986;11:450–469.

30. Booker HE, Darcy B. Serum concentrations of free diphenylhydantoin and their relationship to clinical intoxication. Epilepsia 1973;14:177–184.

31. Conford EM, et al. Increased blood-brain barrier transportation of protein-bound anticonvulsant drugs in the newborn. J Cereb Blood Flow Metabol 1983;3:280–286.

32. Tozer TN, Gambertoglio JG, Furst DE, Avery DS, Holford NH. Volume shifts and protein binding estimates using equilibrium dialysis: application to prednisolone binding in humans. J Pharm Sci 1983;12:1442–1446.

33. Thummel KE, Shen DD. Appendix II: design and optimization of dosage regimens: pharmacokinetic data. In: Hardman JG, eds. Goodman and Gilman's The

Pharmacologic Basis of Therapeutics. 10th Ed. New York: McGraw-Hill, 2001:1917–2023.

34. LeMarie M, Tillement JP. Role of lipoproteins and erythrocytes in the in vitro binding and distribution of cyclosporin A in the blood. J Pharm Pharmacol 1982;34:715–718.

35. Niederberger W, et al. Distribution and binding of cyclosporine in blood and tissue. Transplant Proc 1983;15:2419–2421.

36. Rowland M. Drug administration and regimens. In: Melmon K, Morelli H, eds. Clinical Pharmacology and Therapeutics. 2nd Ed. New York: MacMillan, 1978:25–70.

37. Reuning RH, et al. Role of pharmacokinetics in drug dosage adjustment: I. Pharmacologic effect kinetics and apparent volume of distribution of digoxin. J Clin Pharmacol 1973;13:127.

38. Gibaldi M, Perrier D. Drug distribution and renal failure. J Clin Pharmacol 1972;12:201.

39. Kappel J, Calissi P. Nephrology: 3. Safe drug prescribing for patients with renal insufficiency. CMAJ 2002;1664:473–477.

40. Rowland M, Tozer TN. Clinical Pharmacokinetics: Concepts and Applications. 2nd Ed. Philadelphia: Lea & Febiger, 1989.

41. Benowitz N. Clinical application of the pharmacokinetics of lidocaine. In: Melmon K, ed. Cardiovascular Drug Therapy. Philadelphia: FA Davis, 1974:77–101.

42. Mitenko PA, Ogilvie RI. Rapidly achieved plasma concentration plateaus, with observation on theophylline kinetics. Clin Pharmacol Ther 1972;13:329.

43. Walsh FM, et al. Significance of non-steady state serum digoxin concentrations. Am J Clin Pathol 1975;63:446.

44. Shapiro W, et al. Relationship of plasma digitoxin and digoxin to cardiac response following intravenous digitalization in man. Circulation 1970;42:1065.

45. Sheiner LB, et al. Estimation of population characteristics of pharmacokinetic parameters from routine clinical data. J Pharmacokinet Biopharm 1977;5:445.

46. Barot MH, et al. Individual variation in daily dosage requirement for phenytoin sodium in patients with epilepsy. Br J Clin Pharmacol 1978;6:267.

47. Vogelstein B, et al. The pharmacokinetics of amikacin in children. J Pediatrics 1977;91:333.

48. FDA Drug Bulletin. IV guidelines for theophylline products. 1980;10:4–6.

49. Lack JA, Stuart-Taylor ME. Calculation of drug dosage and body surface area of children. Br J Anesth 1997;5:601–605.

50. Sawyer M, Ratain MJ. Body surface area as a determinant of pharmacokinetics and drug dosing. Invest New Drugs 2001;2:171–177.

51. Diem K, Lentner C, eds. Documentia Geigy: Scientific Tables. 7th Ed. Switzerland: Ciba-Geigy, 1972.

52. Gunn VL, Nechyba C, eds. The Harriet Lane Handbook: A Manual for Pediatric House Officers. 16th Ed. Chicago: Mosby, 2003.

53. Taketomo CK, ed. Pediatric Dosage Handbook. 9th Ed. Hudson, OH: Lexi-Comp, 2002.

54. Ohnhaus EE, et al. Protein binding of digoxin in human serum. Eur J Clin Pharmacol 1972;5:34.

55. Pang SK, Rowland M. Hepatic clearance of drugs: I. Theoretical considerations of a "well-stirred" model and a "parallel tube" model. Influence of hepatic blood flow, plasma and blood cell binding and hepatocellular enzymatic activity on hepatic drug clearance. J Pharmacokinet Biopharm 1977;5:625.

56. Powell JR, et al. Theophylline disposition in acutely ill hospitalized patients. Am Rev Respir Dis 1978;118:229.

57. Terbraak EW, et al. Once-daily dosing regimen for aminoglycoside plus beta-lactam combination therapy for serious bacterial infection: comparative trial with netilmicin plus ceftriaxone. Am J Med 1990;89:58–66.

58. Nicolau D, et al. Experience with a once-daily aminoglycoside program administered to 2,184 adult patients. Antimicrob Agents Chemother 1995;39:650–655.

59. Craig WA, Vogelman B. The post antibiotic effect. [Editorial.] Ann Intern Med 1987;106:900–902.

60. Zeisler JA, et al. Lidocaine therapy: time for re-evaluation. Clin Pharm 1993; 12:527–528.

61. Wilensky AJ, et al. Kinetics of phenobarbital in normal subjects and epileptic patients. Eur J Clin Pharmacol 1982;23:87–92.

62. Chiou WL, et al. Method for rapid estimation of the total body drug clearance and adjustment of dosing regimen in patients during a constant-rate intravenous infusion. J Pharmacokinet Biopharm 1978;6:135–151.

63. Vozeh S, et al. Rapid prediction of steady-state serum theophylline concentration in patients treated with intravenous aminophylline. Eur J Clin Pharmacol 1980;18:473–477.

64. Slattery JT, et al. Prediction of maintenance dose required to attain a desired drug concentration at steady state from a single determination of concentration after an initial dose. Clin Pharmacokinet 1980;5:377.

65. Koup JR. Single-point prediction methods: a critical review. Drug Intell Clin Pharm 1982;16:855.

66. Unadkat JD, et al. Further considerations of the "single-point, single-dose" method to estimate individual maintenance dosage requirements. Ther Drug Monit 1982;4:201.

67. Glazko AJ. Phenytoin: chemistry and methods of determination. In: Levy RH, et al., eds. Antiepileptic Drugs. 3rd Ed. New York: Raven Press,1989:159–176.

68. Steijns LS, Bouw J, van der Weide J. Evaluation of fluorescence polarization assays for measuring valproic acid, phenytoin, carbamazepine and phenobarbital in serum. Ther Drug Monit 2002;24:432–435.

69. Patel JA, et al. Abnormal theophylline levels in plasma by fluorescence polarization immunoassay in patients with renal disease. Ther Drug Monit 1984;6:458–460.

70. Hicks JM, Brett EM. Falsely increased digoxin concentrations in samples from neonates and infants. Ther Drug Monit 1984;6:461–464.

71. Flachsh H, Rasmussen JM. Renal disease may increase apparent phenytoin in serum as measured by enzyme-multiplied immunoassay. [Letter.] Clin Chem 1980;26:361.

72. Frank El, et al. Performance characteristics of four immunoassays for antiepileptic drugs on the IMMULITE 2000 automated analyzer. Am J Clin Pathol 2002;1:124–131.

73. Dasgupta A. Digoxin-like immunoreactive substances in elderly people. Impact on therapeutic drug monitoring of digoxin and digitoxin concentrations. Am J Clin Pathol 2002;118;4:600–604.

74. Steimer W, Muller C, Eber B. Digoxin assays: frequent, substantial and potentially dangerous interference by spironolactone, canrenone, and other steroids. Clin Chem 2002;48:507–516.

75. Somerville AL, Wright DH, Rotschafer JC. Implications of vancomycin degradation products on therapeutic drug monitoring in patients with end-stage renal disease. Pharmacotherapy 1999;702–707.

76. Sym D, Smith C, Meenan G, Lehrer M. fluorescence polarization immunoassay: can it result in an overestimation of vancomycin in patients not suffering from renal failure? Ther Drug Monit 2001;23:441–444.

77. Kingery JR, Sowinski KM, Kraus MA, Klaunig JE, Mueller BA. Vancomycin assay performance in patients with end-stage renal disease receiving hemodialysis. Pharmacotherapy 2000;20:653–656.

78. Drayer E. Pharmacologically active metabolites, therapeutic and toxic activities, plasma and urine data in man, accumulation in renal failure. Clin Pharmacokinet 1976;1:426.

79. Gibson TP. Acetylation of procainamide in man and its relationship to isonicotinic acid-hydrazide acetylation phenotype. Clin Pharmacol Ther 1975;17:395.

80. Kassirer JP. Clinical evaluation of kidney function-glomerular function. N Engl J Med 1971;285:385.

81. Toto RD. Conventional measurement of renal function utilizing serum creatinine, creatinine clearance, inulin and para-aminohippuric acid clearance. Curr Opin Nephrol Hypertens 1995;4:505–509.

82. Manjunath G, Sarnak MJ, Levey AS. Estimating the glomerular filtration rate. Dos and don'ts for assessing kidney function. Postgrad Med 2001:110;55–62.

83. Lott RS, Hayton WL. Estimation of creatinine clearance from serum creatinine concentration: a review. Drug Intell Clin Pharm 1978;12:140.

84. Bjornsson T_D. Use of serum creatinine concentrations to determine renal function. Clin Pharmacokinet 1979;4:200.

85. Daugirdas JT, Blake PG, Ing TS, Handbook of Dialysis. New York: Lippincott Williams & Wilkins, 2001.

86. Henrich W. Principles and Practice of Dialysis. Philadelphia: Lippincott Williams & Wilkins, 1998.

87. Goldman R. Creatinine excretion in renal failure. Proc Soc Biol Med 1954;85:446.

88. Jelliffe RW. Creatinine clearance: bedside estimate. Ann Intern Med 1973;79:604.

89. Siersbaek-Nielson K, et al. Rapid evaluation of creatinine clearance. [Letter.] Lancet 1971;1:1133.

90. Lentner C, Lentner C, Wink A, eds. Geigy Scientific Tables. Body Surface of Children/Adults. West Caldwell, NJ: Ciba-Geigy, 1981:226–227.

91. Cockcroft DW, Gault MH. Prediction of creatinine clearance from serum creatinine. Nephron 1976;16:31.

92. Hernandez de Acevedo L, Johnson CE. Estimation of creatinine clearance in children: comparison of six methods. Clin Pharm 1982;1:158.

93. Devine BJ. Gentamicin therapy. Drug Intell Clin Pharm 1974:7:650–655.

94. Dionne RE, et al. Estimating creatinine clearance in morbidly obese patients. Am J Hosp Pharm 1981;38:841–844.

95. Bauer LA, et al. Influence of weight on aminoglycoside pharmacokinetics in normal weight and morbidly obese patients. Eur J Clin Pharmacol 1983;24:643–647.

96. Robert S, Zarowitz BJ, Peterson EL, Dumler F. Predictability of creatinine clearance estimates in critically ill patients. Crit Care Med 1993;21:1487–1495.

97. Woo MC, Boro MS. Predicting serum aminoglycoside concentrations in patients with low serum creatinine. Hosp Pharm 1998;33:1378–1383.

98. Smythe M, Hoffman J, Kizy K, Dmuchowski C. Estimating creatinine clearance in elderly patients with low serum creatinine concentrations. Am J Hosp Pharm 1994;51:198–204.

99. Bertino JS. Measured versus estimated creatinine clearance in patients with low serum creatinine values. Ann Pharmacother 1993;27:1439–1441.

100. Traub SL, Johnson CE. Comparison of methods of estimating creatinine clearance in children. Am J Hosp Pharm 1980;37:195–200.

101. Schwartz GJ, Haycock GB, Edelmann CM Jr, Spitzer A. A simple estimate of glomerular filtration rate in children derived from body length and plasma creatinine. Pediatrics 1976:104;259–263.

102. Schwartz GJ, Feld LG, Langford DJ. A simple estimate of glomerular filtration rate in full-term infants during the first year of life. J Pediatr 1984;104:849–854.

103. Mitch WE, et al. Creatinine metabolism in chronic renal failure. Clin Sci 1980;58:327.

104. Chow MS, Schweitzer R. Estimation of renal creatinine clearance in patients with unstable serum creatinine concentrations: comparisons of multiple methods. Drug Intell Clin Pharm 1985;19:385–390.

105. Bleiler RE, Schedl HP. Creatinine excretion: variability and relationships to diet and body size. J Lab Clin Med 1962;59:945.

106. Aweeka FT. Appendix: drug reference table. In: Schrier RW, Gambertoglio JG, eds. Handbook of Drug Therapy in Liver and Kidney Disease. Boston: Little, Brown and Co. 1991.

107. Takki S, et al. Pharmacokinetic evaluation of hemodialysis in acute drug overdose. Pharmacokinet Biopharm 1978;6:427.

108. Lee CC, Marbury TC. Drug therapy in patients undergoing haemodialysis. Clinical pharmacokinetic considerations. Clin Pharmacokinet 1984;9:42.

109. Maher JF. Pharmacokinetics in patients with renal failure. Clin Nephrol 1984;21:39–46.

110. Gokal R, Hutchison A. Dialysis therapies for end-stage renal disease. Semin Dial 2002;14:220–226.

111. Nanese DM, et al. Markedly increased clearance of vancomycin during hemodialysis using polysulfone dialyzers. Kidney Int 1989;35:1409–1412.

112. Pollard TA, et al. Vancomycin redistribution: dosing recommendations following high-flux hemodialysis. Kidney Int 1994;45:232–237.

113. Zoer J, Schrander-van der Meer AM, van Dorp WT. Dosage recommendation of vancomycin during haemodialysis with highly permeable membranes. Pharm World Sci 1997;19:191–196.

114. Gloper TA. Continuous arteriovenous hemofiltration in acute renal failure. Am J Kidney Dis 1985;6:373–386.

115. Pattison ME, et al. Continuous arteriovenous hemodiafiltration: an aggressive approach to the management of acute renal failure. Am J Kidney Dis 1988;11:43–47.

116. Bickley SK. Drug dosing during continuous arteriovenous hemofiltration. Clin Pharm 1988;7:198–206.

117. Davies JG, Kingswood JC, Sharpstone P, Street MK. Drug removal in continuous haemofiltration and haemodialysis. Br. J Hosp Med 1995;12:524–528.

118. Bugge JF. Pharmacokinetics and drug dosing adjustments during continuous venovenous hemofiltration or hemodiafiltration in critically ill patients. Acta Anaesthesiol Scand 2001;45:929–934.

119. Bohler J, Donauer J, Keller F. Pharmacokinetic principles during continuous renal replacement therapy: drugs and dosage. Kidney Int Suppl 1999;72:S24–S28.

120. Reetze-Bonorden P, Bohler J, Keller E. Drug dosage in patients during continuous renal replacement therapy: pharmacokinetic and therapeutic considerations. Clin Pharmacokinet 1993;24:362–379.

121. Golper TA, Marx MA. Drug dosing adjustments during continuous renal replacement therapies. Kidney Int Suppl 1998;66:S165–S168.

122. Domoto DT, Brown WW, Bruggensmith P. Removal of toxic levels of N-acetyl procainamide with continuous arteriovenous hemofiltration or continuous arteriovenous hemodiafiltration. Ann Int Med 1987;106:550–552.

123. Lamier N, et al. Peritoneal pharmacokinetics and pharmacological manipulation of peritoneal transport in continuous ambulatory peritoneal dialysis. In: Gokal R, ed. New York: Churchill Livingstone, 1986:56–93.

124. Matzke GR, Millikin SP. Influence of renal function and dialysis on drug disposition. In: Evans WE, Schentag JJ, Jusko WJ, eds. Applied Pharmacokinetics: Principles of Therapeutic Drug Monitoring. 3rd Ed. Vancouver, WA: Applied Therapeutics, 1992.

125. Mars RL, Moles K, Pope K, Hargrove P. Use of bolus intraperitoneal aminoglycosides for treating peritonitis in end-stage renal disease patients receiving continuous ambula-

tory peritoneal dialysis and continuous cycling peritoneal dialysis. Adv Perit Dial 2000;16:280–284.

126. Matzke GR. Vancomycin. In: Evans WE, Schentag JJ, Jusko WJ, eds. Applied Pharmacokinetics: Principles of Therapeutic Drug Monitoring. 3rd Ed. Vancouver, WA: Applied Therapeutics, 1992.

127. O'Brien MA, Mason NA. Systemic absorption of intra-peritoneal antimicrobials in continuous ambulatory peritoneal dialysis. Clin Pharm 1992;11:256.

128. Voinescu CG, Khanna R. Peritonitis in peritoneal dialysis. Int J Artif Organs 2002;25:249–260.

129. Keller E, Reetze P, Schollmeyer P. Drug therapy in patients undergoing continuous ambulatory peritoneal dialysis. Clinical and pharmacokinetic considerations. Clin Pharmacokinet 1990;18:104–117.

130. Keane WF, Everett ED, Golper TA, et al. Peritoneal dialysis-related peritonitis treatment recommendations 1993 update. Perit Dial Int 1993;13:14–28.

PART TWO

Drug Monographs

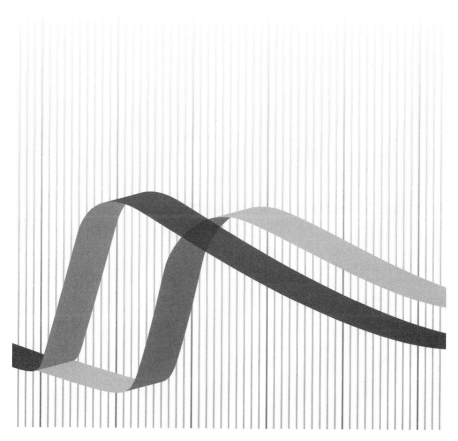

1

AMINOGLYCOSIDE ANTIBIOTICS

Paul Beringer and Michael E. Winter

The aminoglycosides are bactericidal antibiotics used in the treatment of serious gram-negative infections. Because absorption from the gastrointestinal tract is poor, the aminoglycosides must be administered parenterally to achieve therapeutic concentrations in the systemic circulation. In most instances, aminoglycosides are administered by intermittent intravenous (IV) infusions. The choice of an aminoglycoside dose is influenced by the specific agent (e.g., gentamicin versus amikacin), infection (e.g., site and organism), renal function, and weight or body composition of the patient. The three most commonly monitored aminoglycoside antibiotics are gentamicin, tobramycin, and amikacin. The usual dose for gentamicin and tobramycin is 5 to 7 mg/kg/d, administered over 30 to 60 minutes as a single daily dose or in divided doses every 8 to 12 hours; the dose of amikacin is 15 to 20 mg/kg/d, administered over 30 to 60 minutes as a single daily dose or in divided doses every 8 to 12 hours. The clearance, volume of distribution, and half-life of all aminoglycosides are similar.[1] Therefore, the same pharmacokinetic model can be used for all the aminoglycosides, and the principles, which are described in this chapter for any given aminoglycoside generally, apply to the others as well. The aminoglycosides have different ranges of "therapeutic" serum concentrations and have different propensities for interaction with penicillin compounds.

PHARMACODYNAMICS OF AMINOGLYCOSIDES

Traditionally, aminoglycosides have been dosed multiple times a day. Over the past decade, investigations into the pharmacodynamic properties of aminoglycosides have yielded data that favor extended interval administration. Bactericidal activity of the aminoglycosides has been demonstrated to be concentration-dependent [i.e., plasma concentrations that exceed 10 times the minimum inhibitory concentration (MIC) for a given bacteria are more effective than concentrations just above the MIC].[2–5] In addition to the concentration-dependent killing, there is also a postantibiotic effect that results in depressed bacterial growth after plasma concentrations have fallen below the MIC.[2,6,7] Taken together, the pharmacodynamic properties of aminoglycosides suggest that less frequent administration of larger doses can maximize bactericidal activity. In addition, saturable uptake mechanisms within the renal cortex and inner ear indicate that extended interval dosing may also minimize the likelihood of developing nephrotoxicity and ototoxicity.[8-10] Experience from randomized controlled trials suggests that once-daily administration of aminoglycosides results in similar efficacy and perhaps a decreased risk of developing toxicities when compared with traditional dosing.[11,12]

THERAPEUTIC AND TOXIC PLASMA CONCENTRATIONS

Peak plasma concentrations for gentamicin and tobramycin using extended interval dosing (i.e., 5 to 7 mg/kg every 24 hours) are in the range of 20 to 30 mg/L. This peak concentration target is based on the pharmacodynamic goal of achieving a peak to MIC ratio of greater than 10 and the breakpoint for susceptibility of 2 mg/L.[13] Trough concentrations are below the limit of detection by design to provide a drug-free interval, which reduces the risk for development of nephrotoxicity. Peak plasma concentrations following traditional multiple daily dosing regimens are in the range of 5 to 8 mg/L.[14-16] Peak plasma concentrations < 2 to 4 mg/L are likely to be ineffective,[15] and successful treatment of pneumonia may require peak concentrations of 8 mg/L or more.[14] Desirable peak concentrations for amikacin are usually 20 to 30 mg/L; trough concentrations are usually < 10 mg/L.[1]

KEY PARAMETERS: **Aminoglycoside Antibiotics**		
Therapeutic Serum Concentrations		
Gentamicin, Tobramycin	Conventional dosing Peak 5–8 mg/L Trough < 2mg/L	"Once-daily" dosing 20 mg/L Undetectable
Amikacin	Peak 20–30 mg/L Trough < 10 mg/L	60 mg/L Undetectable
V[a]	0.25 L/kg	
Cl Normal Renal Function Functionally Anephric Patients[b] Surgically Anephric Patients[b] Hemodialysis[b]	Equal to Cl_{Cr} 0.0043 L/kg/hr 0.0021 L/kg/hr 1.8 L/hr	
AUC_{24}	70–100 mg · hr/L	
T½ Normal Renal Function Functionally Anephric Patients	2–3 hr 30–60 hr	

[a]Volume of distribution should be adjusted for obesity and/or alterations in extracellular fluid status.
[b]A functionally anephric patient is a dialysis patient with kidneys intact. A surgically anephric patient is a dialysis patient with kidneys removed. Hemodialysis clearance of 1.8 L/hr refers to standard hemodialysis, not high-flux or peritoneal dialysis.

Most available data correlating aminoglycoside concentrations with ototoxicity and nephrotoxicity refer to trough plasma concentrations, although some data suggest a correlation between peak concentrations and toxicity.[17,18] Although gentamicin trough concentrations of > 2 mg/L have been associated with renal toxicity, the high trough concentrations may be the result, and not the cause, of renal dysfunction. In fact, the use of elevated trough concentrations as an indication of early renal damage has been suggested by some investigators.[19,20] Fortunately, most patients who develop renal dysfunction during aminoglycoside therapy appear to regain normal renal function after the drug has been discontinued.[21]

Ototoxicity has been associated with trough plasma concentrations of gentamicin exceeding 4 mg/L for more than 10 days. When the trough concentration is multiplied by the number of days of therapy, the risk of ototoxicity is increased when the product exceeds 40 mg-days/L. Aminoglycoside ototoxicity also seems to be most prevalent in patients who have existing impaired renal function or have received large doses during the course of their treatment.[17–19,22,23]

Although it is the standard practice to use aminoglycoside plasma concentrations as predictors for both efficacy and toxicity, it is controversial whether this is valid.[24] The adoption of once-daily aminoglycoside dosing at many institutions has led to less intensive monitoring of serum concentrations. The nomogram developed by Nicolau and colleagues recommends a single level be drawn 6 to 14 hours after the dose.[13] The nomogram then defines in graphical form whether the dosing interval is appropriate or needs to be extended. This type of approach is much more simplified than the traditional method of determining the individualized pharmacokinetic parameters based on measured peak and trough concentrations; however, it may not provide the same precise control of drug exposure [i.e., peak, area under the curve (AUC)] in patients who exhibit altered pharmacokinetics (i.e., third space fluid, burns, cystic fibrosis, spinal cord injury). Alternatively, Barclay and colleagues have defined a method of dosage individualization of extended interval aminoglycoside dosing based on a measured peak concentration and an estimation of the AUC.[25] This dosing method is based on the assumption that the goal is to provide a similar degree of drug exposure as traditional daily dosing methods (i.e., AUC) to minimize the risk of toxicity but provide a higher peak concentration to maximize the bactericidal activity. The target AUC_{24} range for gentamicin and tobramycin is 70 to 100 mg · hr/L.

BIOAVAILABILITY (F)

The aminoglycoside antibiotics are very water soluble and poorly lipid soluble compounds. As a result, they are poorly absorbed when administered orally and must be administered parenterally for the treatment of systemic infections.

VOLUME OF DISTRIBUTION (V)

The volume of distribution of the aminoglycosides is ≈ 0.25 L/kg, although a relatively wide range of 0.1 to 0.5 L/kg has been reported.[26–32] Since aminoglycosides distribute very poorly into adipose tissue, lean rather than total body weight (TBW) should result in a more accurate approximation of V in obese patients.[33] The aminoglycoside volume of distribution in obese subjects also could be adjusted based on the patient's ideal body weight (IBW) plus 10% of his or her excess weight.[34,35] These adjustments in the estimation of aminoglycoside volumes of distribution in obese patients seem reasonable because aminoglycoside antibiotics appear to distribute into extracellular space, and the extracellular fluid volume of adipose tissue is approximately 10% of total body weight versus 25% for other tissues. Equation 1.1 can be used to approximate the volume of distribution (V) in obese patients:

$$\text{Aminoglycoside V (Obese Patients)} = (0.25 \text{ L/kg})(\text{IBW}) + 0.1(\text{TBW} - \text{IBW}) \qquad \text{[Eq. 1.1]}$$

The non-obese or ideal body weight can be approximated using Equations 1.2 and 1.3 [see Part I: Creatinine Clearance (Cl_{Cr})].

$$\text{Ideal body weight for males in kg} = 50 + (2.3)(\text{Height in Inches} > 60) \qquad \text{[Eq. 1.2]}$$

$$\text{Ideal Body Weight for females in kg} = 45 + (2.3)(\text{Height in Inches} > 60) \qquad \text{[Eq. 1.3]}$$

The volume of distribution of aminoglycosides is increased in patients with ascites, edema, or other enlarged "third space" volume.[36,37] One approach to approximating the increased volume of distribution for patients with ascites or edema is to increase the V by 1 L for each kg of weight gain. This approach is based on the assumption that the volume of distribution of aminoglycoside antibiotics is approximately equal to the extracellular fluid volume. This is consistent with the low plasma protein binding[1] and the fact that aminoglycosides cross membranes very poorly.

$$\text{Aminoglycoside V (L)} = \left(\begin{array}{c}0.25 \text{ L/kg} \times \text{Non-Obese,} \\ \text{Non-Excess Fluid Weight (kg)}\end{array}\right) + 0.1\left(\begin{array}{c}\text{Excess} \\ \text{Adipose} \\ \text{Weight (kg)}\end{array}\right) + \left(\begin{array}{c}\text{Excess Third-} \\ \text{Space Fluid} \\ \text{Weight (kg)}\end{array}\right) \qquad \text{[Eq. 1.4]}$$

The volume of distribution for aminoglycosides can be estimated using Equation 1.4, in which the non-obese, non-excess fluid weight usually can be estimated as the ideal body weight, and the excess adipose weight as the difference between the non-obese weight and the patient's total weight without excess third space fluid. The excess third space fluid weight is estimated clinically. In cases in which a rapid increase in weight has occurred over several days, this weight gain is likely to represent fluid in a third space; it is therefore easily estimated by taking a difference between the initial and current weights. Some patients may exhibit significant third spacing of fluids (apparent as either edema or ascites) on initial evaluation. It is most difficult to estimate an aminoglycoside V in the obese patient with significant third spacing of fluid. As Equation 1.4 illustrates, assigning excess third space fluid to adipose weight could result in a significant underestimation of the volume of distribution. For this reason, it should be recognized that Equation 1.4 only approximates the V, and plasma concentration measurements are needed to make patient-specific adjustments.

Pediatric patients younger than 5 years of age tend to have a volume of distribution of 0.5 L/kg. Between birth and 5 years of age, the volume of distribution probably continues to decline from an initial value of 0.5 L/kg to the adult value of 0.25 L/kg.[38]

$$\text{Aminoglycoside V (L)} \atop \text{in Children 1 to 5 years} = \left(0.5 \text{ L/kg} - \left(\frac{\text{Age in Years}}{5} \times 0.25\right)\right)\left(\frac{\text{Weight}}{\text{in kg}}\right) \quad \text{[Eq. 1.5]}$$

Because the change in volume of distribution is gradual, some clinicians have chosen to use the above algorithm to estimate the volume of distribution for patients between 1 and 5 years of age. After 5 years of age, a V of 0.25 L/kg is generally used. Note that in Equation 1.5, it is assumed that the child's weight in kg represents a weight that is not obese and does contain significant excess third space fluid. Although there are no data on the subject, obese children should have a smaller-than-average volume of distribution for their age and size, and children with significant third spacing of fluid should have a larger-than-average V.

The pharmacokinetics of the aminoglycoside antibiotics has been described by a two- or three-compartment model.[39,40] However, a one-compartment model has been used widely in the clinical setting to facilitate aminoglycoside pharmacokinetic calculations. The initial distribution phase following a gentamicin IV infusion is not considered when the one-compartment model is utilized for gentamicin pharmacokinetic calculations.[40-42] For this reason, reported values for plasma samples obtained near the conclusion of an IV infusion may be higher than expected. In addition, there is some evidence that the length of the distribution phase may be dose-dependent.[43] These reported values probably have no correlation with the therapeutic or toxic effects of the drug; however, they are important in terms of the optimal timing and interpretation of measured serum concentrations. A third distribution phase, or gamma phase, for gentamicin has also been identified.[39] This final volume of distribution phase for gentamicin is large, and because gentamicin clearance is decreased when plasma concentrations are low, the average half-life associated with this third compartment is in excess of 100 hours.[39,40] This large final volume of distribution and long terminal half-life may be significant when evaluating a patient's potential for aminoglycoside toxicity.[44]

Despite the existence of the three-compartment model for the aminoglycosides, pharmacokinetic calculations can be based on a one-compartment model that utilizes the second volume of distribution. The errors encountered when using a single-compartment model for aminoglycosides can be minimized if plasma drug concentrations are obtained at times that avoid the first and third distribution phases and at 24 hours after therapy has been initiated.[45] Aminoglycoside concentrations <1 mg/L should be evaluated cautiously because the influence of the large third compartment will become greater at these low concentrations.[40]

CLEARANCE (Cl)

The aminoglycoside antibiotics are eliminated almost entirely by the renal route.[1,31] Since the aminoglycoside and creatinine clearances are similar over a wide range of renal function, aminoglycoside clearance can be estimated from the formulas used to estimate creatinine clearance (Equations 1.6 and 1.7) when concentrations are within the therapeutic range:[1,26,31,40]

$$Cl_{cr} \text{ for males (mL/min)} = \frac{(140 - \text{Age})(\text{Weight})}{(72)(SCr_{ss})} \qquad \text{[Eq. 1.6]}$$

$$Cl_{cr} \text{ for females (mL/min)} = (0.85)\frac{(140 - \text{Age})(\text{Weight})}{(72)(SCr_{ss})} \qquad \text{[Eq. 1.7]}$$

As presented in Part I, the age is in years, weight is in kg, and serum creatinine is in mg/dL. Correct estimates of creatinine clearance can only be obtained if the patient's weight represents a normal ratio of muscle mass to total body weight and the serum creatinine is at steady state. For this reason, pharmacokinetic calculations for obese patients and patients who have significant third spacing of fluid should take into consideration adjustments for obesity and third spacing. Generally, the ideal body weight for obese subjects calculated from Equations 1.2 and 1.3 can be used; adjustments for ideal body weight in patients who are < 20% overweight are probably unnecessary.

In patients who are morbidly obese (i.e., actual body weight approximately double their ideal body weight), creatinine and aminoglycoside clearances are best estimated by using a weight that falls between the ideal and total body weight.[46,47] For this reason, some clinicians prefer to estimate the non-obese weight by using the following equation:

$$\text{Non-Obese Weight} \approx \text{IBW} + 0.4\,(\text{TBW} - \text{IBW})$$

where IBW is the ideal body weight as estimated by Equations 1.2 and 1.3, and TBW represents the patient's total body weight without the presence of excess third space fluid.

Non-Renal Clearance

Another factor that should be considered when estimating the clearance of aminoglycosides is the non-renal clearance, which is ≈ 0.0021 L/kg/hr (or ≈ 2.5 mL/min/70 kg). The non-renal clearance of aminoglycosides is generally ignored in most patients, but it is significant in patients whose renal function is significantly diminished. In patients who are functionally anephric and receiving intermittent hemodialysis, a clearance value of ≈ 0.0043 L/kg/hr (5 mL/min/70 kg) represents the residual renal clearance and the non-renal clearance. These values, however, are only approximations; serum concentrations of aminoglycosides should be monitored in patients with poor renal function.

Penicillin Interaction

Carbenicillin, ticarcillin, and related extended-spectrum penicillins chemically inactivate gentamicin and tobramycin in vitro. This inactivation can become clinically significant in vivo in patients with renal failure. Although this interaction is usually not considered a route of aminoglycoside clearance, it does act as a mechanism for drug "elimination." This interaction is a function of the specific aminoglycoside, the penicillin compound, the concentration of the penicillin compound, and the temperature. In general, tobramycin and gentamicin interact with penicillins in a similar manner; amikacin is much less likely to interact with these penicillins.[48-53] The newer semisynthetic acylureido penicillins appear to be less reactive than carbenicillin, and the cephalosporins appear to be relatively nonreactive.[54-56] For patients with very poor renal function who are receiving carbenicillin or ticarcillin, the additional gentamicin clearance can be approximated by multiplying the patient's apparent volume of distribution for the aminoglycoside by 0.017 hr^{-1}.

$$\begin{array}{l}\text{Tobramycin, Gentamicin} \\ \text{Clearance by Carbenicillin} \\ \text{or Ticarcillin (L/hr)}\end{array} = (0.017\ \text{hr}^{-1})\left(\begin{array}{c}\text{Volume of Distribution} \\ \text{for Aminoglycosides}\end{array}\right) \quad \text{[Eq. 1.8]}$$

Liverpool John Moores University
Avril Robarts LRC

03/02/05   09:21 pm

Basic clinical pharmacokinetics /
31111010536348   24/02/2005 Due Date:
23:59

21111061211116

Thank You for using
the 3M SelfCheck System!

Liverpool John Moores University
Avril Robarts LRC

03/02/05   09:21 pm

Basic clinical pharmacokinetics /
31111010536348   24/02/2005 Due Date:
                                    23:59

21111061211116

Thank You for using
the 3M SelfCheck System!

The elimination rate constant (K) of 0.017 hr^{-1} represents the approximate in vitro elimination rate for aminoglycosides exposed to carbenicillin concentrations of 250 to 500 mg/L at a temperature of 37°C. This clearance by carbenicillin is only an approximation and should not be used for amikacin, because the interaction between amikacin and carbenicillin is relatively minor. The additional clearance secondary to inactivation by carbenicillin or other penicillins is not clinically relevant in patients with reasonably normal renal function. Enhancement of gentamicin clearance by this interaction is small and usually of consequence only in anephric patients (0.3 L/hr or 5 mL/min). Because the third-generation cephalosporin antibiotics have, to a large degree, replaced the use of penicillin derivatives, the interaction between aminoglycoside antibiotics and penicillin derivatives is encountered infrequently in most clinical practices.

ELIMINATION HALF-LIFE

The elimination half-life of aminoglycoside antibiotics from the body is a function of the volume of distribution and clearance. Since renal function varies considerably among individuals, the half-life is also variable. For example, a 70-kg, 25-year-old man with a serum creatinine of 0.8 mg/dL might have an aminoglycoside clearance of 100 mL/min or more. If his volume of distribution is 0.25 L/kg, the corresponding elimination half-life will be approximately 2 hours. In contrast, a 75-year-old man with a similar V and a serum creatinine of 1.4 mg/dL might have an aminoglycoside clearance of $\approx$35 mL/min and a half-life of approximately 6 hours. For this reason, the initial aminoglycoside dose and dosing interval should be selected with care. Although initial estimates of the patient's aminoglycoside pharmacokinetic parameters may be highly variable, it is hoped that pharmacokinetic adjustments will optimize the achievement of therapeutic, yet nontoxic, concentrations of aminoglycoside antibiotics.

NOMOGRAMS AND COMPUTERS

The wide availability of nomograms to dose aminoglycosides may lead one to question the necessity for pharmacokinetic calculations.[10] These nomograms, however, are usually designed to achieve fixed peak and trough serum concentrations, and they do not allow the clinician to individualize the dosing regimens to account for the type of infection treated or the benefit-to-risk ratio for the individual patient. Furthermore, nomograms are based on average pharmacokinetic parameters and do not provide a method for dose adjustment for unique patients (e.g., obese individuals or those who have significant third spacing of fluid). Patient-specific adjustments based on measured plasma concentrations also cannot be extrapolated from these nomograms. An understanding of the basic pharmacokinetic principles used to individualize aminoglycoside doses, coupled with a rational clinical approach, will enable the clinician to provide optimal therapy for the patient.

A number of computer programs are available to help clinicians dose aminoglycosides and other therapeutic agents. Computers tend to be more flexible than nomograms in that the user often can select dosing intervals and peak or trough concentrations based on clinical judgment. In addition, they enable dosage determination based on data (including multiple sets of measurements) obtained under nonsteady-state conditions, which is particularly important in patients with changing renal function. Bayesian analysis has been incorporated into most computerized pharmacokinetic programs and has been proven to provide very precise estimates of the pharmacokinetic parameters. One potential pitfall, however, is that the user must be familiar with the algorithms initially used to define the expected pharmacokinetic parameters and how patient-specific parameters are revised when plasma concentrations and dosing histories are supplied. In the revision process, the user must be able to recognize data that are obviously wrong and to interpret the computer output to ensure that the parameters and dosing recommendations are reasonable. The computer should be viewed as a labor-saving device, not as a substitute for a thorough understanding of the pharmacokinetic process.

TIME TO SAMPLE

Correct timing of the sample collection is important because aminoglycoside antibiotics have a relatively short half-life and a small but significant distribution phase. The most widely accepted guidelines recommend that samples for peak serum concentrations be obtained 1 hour after the maintenance dose has been initiated. This recommendation assumes that the drug is infused over about 30 minutes; an acceptable range for the infusion period is 20 to 40 minutes. If it is longer than 40 minutes, peak concentrations should be obtained approximately 30 minutes after the end of the infusion to ensure that distribution is complete. Others have suggested that peak measurements should be obtained later in the dosing interval to avoid the distribution phase, particularly with extended interval dosing due to the potential dose-dependent distribution phase.[43] Trough concentrations generally should be obtained within the half-hour before the administration of the next maintenance dose. In cases in which the trough concentrations are expected to be lower than the assay sensitivity (particularly with extended interval dosing), an earlier sampling time may be appropriate so that measurable trough concentrations can be obtained and patient-specific pharmacokinetic parameters derived. Ideally, the interval between the two concentration measurements should be two to four half-lives to provide more precise estimates of the half-life and reduce the potential for the later concentration to fall below the level of assay sensitivity. In all cases, the exact time of sampling and dose administration should be recorded.

When aminoglycoside plasma concentrations are sampled at a time that extends beyond the expected peak, it is possible to calculate the plasma concentration at the earlier time by simply rearranging

$$C = C^{o}e^{-Kt}$$ [Eq. 1.9]

where C^{o} is the initial plasma concentration, C is a concentration at some time t later, to

$$C^{o} = \frac{C}{e^{-Kt}}$$ [Eq. 1.10]

In the above equation, t represents the time from the measured plasma concentration (C) to the earlier plasma concentration (C^{o}). This equation is used to back-extrapolate a plasma concentration to the "clinical peak," which is 1 hour after the start of the infusion. The "clinical peak" concentration has generally been used as a guide to aminoglycoside efficacy.

The optimal time to sample within the first 24 hours of therapy is difficult to determine. For patients who are critically ill, a peak and subsequent trough (or midpoint for extended interval dosing) serum aminoglycoside concentration obtained after the initial loading dose allows for the most rapid evaluation of patient-specific parameters and subsequent dose adjustment, if necessary. In a large number of cases, however, this early sampling may not be necessary, particularly if the expected duration of therapy is relatively short (i.e., 3 to 5 days). The standard of practice in many institutions has been to obtain the first aminoglycoside samples after three or four doses of aminoglycoside have been administered. The majority of patients will be approaching steady state by this time; however, with the wide availability of computers and pharmacokinetic software programs, it is not absolutely necessary to wait until steady state is achieved. With extended interval dosing there should be no significant accumulation with multiple dosing; therefore, measurements can be obtained after any dose.

Although one can estimate patient-specific pharmacokinetic parameters more accurately with three or four aminoglycoside plasma concentrations (particularly using a multi-compartment model), reasonable pharmacokinetic parameters can be estimated using a one-compartment model and two plasma samples in most cases.

When aminoglycoside antibiotics are administered intramuscularly (IM), the time for absorption or drug input is less predictable; however, in most patients, plasma concentrations peak about 1 hour after the IM injection.[57] For this reason, a peak plasma concentration should be obtained 1 hour after the IM dose is administered. Because the rate of absorption is uncertain, it is difficult to know whether unusual plasma concentrations following IM administration represent delayed absorption or unusual pharmacokinetic parameters (e.g., a large volume of distribution).

Question #1. *R.W. is a 30-year-old, 70-kg, non-obese woman with a serum creatinine of 0.9 mg/dL. An initial gentamicin dose of 140 mg was infused intravenously over 30 minutes. Calculate the plasma concentration of gentamicin 1 hour after the infusion was started (i.e., one-half hour after the infusion was completed).*

A rough estimate of the peak gentamicin concentration can be calculated using Equation 1.11 by treating the 60-minute infusion as a bolus dose. The 140-mg dose would be divided by the literature value for the volume of distribution ($\approx$0.25 L/kg or 17.5 L) in this 70-kg woman.

$$C_1 = \frac{(S)(F)(\text{Loading Dose})}{V} \qquad \text{[Eq. 1.11]}$$

$$= \frac{(1)(1)(140 \text{ mg})}{17.5}$$

$$= 8.0 \text{ mg/L}$$

The salt form (S) and bioavailability (F) were both assumed to be 1.0, and the plasma concentration of 8.0 mg/L is an approximation that assumes absorption was very rapid and that no significant drug elimination took place during the time of administration. In addition, it is assumed that the drug is distributed into a single compartment. Even though there is clearly a distribution phase associated with the IV injection of aminoglycosides, the initially high drug concentration can be ignored as long as plasma sampling is avoided during this distribution phase.[30,31,41]

A more precise calculation of the plasma concentration 1 hour after the half-hour infusion has been initiated would take into account the decay of gentamicin levels from the peak concentration as calculated by Equation 1.9. In Equation 1.12 for C_1 below, t_1 is the time elapsed from the beginning of the IV infusion to the time of sampling at 1 hour, and the elimination rate constant (K) represents the clearance of gentamicin divided by its volume of distribution (V) (Equation 1.13).

$$C_1 = \frac{(S)(F)(\text{Loading Dose})}{V}(e^{-Kt_1}) \qquad \text{[Eq. 1.12]}$$

$$K = \frac{Cl}{V} \qquad \text{[Eq. 1.13]}$$

A creatinine clearance (and therefore gentamicin clearance) of approximately 101 mL/min or 6.06 L/hr can be calculated for R.W., using Equation 1.7:

$$Cl_{cr} \text{ for females (mL/min)} = (0.85)\frac{(140 - \text{Age})(\text{Weight})}{(72)(SCr_{ss})}$$

$$= (0.85)\left[\frac{(140 - 30)(70)}{(72)(0.9)}\right]$$

$$= 101 \text{ mL/min}$$

$$Cl_{cr} \text{ (L/hr)} = \left[(101 \text{ mL/min})\left(\frac{60 \text{ min/hr}}{1000 \text{ mL/L}}\right)\right]$$

$$= 6.06 \text{ L/hr}$$

Using this clearance of approximately 6 L/hr and the apparent volume of distribution of 17.5 L, an elimination rate constant of 0.346 hr^{-1} can be calculated using Equation 1.13. This elimination rate constant, when used in Equation 1.12 to calculate the gentamicin concentration 1.0 hour after the dose, results in a predicted concentration of 5.7 mg/L.

$$K = \frac{Cl}{V}$$

$$= \frac{6.06 \text{ L/hr}}{17.5 \text{ L}}$$

$$= 0.346 \text{ hr}^{-1}$$

$$C_1 = \frac{(S)(F)(\text{Loading Dose})}{V}(e^{-Kt_1})$$

$$= [8 \text{ mg/L}][e^{-(0.346 \text{ hr}^{-1})(1 \text{ hr})}]$$

$$= (8 \text{ mg/L})(0.71)$$

$$= 5.7 \text{ mg/L}$$

To evaluate whether the IV bolus dose model is appropriate, the duration of infusion (one-half hour) should be compared to the apparent drug half-life. When the duration of infusion or absorption is less than one-sixth of the half-life, then the bolus dose model can be used (see Part I: Selecting the Appropriate Equation). If, however, the duration of drug input is greater than one-sixth of the half-life, then an infusion model should be used. Using Equation 1.14 and the elimination rate constant of 0.346 hr^{-1}, R.W.'s half-life is calculated to be approximately 2 hours as follows:

$$t\frac{1}{2} = \frac{0.693}{K} \qquad \text{[Eq. 1.14]}$$

$$= \frac{0.693}{0.346 \ hr^{-1}}$$

$$= 2.0 \ hr$$

Since the duration of infusion was one-half hour, the absorption time was approximately one-fourth of the half-life. In practice, an infusion time of greater than one-sixth of the half-life is often used as the criterion for requiring the infusion model (see Part I: Selecting the Appropriate Equation).

Question #2. *Using the clearance of 6.06 L/hr, the volume of distribution of 17.5 L, the elimination rate constant of 0.346 hr^{-1}, and the short infusion model, calculate the expected gentamicin concentration for R.W. 1 hour after initiating the one-half hour infusion of a 140-mg dose.*

Equation 1.15 represents the short infusion model and can be used to calculate the plasma concentration 1 hour after starting the half-hour infusion. The duration of infusion or t_{in} would be 0.5 hours, and t_2, or the time of decay from the end of the infusion, would be 0.5 hours. Using these values, the plasma concentration 1 hour after initiation of the half-hour infusion would be 6.2 mg/L.

$$C_2 = \frac{(S)(F)(Dose/t_{in})}{Cl} (1 - e^{-Kt_{in}})(e^{-Kt_2}) \qquad [Eq. \ 1.15]$$

$$= \frac{(1)(1)(140 \ mg/0.5 \ hr)}{6.06 \ L/hr} (1 - e^{-(0.346 \ hr^{-1})(0.5 \ hr)})(e^{-(0.346 \ hr^{-1})(0.5 \ hr)})$$

$$= (46.2 \ mg/L)(0.16)(0.84)$$

$$= (7.4 \ mg/L)(0.84)$$

$$= 6.2 \ mg/L$$

Note that the plasma concentration of 7.4 mg/L at the end of the half-hour infusion is lower than the calculated peak concentration of 8 mg/L following a bolus dose (see Question 1). This lower concentration at the end of the infusion reflects the clearance of drug during the infusion process. Also note that the plasma concentration of 6.2 mg/L at 1 hour calculated by the infusion model is greater than the comparable plasma concentration (5.7 mg/L) calculated by the bolus dose model in Question 1. Less drug remains in the body at this time when the bolus dose model is used, because this model assumes that the entire dose entered the body at the beginning of the infusion. The total dose, therefore, has been exposed to the body's clearing mechanisms for a longer time.

Question #3. *In what types of patients is it more appropriate to use the infusion equation for the prediction of aminoglycoside concentrations? When can the bolus dose model be used satisfactorily?*

Since the difference between the results obtained from these two approaches is primarily related to the amount of drug cleared from the body during the infusion period, it is reasonable to assume that in patients with decreased renal function and longer aminoglycoside half-lives, the bolus dose model could be used satisfactorily. In patients with good renal function (e.g., young adults and children), use of the infusion model is more appropriate because these patients often have very short aminoglycoside half-lives.

Question #4. *R.W., the 70-kg woman described in Question 1, was given 140 mg of gentamicin over one-half hour every 8 hours. Predict her peak and trough plasma concentrations at steady state.*

Again, one could treat this problem as if R.W. were receiving intermittent IV boluses or as if she were receiving one-half hour infusions every 8 hours. If the bolus dose model is applied, Equation 1.16 can be used to predict the peak levels, where t_1 represents the time interval between the start of the infusion and the time at which the "peak concentration" is sampled (1 hour) and τ is the interval between the doses (8 hours). Using the volume of distribution of 17.5 L and the elimination rate constant of 0.346 hr^{-1}, the calculated peak concentration would be 6.1 mg/L.

$$Css_1 = \frac{\dfrac{(S)(F)(Dose)}{V}}{(1 - e^{-K\tau})} e^{-Kt_1} \qquad \text{[Eq. 1.16]}$$

$$= \frac{\dfrac{(1)(1)(140 \text{ mg})}{17.5 \text{ L}}(e^{-(0.346 \text{ hr}^{-1})(1 \text{ hr})})}{[1 - e^{-(0.346 \text{ hr}^{-1})(8 \text{ hr})}]}$$

$$= \left[\frac{8 \text{ mg/L}}{1 - 0.063} \right][0.71]$$

$$= \left[\frac{8 \text{ mg/L}}{0.937} \right][0.71]$$

$$= [8.5 \text{ mg/L}][0.71]$$

$$= 6.1 \text{ mg/L}$$

The trough concentration also can be calculated using Equation 1.16, where t_1 is the time interval between the start of the infusion and the time at which trough level is sampled (8 hours). If the trough sample is obtained just before the start of the next infusion, then Equation 1.17 for Css min also can be used. Using the appropriate values for volume of distribution, elimination rate constant, and dosing interval, the calculated trough concentration would be 0.54 mg/L:

$$\text{Css min} = \frac{\dfrac{(S)(F)(Dose)}{V}}{(1 - e^{-K\tau})} e^{-K\tau} \qquad \text{[Eq. 1.17]}$$

$$= \frac{\dfrac{(1)(1)(140 \text{ mg})}{17.5 \text{ L}}(e^{-(0.346 \text{ hr}^{-1})(8 \text{ hr})})}{[1 - e^{-(0.346 \text{ hr}^{-1})(8 \text{ hr})}]}$$

$$= \frac{8 \text{ mg/L}}{(0.937)}(0.063)$$

$$= 0.54 \text{ mg/L}$$

If the infusion input model,

$$C_{t_{in}} = \frac{(S)(F)(Dose/t_{in})}{Cl}(1 - e^{-Kt_{in}}) \qquad \text{[Eq. 1.18]}$$

where t_{in} is the duration of the infusion, and is used to replace the bolus dose model

$$\frac{(S)(F)(Dose)}{V} \qquad \text{[Eq. 1.19]}$$

in Equations 1.16 and 1.17, the resultant substitution results in an equation describing the intermittent infusion steady-state model (also see Part I: Selecting the Appropriate Equation).

$$\text{Css}_2 = \frac{\dfrac{(S)(F)(Dose/t_{in})}{Cl}(1 - e^{-Kt_{in}})}{(1 - e^{-K\tau})}(e^{-Kt_2}) \qquad \text{[Eq. 1.20]}$$

where τ is the dosing interval and t_2 is the time interval between the end of the infusion and the time at which the concentration is measured. That is, when peak concentrations are measured 1 hour after the initiation of a half-hour infusion, t_2 is 0.5 hours. For trough concentrations that are sampled just before the start of a subsequent infusion (i.e., administered on an 8-hour schedule, t_2 is 7.5 hours).

Again, assuming S and F to be 1.0, the infusion time to be 0.5 hours, the dosing interval (τ) to be 8 hours, the clearance (Cl) and the elimination rate constant (K) to be 6.06 L/hr and 0.346 hr^{-1}, respectively, the "peak" concentration 1 hour after starting the half-hour infusion would be calculated using Equation 1.20 as follows:

$$Css_2 = \frac{\frac{(S)(F)(Dose/t_{in})}{Cl}(1 - e^{-Kt_{in}})}{(1 - e^{-K\tau})}(e^{-Kt_2})$$

$$= \frac{\frac{(1)(1)(140\ mg/0.5\ hr)}{6.06\ L/hr}(1 - e^{-(0.346\ hr^{-1})(0.5\ hr)})}{(1 - e^{-(0.346\ hr^{-1})(8\ hr)})}(e^{-(0.346\ hr^{-1})(0.5\ hr)})$$

$$= \frac{(46.2\ mg/L)(0.16)}{0.937}(0.84)$$

$$= (7.9\ mg/L)(0.84)$$

$$= 6.6\ mg/L$$

Note that this steady-state "peak concentration" is not the true peak value which would occur at the end of the infusion, but a concentration that is obtained 1 hour after starting the infusion. It is this 1-hour value that is traditionally used to make the clinical correlation with aminoglycoside efficacy. Concentrations measured earlier may be considerably higher due to the two-compartment modeling associated with the IV administration of the aminoglycosides.

If the trough concentration is sampled just before the start of an infusion, a modification of Equation 1.20 can be used, where t_2 is represented by ($\tau - t_{in}$). A trough concentration of 0.59 mg/L is calculated, making the appropriate substitution of 8 hours for τ and 0.5 hours for t_{in} (Fig. 1.1).

$$Css\ min = \frac{\frac{(S)(F)(Dose/t_{in})}{Cl}(1 - e^{-Kt_{in}})}{(1 - e^{-K\tau})}(e^{-K(\tau - t_{in})}) \qquad \text{[Eq. 1.21]}$$

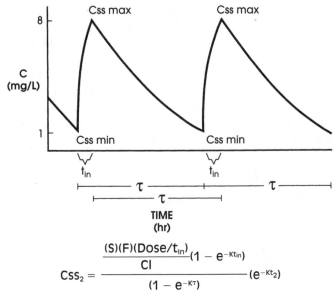

$$Css_2 = \frac{\dfrac{(S)(F)(Dose/t_{in})}{Cl}(1 - e^{-Kt_{in}})}{(1 - e^{-K\tau})}(e^{-Kt_2})$$

FIGURE 1.1. Intermittent intravenous infusion at steady state. The infusion is administered over t_{in} hours, and τ is the dosing interval; t_2 represents the time from the end of the infusion to the time of sampling.

$$= \frac{\dfrac{(1)(1)(140 \text{ mg}/0.5 \text{ hr})}{6.06 \text{ L/hr}}(1 - e^{-(0.346 \text{ hr}^{-1})(0.5 \text{ hr})})}{(1 - e^{-(0.346 \text{ hr}^{-1})(8 \text{ hr})})}(e^{-(0.346 \text{ hr}^{-1})(8 \text{ hr}-0.5 \text{ hr})})$$

$$= (7.9 \text{ mg/L})(e^{-(0.346 \text{ hr}^{-1})(7.5 \text{ hr})})$$

$$= (7.9 \text{ mg/L})(0.075)$$

$$= 0.59 \text{ mg/L}$$

Note that if the trough concentration is obtained at a time earlier than just before the next dose, Equation 1.21 should not be used. Instead, Equation 1.20 should be used where t_2 represents the time interval from the end of the infusion to the time of sampling. For example, if the trough concentration were obtained one-half hour before the next dose, then t_2 in Equation 1.20 would be 7 hours rather than 7.5 hours in Equation 1.21.

Trough concentrations can also be calculated by multiplying the peak concentration 1 hour after the dose by the fraction of drug remaining at the time the trough level is sampled (Equation 1.9):

$$C = C^0 e^{-Kt}$$

where C^o represents the peak concentration 1 hour after the dose, and t is the time from the peak concentration to the time of the trough sampling (7 hours if trough samples are obtained just before a dose, and 6.5 hours if trough samples are obtained one-half hour before a dose administered at a dosing interval of 8 hours).

Question #5. *When aminoglycosides are administered intramuscularly, how should the steady-state peak and trough plasma concentrations be calculated?*

Although the time required to achieve peak plasma concentrations following IM injection varies, aminoglycoside concentrations peak after approximately 1 hour in most patients.[15,31,40] Since it is difficult to estimate the rate of absorption from the site of injection, IM injections can be approached as though the patient were given an IV infusion over 1 hour. Therefore, the intermittent infusion model (Equation 1.20) can be used, with a t_{in} of 1 hour and t_2 of 0 hours. As noted earlier, unusual measured plasma concentrations will be difficult to evaluate in this situation because one cannot determine whether they represent unusual aminoglycoside absorption characteristics or pharmacokinetic parameters.

Question #6. *If R.W. was given tobramycin 7 mg/kg QD, what would be the calculated steady-state peak concentration 1 hour after starting the half-hour infusion? Also predict subsequent steady-state plasma concentrations 12 hours after starting the infusion and at the trough.*

Using the previously calculated gentamicin pharmacokinetic parameters of 6.06 L/hr for clearance, 17.5 L for volume, and 0.346 hr^{-1} for K, the expected steady-state peak concentration one-half hour after the half-hour infusion would be ≈ 21 mg/L as calculated from Equation 1.20.

$$Css_2 = \frac{\dfrac{(S)(F)(Dose/t_{in})}{Cl}(1 - e^{-Kt_{in}})}{(1 - e^{-K\tau})}(e^{-Kt_2})$$

$$= \frac{\dfrac{(1)(1)(480 \text{ mg}/0.5 \text{ hr})}{6.06 \text{ L/hr}}(1 - e^{-0.346(0.5)})}{(1 - e^{-0.346(24)})}(e^{-0.346(0.5)})$$

$$= \frac{161.7 \text{ mg/L}(1 - 0.84)}{(1 - 0.0002)}(0.84)$$

$$= 21.6 \text{ mg/L}$$

The plasma concentrations at 12 and 24 hours can be estimated using Equation 1.9, where C^o would be approximately 21 mg/L, and t would be 11 hours for the mid-concentration and 23 hours for the trough concentration.

$$C = C^0 e^{-Kt}$$

$$= (21 \text{ mg/L})(e^{-(0.346)(11 \text{ hr})})$$

$$= (21 \text{ mg/L})(0.022)$$

$$= 0.47 \text{ mg/L}$$

12 hours after starting the infusion and

$$C = (21 \text{ mg/L})(e^{-(0.346)(23 \text{ hr})})$$

$$= (21 \text{ mg/L})(0.00035)$$

$$= 0.007 \text{ mg/L } \textit{at the trough}$$

These calculations show that the initial plasma concentrations are well above the usual accepted therapeutic range for tobramycin, and the mid-interval and trough concentrations are very low. As previously discussed, administration of aminoglycosides as a total daily dose once every 24 hours appears in most cases to be as efficacious as the usual 8-hour divided dose and may reduce the risk for development of nephrotoxicity. Most institutions have guidelines for use of high-dose, once-daily aminoglycoside therapy. This type of regimen is usually restricted to patients who have reasonable renal function (e.g., $Cl_{Cr} > 60$ mL/min) and reasonably normal body composition (e.g., not excessively obese or having excessive third space fluid).

One common question is whether aminoglycoside plasma concentrations should be monitored in patients receiving the drug once daily. In most cases, peak concentrations will have little meaning because they are likely to be well above the usual therapeutic range: ≈20 mg/L for gentamicin and tobramycin and about three times that value for amikacin. Trough plasma concentrations do not appear to be useful in that they are likely to be well below the usual detectable range. In patients with diminished renal function, plasma level monitoring may be warranted to guard against excessive drug accumulation. One method that has been described is the peak-AUC method of dosing. With this method, serum concentrations are obtained at a peak and approximately two to four half-lives later. The two levels are then used to calculate the 24-hour AUC and the extrapolated peak concentration at 1 hour into the dosing interval. The assumption with this method is that the level of drug exposure with extended interval dosing should be the same as conventional multiple daily dosing regimens (i.e., AUC_{24} 70 to 100 mg·hr/L).[25]

Question #7. *Y.B., a 70-kg, 38-year-old patient with a serum creatinine of 1.8 mg/dL, has been receiving IV tobramycin, 100 mg over one-half hour every 8 hours, for several days. A peak plasma concentration obtained 1 hour after the start of an infusion was 8 mg/L, and a trough concentration obtained just before the initiation of a dose was 3 mg/L. Estimate the apparent elimination rate constant (K), clearance (Cl), and volume of distribution (V) for tobramycin in Y.B.*

The two reported plasma concentrations were measured from samples obtained during the elimination phase of the plasma concentration-versus-time curve. Since the 7-hour time interval between samples exceeds the half-life of tobramycin in Y.B. (i.e., the trough concentration is less than one-half the measured peak concentration), the two concentrations can be used to estimate the elimination rate constant [see Part I: Elimination Rate Constant (K) and Half-Life ($t_{1/2}$) and Equation 1.22].

$$K = \frac{\ln\left(\frac{C_1}{C_2}\right)}{t} \qquad \text{[Eq. 1.22]}$$

$$= \ln\frac{\left(\frac{8.0}{3.0}\right)}{7 \text{ hr}}$$

$$= \frac{0.98}{7 \text{ hr}}$$

$$= 0.14 \text{ hr}^{-1}$$

Using the elimination rate constant of 0.14 hr^{-1}, the observed peak concentration of 8 mg/L, and the dosing regimen of 100 mg administered over one-half hour every 8 hours, Y.B.'s volume of distribution can be calculated by rearranging Equation 1.16 for Css_1 where τ is 8 hours and the sample is obtained 0.5 hours after the end of the 0.5-hr infusion making t_1 1 hour.

$$Css_1 = \frac{\frac{(S)(F)(Dose)}{V}}{(1 - e^{-K\tau})}e^{-Kt_1}$$

$$V = \frac{\dfrac{(S)(F)(Dose)}{Css_1}}{(1 - e^{kt_1})} e^{-K\tau} \qquad [Eq.\ 1.23]$$

$$V = \frac{\dfrac{(1)(1)(100\ mg)}{8\ mg/L}}{(1 - e^{-(0.14\ hr^{-1})(8\ hr)})}(e^{-(0.14\ hr^{-1})(1\ hr)})$$

$$= \frac{12.5\ L}{0.67}(0.87)$$

$$= 16.2\ L$$

and the clearance can be calculated using a rearrangement of Equation 1.13.

$$K = \frac{Cl}{V}$$

to solve for Cl.

$$Cl = (K)(V) \qquad [Eq.\ 1.24]$$

$$= (0.14\ hr^{-1})(16.2\ L)$$

$$= 2.3\ L/hr$$

This volume of distribution of 16.2 L corresponds to about 0.23 L/kg. The value of calculating tobramycin pharmacokinetic parameters that are specific for Y.B. is that they may now be used to calculate a dosing regimen that will produce any desired peak and trough concentrations.

Question #8. *The microbiology report reveals Pseudomonas aeruginosa with a MIC of 1 mcg/mL. Calculate a dosing regimen for Y.B. that will achieve a peak concentration of > 10 mg/L (peak:MIC > 10:1) and a AUC_{24} in the range of 70 to 100 mg · hr/L.*

As before, the dose required to achieve a specific peak concentration can be calculated from Equation 1.16. To select an appropriate dosing interval, however, one should first consider Y.B.'s apparent half-life, which can be calculated using Equation 1.14 and the elimination rate constant of 0.14 hr^{-1}.

$$t\tfrac{1}{2} = \frac{0.693}{K}$$

$$= \frac{0.693}{0.14\ hr^{-1}}$$

$$= 4.9\ hr$$

As presented earlier, a dosing interval of approximately four to five half-lives is desirable to maximize the peak concentration and bactericidal activity while minimizing drug accumulation and potential nephrotoxicity and ototoxicity. Because Y.B.'s tobramycin half-life is approximately 5 hours, the most convenient dosing interval is 24 hours. Using this dosing interval and the appropriate volume of distribution and elimination rate constant, Equation 1.25 (a rearrangement of Equation 1.16 to solve for Dose) indicates that a dose of 200 mg administered every 24 hours should result in a peak concentration of ≈10 mg/L 1 hour after the start of a half-hour infusion.

$$\text{Dose} = \frac{(Css_1)(V)(1 - e^{-K\tau})}{(S)(F)(e^{-Kt_1})} \qquad \text{[Eq. 1.25]}$$

$$\text{Dose} = \frac{(10 \text{ mg/L})(17.5 \text{ L})(1 - e^{-(0.14 \text{ hr}^{-1})(24 \text{ hr})})}{(1)(1)(e^{-(0.14 \text{ hr}^{-1})(1 \text{ hr})})}$$

$$= \frac{(10 \text{ mg/L})(17.5 \text{ L})(0.97)}{(1)(1)(0.87)}$$

$$= 195.1 \text{ mg or } \approx 200 \text{ mg}$$

Equation 1.9 can be used to determine the trough concentration. A "t" of 23 hours and a C° of 10 mg/L should be used.

$$C = C^\circ e^{-Kt}$$

$$= (10 \text{ mg/L})(e^{-(0.14 \text{ hr}^{-1})(23 \text{ hr})})$$

$$= (10 \text{ mg/L})(0.04)$$

$$= 0.4 \text{ mg/L}$$

To confirm whether the level of drug exposure is in the desirable range, Equation 1.26 can be used to calculate the AUC_{24}.

$$AUC_{24} = \frac{\text{Dose}_{24} \text{ (mg)}}{\text{Cl (L/hr)}} \qquad \text{[Eq. 1.26]}$$

$$= \frac{(200 \text{ mg})}{2.3 \text{ L/hr}}$$

$$= 87 \text{ mg} \cdot \text{hr/L}$$

Question #9. *C.I. is a 50-year-old, 60-kg man with a serum creatinine of 1.5 mg/dL, who is receiving 350 mg of amikacin IV over one-half hour every 8 hours at midnight, 8:00 a.m., and 4:00 p.m. He had a trough concentration of 6 mg/L obtained just before the 8:00 a.m.*

dose, and a peak concentration of 15 mg/L obtained at 9:00 a.m. Assuming these peak and trough concentrations represent steady-state levels, calculate C.I.'s elimination rate constant, clearance, and volume of distribution. Evaluate whether these parameters seem reasonable and should be used to adjust C.I.'s amikacin maintenance dose.

The approach to calculating the revised pharmacokinetic parameters for C.I. is essentially the same as that used in the previous questions. First, the elimination rate constant of 0.13 hr^{-1} can be calculated using Equation 1.22 and the 7-hour time interval between the peak and trough concentrations (Fig. 1.2):

$$K = \frac{\ln\left(\dfrac{C_1}{C_2}\right)}{t}$$

$$= \frac{\ln\left(\dfrac{15}{6}\right)}{7 \text{ hr}}$$

$$= 0.13 \text{ hr}^{-1}$$

Next, the volume of distribution can be calculated by using Equation 1.23. A dose of 350 mg and a "τ" of 8 hours can be used. The latter t_1 represents the time from the beginning of the infusion to the "peak concentration" sampling time ($t_1 = 1$ hr).

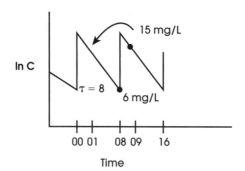

FIGURE 1.2. Calculating K by transposing Css max into the same interval as Css min. Note that steady state must have been achieved (same dose, same interval for greater than 3 to 5 t½'s). Also, the Css max is moved to the same time within the interval relative to the preceding dose (i.e., from 09:00 in one interval to 01:00 in the preceding interval). The intermittent bolus dose model has been used for the input model and the concentrations are ln concentrations so that the decay phase is a straight line.

$$V = \frac{\dfrac{(S)(F)(Dose)}{Css_1}}{(1 - e^{-K\tau})} e^{-Kt_1}$$

$$= \frac{\dfrac{(1)(1)(350 \text{ mg})}{15 \text{ mg/L}}}{(1 - e^{-(0.13 \text{ hr}^{-1})(8 \text{ hr})})} (e^{-(0.13 \text{ hr}^{-1})(1 \text{ hr})})$$

$$= \frac{(23.3 \text{ L})(0.88)}{(0.65)}$$

$$= 31.5 \text{ L}$$

Using the calculated volume of distribution of 31.5 L and the elimination rate constant of 0.13 hr^{-1}, a clearance value of 4.1 L/hr can be calculated using Equation 1.24.

$$Cl = (K)(V)$$

$$Cl = (0.13 \text{ hr}^{-1})(31.5 \text{ L})$$

$$= 4.1 \text{ L/hr}$$

Before these parameters are used to calculate an adjusted amikacin dosing regimen that will bring C.I.'s peak concentration into the range of 20 to 30 mg/L and the trough concentration below 10 mg/L, care should be taken to evaluate whether these parameters appear reasonable. The calculated clearance of 4.1 L/hr is slightly greater than the expected clearance of 3 L/hr, which would be calculated using Equation 1.6 and C.I.'s age, weight, and serum creatinine.

$$Cl_{cr} \text{ for males (mL/min)} = \frac{(140 - Age)(Weight)}{(72)(SCr_{ss})}$$

$$= \frac{(140 - 50)(60 \text{ kg})}{(72)(1.5 \text{ mg/dL})}$$

$$= 50 \text{ mL/min}$$

or

$$Cl_{cr}(\text{L/hr}) = (50 \text{ mL/min})\left(\frac{60 \text{ min/hr}}{100 \text{ mL/L}}\right)$$

$$= 3 \text{ L/hr}$$

While this clearance value is greater than expected, it is not so unusual as to be considered unrealistic.

The volume of distribution value of 0.53 L/kg (31.5L/60 kg), however, is unusually large. In general, volumes of distribution > 0.35 L/kg are only observed in patients who have significant third spacing of fluid (e.g., ascites or edema). If there is no evidence of any third spacing in C.I., then the volume of distribution would be unrealistically large. Therefore, the dosing history or the measured plasma concentrations are probably in error. If C.I. had received tobramycin or gentamicin, the possibility of a penicillin interaction resulting in spuriously low plasma concentrations would have to be considered; however, amikacin does not interact with penicillins to a significant extent. Therefore, this is an unlikely explanation for the unusually large volume of distribution.

In any case, when pharmacokinetic calculations lead to parameters that are very different from those expected, there may be an error in the time of sampling, assay results, or dosing history. In such cases, it may be more prudent to use the expected rather than the calculated parameters to adjust doses. In some cases, however, the patient may actually have unusual parameters. When this is suspected, the dosing history should be reevaluated and another set of plasma drug concentrations should be obtained, with special attention to precise sampling times and the dosing history.

Question #10. *D.H., a 40-year-old man, was admitted to the hospital following an automobile accident. He is 5 feet 5 inches tall and on admission weighed 85 kg. He was taken for abdominal surgery and postoperatively became hypotensive and required large volumes of fluid to maintain his blood pressure. Currently, he weighs 105 kg and has a serum creatinine of 2 mg/dL. D.H. is to receive gentamicin empirically after his abdominal surgery. Estimate his pharmacokinetic parameters and dose to achieve peak gentamicin concentrations > 10 mg/L and an AUC_{24} between 70 and 100 mg · hr/L.*

To calculate D.H.'s pharmacokinetic parameters, it is first necessary to identify his non-obese, excess adipose and excess third space fluid weight. Using Equation 1.2, D.H.'s ideal body weight is calculated to be ≈61.5 kg.

$$\text{Ideal body weight for males in kg} = 50 + (2.3)(\text{Height in Inches} > 60)$$

$$= 50 + 2.3(5 \text{ Inches})$$

$$= 61.5 \text{ kg}$$

Assuming D.H. did not have any excess third space fluid on admission, his excess adipose weight is ≈23.5 kg (estimated by subtracting his ideal body weight of 61.5 kg from his admission weight of 85 kg). D.H.'s excess third space fluid weight of 20 kg can be estimated by subtracting his initial weight of 85 kg from his current weight of 105 kg. Using these weight estimates for his body composition, Equation 1.4 can be used to estimate an aminoglycoside volume of distribution of ≈38 L:

$$\text{Aminoglycoside V (L)} = \left(\begin{array}{c} 0.25 \text{ L/kg} \times \text{Non-Obese,} \\ \text{Non-Excess Fluid Weight (kg)} \end{array} \right) +$$

$$0.1 \left(\begin{array}{c} \text{Excess} \\ \text{Adipose} \\ \text{Weight (kg)} \end{array} \right) + \left(\begin{array}{c} \text{Excess Third-} \\ \text{Space Fluid} \\ \text{Weight (kg)} \end{array} \right)$$

$$= (0.25 \text{ L/kg} \times 61.5 \text{ kg}) + 0.1(23.5 \text{ kg}) + (20 \text{ kg}) = 37.7 \text{ L or } 38 \text{ L}$$

To estimate D.H.'s gentamicin clearance, one would use Equation 1.6, his IBW of 61.5 kg, and his current serum creatinine of 2 mg/dL.

$$\text{Cl}_{cr} \text{ for males (mL/min)} = \frac{(140 - \text{Age})(\text{Weight})}{(72)(\text{SCr}_{ss})}$$

$$= \frac{(140 - 40 \text{ yr})(61.5 \text{ kg})}{(72)(2 \text{ mg/dL})}$$

$$= 42.7 \text{ mL/min}$$

$$= 42.7 \text{ mL/min} \times \frac{60 \text{ min/hr}}{1000 \text{ mL/L}}$$

$$= 2.56 \text{ L/hr}$$

Using the estimated creatinine clearance of 2.56 L/hr as the gentamicin clearance and the volume of distribution of 38 L, the elimination rate constant (Equation 1.13) and half-life (Equation 1.14) are calculated to be 0.067 hr^{-1} and 10.34 hr, respectively:

$$K = \frac{\text{Cl}}{V}$$

$$= \frac{2.56 \text{ L/hr}}{38 \text{ L}}$$

$$= 0.067 \text{ hr}^{-1}$$

$$t\frac{1}{2} = \frac{0.693}{K}$$

$$= \frac{0.693}{0.067 \text{ hr}^{-1}}$$

$$= 10.34 \text{ hr}$$

Given D.H.'s half-life of approximately 10 hours and an infusion time of one-half hour, Equation 1.25, the steady-state bolus dose model, can be used to calculate his regimen.

$$\text{Dose} = \frac{(\text{Css}_1)(V)(1 - e^{-K\tau})}{(S)(F)(e^{-Kt_1})}$$

Because aminoglycoside dosing intervals are now typically greater than four to five half-lives, a dosing interval of 48 hours is reasonable given D.H.'s half-life of approximately 10 hours. Making the appropriate substitution in the rearranged equation where Css$_1$ is assumed to be 10 mg/L, t$_1$ is 1 hour (indicating that the peak concentration is to be obtained 1 hour after the start of the infusion), a dose of ≈400 mg is calculated.

$$\text{Dose} = \frac{(10 \text{ mg/L})(38 \text{ L})(1 - e^{-(0.067 \text{ hr}^{-1})(48 \text{ hr})})}{(1)(1)(e^{-(0.067 \text{ hr}^{-1})(1 \text{ hr})})}$$

$$= \frac{(10 \text{ mg/L})(38 \text{ L})(1 - 0.04)}{(1)(1)(0.94)}$$

$$= 388 \text{ mg or} \approx 400 \text{ mg}$$

Although a dose of 400 mg appears to be large, this is due in part to the extensive third spacing fluid and large volume of distribution. In many cases, a somewhat lower dose might be employed; however, the peak concentration would be proportionately decreased. Also, although the dose of 400 mg seems large, D.H. is receiving this dose only every other day and based on his non-obese or ideal body weight of 61.5 kg, this equates to ≈3.0 mg/kg/day, which is below the lower end of the usual range (5 to 7 mg/kg/day). It is also important to ensure that AUC_{24} is in the desired range (70 to 100 mg · hr/L).

$$AUC_{24} = \frac{\text{Dose}_{24} \text{ (mg)}}{\text{Cl (L/hr)}}$$

$$= \frac{200 \text{ mg}}{2.56 \text{ L/hr}}$$

$$= 78 \text{ mg · hr/L}$$

The AUC_{24} value of 78 mg · hr/L is in the lower end of the desired range (70 to 100 mg · hr/L), indicating that the dose could be increased if necessary depending on the severity of the infection. If the dosing interval remains 48 hours, an increase in dose will result in a proportional increase in AUC_{24} and peak concentration (see Equations 1.16 and 1.26). For example, a 30% increase in dose would result in an AUC_{24} of approximately 100 mg · hr/L and a peak concentration of 13 mg/L.

Question #11. *D.L., a 38-year-old, 70-kg patient with renal failure, is receiving gentamicin and ticarcillin for treatment of a fever of unknown origin. How might the concurrent administration of ticarcillin influence the pharmacokinetics of gentamicin? Are there other antibiotic combinations that may influence gentamicin dosing?*

The beta lactam ring of the penicillin compounds interacts in vivo and in vitro with one of the primary amines on both gentamicin and tobramycin to form an inactive amide.[48–50] The rate of gentamicin and tobramycin inactivation by penicillins is slow, however, and this interaction probably is significant only in patients with severely impaired renal function.[49–51] In these patients, the concurrent administration of carbenicillin or ticarcillin can decrease the half-life of gentamicin from approximately

46 to 22 hours. It has been recommended that the penicillin compounds and aminoglycosides be administered separately, and that in the case of carbenicillin, the dose be decreased to avoid excessive accumulation in patients with poor renal function. To estimate the degree to which this interaction affects gentamicin clearance, Equation 1.8 can be used to calculate an apparent ticarcillin-related clearance value for D.H. Using a standard volume of distribution of 0.25 L/kg for this 70-kg patient and the apparent rate constant for the in vitro interaction between ticarcillin and gentamicin of 0.017 hr^{-1}, a clearance value of 0.3 L/hr can be calculated:

$$\begin{matrix} \text{Tobramycin, Gentamicin} \\ \text{Clearance by Carbenicillin} \\ \text{or Ticarcillin (L/hr)} \end{matrix} = (0.017 \text{ hr}^{-1}) \begin{pmatrix} \text{Volume of Distribution} \\ \text{for Aminoglycosides} \end{pmatrix}$$

$$= (0.017 \text{ hr}^{-1})(0.25 \text{ L/kg})(70 \text{ kg}) = 0.3 \text{ L/hr}$$

This clearance value of 0.3 L/hr would be added to the estimated gentamicin clearance associated with D.H.'s residual renal function and nonrenal clearance (0.0043 L/kg/hr). This is only an estimate, however, and plasma levels must be monitored to make patient-specific adjustments.

Plasma samples for patients receiving aminoglycosides and penicillins concurrently must be obtained at a time when the in vitro interaction is minimal. Plasma samples for assay of aminoglycoside concentrations should be obtained when the penicillin is at its lowest concentration and assayed as soon as possible. If storage is required, samples should be frozen to minimize the continual in vitro effect of this interaction. Amikacin appears to be more resistant to degradation by penicillins.[48] Some of the more recent penicillin compounds (e.g., azlocillin, mezlocillin) appear to interact with gentamicin and tobramycin similarly but to a lesser extent than carbenicillin and ticarcillin.[54] Furthermore, the in vitro interaction between the cephalosporins (e.g., cefazolin, cefamandole) and the aminoglycoside antibiotics appears to be minimal.[54,56]

Although somewhat debatable, the combined use of cephalosporins and aminoglycosides may place patients at a greater risk for nephrotoxicity.[58,59]

Question #12. *What is the significance of a changing serum creatinine in a patient receiving gentamicin?*

A rising serum creatinine in a patient always raises the question of gentamicin-induced nephrotoxicity. In this event, the drug may be discontinued, the plasma concentration reevaluated, and/or the dose adjusted, since gentamicin may accumulate substantially when renal function is impaired. Dose modification should be based on plasma gentamicin levels rather than serum creatinine levels, because serum creatinine concentrations that are not at steady state can be misleading [see Part I: Creatinine Clearance (Cl$_{Cr}$)]. The reason for this is that despite the similarity between gentamicin and creatinine clearances,[31,40] their volumes of distribution differ. Gentamicin's V of 0.25 L/kg is smaller than that of creatinine, which is 0.5 L/kg.[26,27,32,60] Since the half-life is determined by the clearance and volume of distribution (see Equation 1.27 below), the half-life for creatinine is approximately twice as long as that of gentamicin and the other aminoglycosides. It will, therefore, take creatinine a longer time to arrive at a new steady-state concentration after a change in renal function.

$$t\frac{1}{2} = \frac{(0.693)(V)}{Cl} \qquad \text{[Eq. 1.27]}$$

When the serum creatinine is rising (i.e., not at steady state), the renal function is worse than would be predicted by use of the serum creatinine, and any gentamicin dose calculated using the serum creatinine would be overestimated. Conversely, when the serum creatinine is falling, renal function may be better than that reflected by the serum creatinine, and the doses calculated on the basis of these levels would be underestimated.

Question #13. *D.W., a 20-year-old, 60-kg man, is receiving 80 mg of tobramycin infused IV over a 30-minute period every 8 hours. His serum creatinine has increased from 1 mg/dL to 2 mg/dL over the past 24 hours. Because his renal function appears to be decreasing, three plasma samples were obtained to monitor serum gentamicin concentrations as follows: just before a dose, 1 hour after that same dose, and 8 hours after that dose (two troughs and one peak level). The serum gentamicin concentrations at these times were 4 mg/L, 8 mg/L, and 5 mg/L, respectively. Calculate the volume of distribution, elimination rate constant, and clearance of tobramycin for D.W.*

Since the second trough concentration of tobramycin is higher than the first, it is apparent that the drug is accumulating. Therefore, steady-state equations should not be used to calculate D.W.'s pharmacokinetic parameters. The first step that should be taken to resolve this dilemma is to calculate the elimination rate constant from the two plasma concentrations that were obtained during the elimination phase (8 mg/L and 5 mg/L). Equation 1.22 can be used to estimate the elimination rate constant; however, this K should only be used as an estimate since the two plasma concentrations were obtained less than one half-life apart.

$$K = \frac{\ln\left(\frac{C_1}{C_2}\right)}{t}$$

$$= \frac{\ln\left(\frac{8 \text{ mg/L}}{5 \text{ mg/L}}\right)}{7 \text{ hr}}$$

$$= 0.067 \text{ hr}^{-1}$$

This elimination rate constant of 0.067 hr^{-1} was calculated by assuming that the peak concentration of 8 mg/L was obtained 1 hour after the start of the tobramycin infusion and that the trough concentration was obtained just before the next dose, resulting in a time interval of 7 hours. The elimination rate constant of 0.067 hr^{-1} corresponds to a half-life of 10.3 hours (Equation 1.14):

$$t\frac{1}{2} = \frac{0.693}{K}$$

$$= \frac{0.693}{0.067 \text{ hr}^{-1}}$$

$$= 10.3 \text{ hr}$$

This half-life of 10.3 hours suggests that relatively little drug is lost during the infusion period; therefore, a bolus model is most appropriately used in this situation. The volume of distribution can be estimated by assuming that the bolus dose is administered instantaneously and calculating the theoretical peak concentration using Equation 1.10. C is the measured concentration of 8 mg/L, t is the 1-hour interval between the start of the infusion and the time of sampling, and C° is the theoretical peak concentration for an IV bolus.

$$C° = \frac{C}{e^{-Kt}}$$

$$= \frac{8 \text{ mg/L}}{e^{-(0.067 \text{ hr}^{-1})(1 \text{ hr})}}$$

$$= \frac{8 \text{ mg/L}}{0.94}$$

$$= 8.5 \text{ mg/L}$$

Since the change in concentration (peak minus trough) is the result of the dose administered and the volume of distribution, the V can be calculated using Equation 1.28 below.

$$V = \frac{Dose}{(C_{peak} - C_{min})} \qquad \text{[Eq. 1.28]}$$

$$V = \frac{80 \text{ mg}}{(8.5 \text{ mg/L} - 4 \text{ mg/L})}$$

$$= 17.8 \text{ L}$$

This volume of distribution of 17.8 L can then be used with the elimination rate constant of 0.067 hr^{-1} in Equation 1.24 to calculate D.W.'s clearance of 1.2 L/hr or 20 mL/min:

$$Cl = (K)(V)$$

$$= (0.067 \text{ hr}^{-1})(17.8 \text{ L})$$

$$= 1.2 \text{ L/hr } or \text{ 20 mL/min}$$

Question #14. *Using the pharmacokinetic parameters calculated for D.W. in Question 13, develop a dosing regimen that will produce reasonable peak and trough concentrations of tobramycin.*

Because D.W.'s tobramycin clearance is low (1.2 L/hr), it will be necessary to reduce his maintenance dose. There are two alternatives: 1) reduce the dose and maintain the same dosing interval, or 2) adjust both the dose and the dosing interval such that the peak concentration and AUC$_{24}$ will be approximately 10 mg/L and 70 to 100 mg · hr/L, respectively.

Reduce the Dose and Maintain the Same Dosing Interval. This method is not acceptable for D.W. because he has such a long half-life ($\approx$10 hours). If a dose that achieves a maximum concentration of 8 mg/L is used and the dosing interval of 8 hours is maintained, the trough level will be $\approx$4.7 mg/L.

$$Css \text{ min} = (Css \text{ max})(e^{-K\tau}) \qquad \text{[Eq. 1.29]}$$

$$Css \text{ min} = (8 \text{ mg/L})(e^{-(0.067 \text{ hr}-1)(8 \text{ hr})})$$

$$= 4.68 \text{ mg/L}$$

This level may place D.W. at risk for tobramycin toxicity.

Adjust Both the Dose and Dosing Interval to Achieve Reasonable Peak Concentration and AUC$_{24}$ values. The only potential limitation to this approach is that most clinicians prefer to avoid prolonged periods during which the gentamicin concentration is below the MIC of the pathogen, because of the possibility of organism regrowth. Clinical experience with dosing intervals in excess of 48 hours is limited. Nevertheless, some animal data suggest that doses which result in high peak and low trough concentrations are less likely to produce renal toxicity than the same dose administered as a continuous IV infusion (i.e., the same average levels).[61] A first estimate of the dosing interval can be made by examining D.W.'s tobramycin half-life of $\approx$10 hours. If an interval of four to five half-lives is chosen, a dosing interval of 48 hours can be used. Since the half-life of tobramycin is long relative to the infusion time of one-half hour, the bolus dose model can be used. As previously stated, Equation 1.26 can be used to calculate a dose required to achieve a specific AUC_{24}. Using Equation 1.26 with the previously derived pharmacokinetic parameters and a dosing interval of 48 hours, a dose of $\approx$240 mg is calculated. A peak concentration that occurs 1 hour after the infusion has been initiated is also assumed (i.e., $t_1 = 1$ hour).

$$AUC_{24} = \frac{Dose_{24} \text{ (mg)}}{Cl \text{ (L/hr)}}$$

$$Dose_{24} = (AUC_{24})(Cl)$$

$$= 100 \text{ mg} \cdot \text{hr/L } (1.2 \text{ L/hr})$$

$$= 120 \text{ mg or 240 mg Q 48h}$$

The peak concentration can be calculated using the bolus dose model (Equation 1.16).

$$Css_1 = \frac{\dfrac{(S)(F)(Dose)}{V}}{(1 - e^{-K\tau})} e^{-Kt_1}$$

$$= \frac{\dfrac{(1)(1)(240 \text{ mg})}{17.8 \text{ L}}}{(1 - e^{-(0.067 \text{ hr}^{-1})(48 \text{ hr})})} (e^{-(0.067 \text{ hr}^{-1})(1 \text{ hr})})$$

$$= \frac{13.4 \text{ mg/L}}{0.96} (0.94)$$

$$= 13.96 \text{ mg/L}(0.94)$$

$$= 13.1 \text{ mg/L}$$

The trough concentration, calculated using Equation 1.29, would be 0.6 mg/L.

$$Css \text{ min} = (Css \text{ max})(e^{-K\tau})$$

$$Css \text{ min} = (13.96 \text{ mg/L})(e^{-(0.067 \text{ hr}^{-1})(48 \text{ hr})})$$

$$= 0.6 \text{ mg/L}$$

Question #15. *M.S., a 70-kg non-obese female, undergoes 4 hours of hemodialysis every 48 hours. She is functionally (not surgically) anephric, and gentamicin is to be started. Calculate a dosing regimen that achieves a peak concentration of 6 mg/L and then maintains average levels of 3.5 mg/L.*

Because the gentamicin half-life for a patient who is functionally anephric is probably in excess of 30 hours, very little drug will be eliminated from the body over the 1-hour period following initiation of the infusion. Therefore, the loading dose may be calculated as though it were a bolus (Equation 1.30). Assuming S and F to be 1 and the volume of distribution to be 17.5 L (0.25 L/kg), a loading dose of ≈100 mg would be calculated as follows:

$$\text{Loading Dose} = \frac{(V)(C)}{(S)(F)} \qquad \text{[Eq. 1.30]}$$

$$= \frac{(17.5 \text{ L})(6 \text{ mg/L})}{(1)(1)}$$

$$= 105 \text{ mg}$$

Since gentamicin elimination in M.S. will be irregular, occurring at higher rates during the dialysis, the usual maintenance dose equation cannot be used. As presented in Part I: Dialysis of Drugs, there are two possible approaches to the resolution of this problem. One approach is to administer a daily dose such that average concentrations are maintained and then to calculate a replacement dose postdialysis. A second approach is to administer the drug after dialysis only. The dose used is the amount of drug lost during the interdialysis and intradialysis period. In both cases, the use of the patient's clearance (Cl_{pat}), dialysis clearance (Cl_{dial}), and the volume of distribution will be required. The reported clearance for aminoglycosides in functionally anephric patients is ≈0.0043 L/kg/hr,[27,62] and aminoglycoside clearance by standard hemodialysis is 20 to 40 mL/min, with an average value of ≈30 mL/min.[27,62–64]

If the approach of giving daily and postdialysis doses is taken, then the maintenance dose on non-dialysis days can be calculated using Equation 1.31, with a patient clearance of 0.3 L/hr (0.0043 L/hr/kg × 70 kg) and a dosing interval of 24 hours. In most dialysis patients, a gentamicin concentration between 3 to 4 mg/L (average: 3.5 mg/L) is set as a goal. Therefore, a dose of ≈25 mg would be appropriate:

$$\text{Dose} = \frac{(\text{Css ave})(Cl_{pat})(\tau)}{(S)(F)} \qquad \text{[Eq. 1.31]}$$

$$\text{Dose} = \frac{(3.5 \text{ mg/L})(0.3 \text{ L/hr})(24 \text{ hr})}{(1)(1)}$$

$$= 25.2 \text{ mg or} \approx 25 \text{ mg}$$

If the patient had been surgically anephric, the Cl_{pat} would have been approximately halved, and the corresponding maintenance dose would also have been one-half or ≈ 13 mg/day. Equation 1.32 can be used to calculate the postdialysis replacement dose. Using the average C_{dial} and a dialysis time (T_d) of 4 hours, the replacement dose is calculated to be ≈ 25 mg.

$$\text{Post Dialysis Replacement Dose} = (V)(\text{Css ave})\left(1 - e^{-\left(\frac{Cl_{pat} + Cl_{dial}}{V}\right)(T_d)}\right) \quad \text{[Eq. 1.32]}$$

$$= [17.5\ L][3.5\ mg/L]\left[1 - e^{-\frac{(0.3\ L/hr + 1.8\ L/hr)}{17.5\ L}(4\ hr)}\right]$$

$$= [17.5\ L][3.5\ mg/L][1 - 0.62]$$

$$= 23.3\ mg\ or\ \approx 25\ mg$$

Note that the dialysis clearance of 1.8 L/hr represents a clearance of ≈ 30 mL/min and that this is the primary route of elimination during the intradialysis period. Also, the postdialysis dose of 25 mg can be added to the maintenance dose of ≈ 25 mg, resulting in a gentamicin dose on dialysis days of 50 mg.

If it is decided to administer the aminoglycoside only after dialysis, Equation 1.33 can be used to calculate the postdialysis replacement dose. In this situation, a steady-state peak concentration of ≈ 4 to 5 mg/L is set as a goal (peak concentrations of 6 to 8 mg/L would expose M.S. to continuously elevated concentrations of gentamicin).

Using Equation 1.33, a Css peak of 5.0 mg/L, a patient clearance of 0.3 L/hr, and a t_1 of 44 hours [derived from a 48-hour interval between the dialyses and a dialysis time (T_d) of 4 hours], the postdialysis replacement dose is 62 mg.

$$\text{Post Dialysis Replacement Dose} = (V)(\text{Css peak})\left(1 - \left[\left(e^{-\left(\frac{Cl_{pat}}{V}\right)(t_1)}\right)\left(e^{-\left(\frac{Cl_{pat} + Cl_{dial}}{V}\right)(T_d)}\right)\right]\right)$$

$$\text{[Eq. 1.33]}$$

$$= [17.5\ L][5\ mg/L]\left[1 - \left(e^{-\left(\frac{0.3\ L/hr}{17.5\ L}\right)(44\ hr)}\right)\left(e^{-\left(\frac{0.3\ L/hr + 1.8\ L/hr}{17.5\ L}\right)(4\ hr)}\right)\right]$$

$$= (17.5\ L)(5\ mg/L)[(1 - (0.47)(0.62)]$$

$$= (17.5\ L)(5\ mg/L)(1 - 0.29)$$

$$= 62\ mg$$

To ensure that trough concentrations just before dialysis are not excessively low, the predialysis drug concentration should be calculated using Equation 1.34:

$$\text{Predialysis Drug Concentration} = [\text{Csspeak}]\left[e^{-\left(\frac{Cl_{pat}}{V}\right)(t_1)} \right] \qquad [\text{Eq. 1.34}]$$

$$= (5\ \text{mg/L})\left[e^{-\left(\frac{0.3\ \text{L/hr}}{17.5\ \text{L}}\right)(44\ \text{hr})} \right]$$

$$= (5\ \text{mg/L})(0.47)$$

$$= 2.35\ \text{mg/L}$$

This predialysis concentration of ≈ 2.4 mg/L is higher than usually desired; however, because the gentamicin half-life is unusually long, it will be difficult to maintain peak levels in the range of 5 mg/L and predialysis trough concentrations of < 2 mg/L. Unfortunately, the persistence of relatively high concentrations between dialysis periods will place M.S. at greater risk for ototoxicity.[65] In addition, although postdialysis concentrations can be calculated, these lower concentrations are transient and probably do not correlate well with the incidence of ototoxicity in dialysis patients. If postdialysis concentrations are to be measured, time should be allowed for equilibration between the plasma compartment (in which concentrations have been lowered during the dialysis period) and the extracellular fluid compartment.[66]

Question #16. *How would the above situation have differed if peritoneal dialysis rather than hemodialysis had been used?*

Peritoneal dialysis is much less effective in removing gentamicin; the usual clearance value is ≈ 4 mL/min/m^2, with an average value of 5 to 10 mL/min for the 70-kg patient. Nonetheless, the total amount of drug removed during dialysis may be as much as 30% or more because acute intermittent peritoneal dialysis is usually continued for ≈ 36 hours.[62,67]

Aminoglycosides can be administered either parenterally or intraperitoneally to achieve systemic plasma concentrations. When administered intraperitoneally, an initial loading dose of ≈ 2 to 3 mg/kg is added to the first peritoneal dialysis exchange. Then, 1.2 mg/kg/day is added to one exchange daily (usually the night-time exchange), or a dose that produces a dialysate concentration of ≈ 6 to 10 mg/L is added to each dialysate exchange. Both of these regimens result in steady-state plasma concentrations of ≈ 3 mg/L with relatively little fluctuation.[68] When aminoglycoside antibiotics are placed in each peritoneal exchange, many clinicians estimate the steady-state plasma concentration to be $\approx 40\%$ of the peritoneal dialysate concentration. As an example, if 16 mg were added to each 2 L peritoneal exchange volume (8 mg/L), the steady-state plasma concentration would be ≈ 3.2 mg/L, or 40% of the 8 mg/L concentration in the dialysate exchanges.[69,70]

Question #17. *A patient with meningitis is being considered for treatment with intrathecal (IT) or intraventricular gentamicin. Which of these routes is preferred and what pharmacokinetic parameters are expected?*

Gentamicin does not cross the blood-brain barrier very effectively, and cerebrospinal fluid (CSF) levels are usually subtherapeutic unless IT or intraventricular injections are given.[71-73] The intraventricular route is preferred to ensure adequate ventricular levels and uniform concentration throughout the subarachnoid space.[71,73] The apparent CSF half-life of aminoglycosides is approximately 6 hours.[71,72] The usual intraventricular dose of aminoglycosides is 5 to 10 mg and is usually repeated on a daily basis. This dosing regimen is similar for gentamicin, tobramycin, and amikacin, even though doses administered systemically vary considerably. If the intraventricular route is to be used, neurosurgery will be required to insert a special access shunt that allows daily administration. CSF peak concentrations measured soon after intraventricular injection approach 100 mg/L or higher; trough concentrations 24 hours later are usually 5 to 15 mg/L.[73]

Question #18. *T.C. is receiving tobramycin 360 mg IV over one-half hour every 24 hours at 9:00 a.m. Levels drawn at 11:00 a.m. and 9:00 p.m. were 15.0 mg/L and 0.9 mg/L, respectively. Calculate the peak concentration expected at 10:00 a.m., or 1 hour after starting the 9:00 a.m. tobramycin infusion, and the AUC_{24} to determine the appropriateness of the current dosing regimen.*

The time interval between 11:00 a.m. and 9:00 p.m. is 10 hours, and Equation 1.22 can be used to determine the elimination rate constant for T.C.

$$K = \frac{\ln\left(\frac{C_1}{C_2}\right)}{t}$$

$$= \frac{\ln\left(\frac{15 \text{ mg/L}}{0.9 \text{ mg/L}}\right)}{10 \text{ hr}}$$

$$= \frac{2.8}{10 \text{ hr}}$$

$$= 0.28 \text{ hr}^{-1}$$

This patient-specific elimination rate constant of 0.28 hr^{-1} can be used in Equation 1.10 to calculate the expected plasma concentration at

10:00 a.m. (1 hour after the start of the infusion) or 1.0 hour before the observed peak of 15 mg/L.

$$C^0 = \frac{C}{e^{-Kt}}$$

$$= \frac{15 \text{ mg/L}}{e^{-(0.28 \text{ hr}^{-1})(1 \text{ hr})}}$$

$$= \frac{15 \text{ mg/L}}{0.76}$$

$$= 19.8 \text{ mg/L}$$

The steady-state infusion model (Equation 1.20)

$$Css_2 = \frac{\frac{(S)(F)(Dose/t_{in})}{Cl}(1 - e^{-Kt_{in}})}{(1 - e^{-K\tau})}(e^{-Kt_2})$$

can be rearranged to solve for clearance: $(t_{in} > \frac{1}{6} t\frac{1}{2})$

$$Cl = \frac{\frac{(S)(F)(Dose/t_{in})}{Css_2}(1 - e^{-Kt_{in}})}{(1 - e^{-K\tau})}(e^{-Kt_2}) \qquad \text{[Eq. 1.35]}$$

$$Cl = \frac{\frac{(1)(1)(360 \text{ mg}/0.5 \text{ hr})}{0.9 \text{ mg/L}}(1 - e^{-(0.28 \text{ hr}^{-1})(0.5 \text{ hr})})}{(1 - e^{-(0.28 \text{ hr}^{-1})(24 \text{ hr})})}(e^{-(0.28 \text{ hr}^{-1})(11.5 \text{ hr})})$$

$$= \frac{(800 \text{ L/hr})(0.13)}{(0.99)}(0.04)$$

$$= 4.2 \text{ L/hr}$$

The AUC_{24} can then be calculated using Equation 1.26.

$$AUC_{24} = \frac{Dose_{24} \text{ (mg)}}{Cl \text{ (L/hr)}}$$

$$= \frac{360 \text{ mg}}{4.2 \text{ L/hr}}$$

$$= 86 \text{ mg} \cdot \text{hr/L}$$

This peak concentration of 19.8 mg/L represents a concentration that is within the target range (peak/MIC > 10) based on the breakpoint for susceptibility (2 mcg/mL). The AUC_{24} is also in the target range (70 to

100 mg · hr/L) and suggests that T.C.'s tobramycin does not require dose adjustment.

Question #19. *J.H. is a 25-year-old man (height, 5'5"; weight, 55 kg) with cystic fibrosis who is admitted for treatment of an acute pulmonary exacerbation. His serum creatinine is 0.6 mg/dL. His treatment is initiated with tobramycin 180 mg infused over 30 minutes every 8 hours. Calculate the predicted steady-state peak and trough concentrations.*

The pharmacokinetics of a number of compounds, including the aminoglycoside antibiotics, have been shown to be altered in patients with cystic fibrosis. In particular, the volume of distribution appears to be larger (0.3 to 0.35 L/kg) and the clearance is faster than age-matched control subjects.[74] Currently, there is no clear physiologic rationale for the altered pharmacokinetics. J.H.'s V and Cl can be calculated using a V of 0.3 L/kg and Equation 1.6 to calculate creatinine clearance.

$$V = (0.3 \text{ L/kg})(55 \text{ kg})$$

$$= 16.5 \text{ L}$$

$$\text{Cl}_{cr} \text{ for males (mL/min)} = \frac{(140 - \text{Age})(\text{Weight})}{(72)(\text{SCr}_{ss})}$$

$$= \frac{(140 - 25 \text{ yr})(55 \text{ kg})}{(72)(0.6 \text{ mg/dL})}$$

$$= 146 \text{ mL/min}$$

$$= 146 \text{ mL/min} \times \frac{60 \text{ min/hr}}{1000 \text{ mL/L}}$$

$$= 8.8 \text{ L/hr}$$

Using the estimated creatinine clearance of 8.8 L/hr as the tobramycin clearance and the volume of distribution of 16.5 L, the elimination rate constant (Equation 1.13) and half-life (Equation 1.14) are calculated to be 0.53 hr^{-1} and 1.3 hr, respectively:

$$K = \frac{\text{Cl}}{V}$$

$$= \frac{8.8 \text{ L/hr}}{16.5 \text{ L}}$$

$$= 0.53 \text{ hr}^{-1}$$

$$t\frac{1}{2} = \frac{0.693}{K}$$

$$= \frac{0.693}{0.53 \text{ hr}^{-1}}$$

$$= 1.3 \text{ hr}$$

The steady-state peak and trough concentrations can be calculated using the short infusion model (Equation 1.20):

$$Css_2 = \frac{\frac{(S)(F)(Dose/t_{in})}{Cl}(1 - e^{-Kt_{in}})}{(1 - e^{-K\tau})}(e^{-Kt_2})$$

$$Css_2 = \frac{\frac{(1)(1)(180\ mg/0.5\ hr)}{8.8\ L/hr}(1 - e^{-(0.53\ hr^{-1})(0.5\ hr)})}{(1 - e^{-(0.53\ hr^{-1})(8\ hr)})}(e^{-(0.53\ hr^{-1})(0.5\ hr)})$$

$$= \frac{(40.9\ mg/L)(0.23)}{(0.99)}(0.77)$$

$$= 7.3\ mg/L$$

The trough concentration could be calculated using the short infusion model as shown above, or by decaying down the peak concentration using Equation 1.9, where "t" is the time between the two drug levels.

$$C = C^o e^{-Kt}$$

$$C = (7.3\ mg/L)(e^{-(0.53\ hr^{-1})(7\ hr)})$$

$$= (7.3\ mg/L)(0.024)$$

$$= 0.18\ mg/L$$

Therefore, although the dose of tobramycin appears quite high (10 mg/kg/day), the altered pharmacokinetics result in predicted serum concentrations that are not different than the target concentrations in other patients. Because of the relatively short elimination half-life in these patients, the use of "once-daily" aminoglycoside regimens cannot be routinely recommended. There are two large clinical trials currently being conducted to determine the comparative efficacy and safety of these regimens in patients with cystic fibrosis.

REFERENCES

1. Pechere J. Clinical pharmacokinetics of aminoglycoside antibiotics. Clin Pharmacokinet 1979;4:170.
2. Craig W, Ebert, SC. Killing and regrowth of bacteria in vivo: a review. Scand J Infect Dis 1991;74:63–71.
3. Kapusnik J, et al. Single, large, daily dosing versus intermittent dosing of tobramycin for treating experimental pseudomonas pneumonia. J Infect Dis 1988;158:7–22.
4. Leggett J, et al. Comparative antibiotic dose-effect relations at several dosing intervals in murine pneumonitis and thigh-infection models. J Infect Dis 1989;159:281–292.

5. Moore R, et al. Clinical response to aminoglycoside therapy: importance of the ratio of peak concentration to minimal inhibitory concentration. J Infect Dis 1987;155:93–99.

6. Craig W, Vogelman, B. The post-antibiotic effect. Ann Intern Med 1987;106:900–902.

7. Craig W, Redington J, Ebert SC. Pharmacodynamics of amikacin in vitro and in mouse thigh and lung infections. J Antimicrob Chemother 1991;27(Suppl C):29–40.

8. Powell S, et al. Once-daily vs. continuous aminoglycoside dosing: efficacy and toxicity in animal and clinical studies of gentamicin, netilmicin, and tobramycin. J Infect Dis 1983;5:918–932.

9. Verpooten G, Giuliano, RA, Verbist, L, et al. Once-daily dosing decreases renal accumulation of gentamicin and netilmicin. Clin Pharmacol Ther 1989;45:22–27.

10. Rybak M, et al. Prospective evaluation of the effect of an aminoglycoside dosing regimen on rates of observed nephrotoxicity and ototoxicity. Antimicrob Agents Chemother 1999;43:1549–1555.

11. Barza M, Ioannidis, JP, Cappelleri, JC, Lau, J. Single or multiple daily doses of aminoglycosides: a meta-analysis. BMJ 1996;312:338–345.

12. Hatala R, Dinh, T, Cook, DJ. Once-daily aminoglycoside dosing in immunocompetent adults: a meta-analysis. Ann Intern Med 1996;124:717–725.

13. Nicolau D, et al. Experience with a once-daily aminoglycoside program administered to 2,184 adult patients. Antimicrob Agents Chemother 1995;39:650–655.

14. Noone P, et al. Experience in monitoring gentamicin therapy during treatment of serious gram-negative sepsis. Br Med J 1979;1:477.

15. Jackson G, Riff, LF. Pseudomonas bacteremia: pharmacologic and other basis for failure of treatment with gentamicin. J Infect Dis 1971;124:185.

16. Klastersky J, et al. Antibacterial activity in serum and urine as a therapeutic guide in bacterial infections. J Infect Dis 1974;129:187.

17. Cox C. Gentamicin: a new aminoglycoside antibiotic: clinical and laboratory studies in urinary tract infections. J Infect Dis 1969;119:486.

18. Jackson G, Arcieri, G. Ototoxicity of gentamicin in man: a survey and controlled analysis of clinical experience in the United States. J Infect Dis 1971;124:130.

19. Goodman E, et al. Prospective comparative study of variable dosage and variable frequency regimens for administrations of gentamicin. Antimicrob Agents Chemother 1975;8:434.

20. Schentag J, et al. Clinical and pharmacokinetic characteristics of aminoglycoside nephrotoxicity in 201 critically ill patients. Antimicrob Agents Chemother 1982;5:721.

21. Wilfret J, et al. Renal insufficiency associated with gentamicin therapy. J Infect Dis 1971;124(Suppl):148.

22. Mawer G. Prescribing aids for gentamicin. Br J Clin Pharmacol 1974;1:45.

23. Federspil P, et al. Pharmacokinetics and ototoxicity of gentamicin, tobramycin, and amikacin. J Infect Dis 1976;134(Suppl):200.

24. McCormack J, Jewesson PJ. A critical re-evaluation of the "therapeutic range" of aminoglycosides. Clin Infect Dis 1992;14:320–339.

25. Barclay M, Duffull SB, Begg EJ, Buttimore RC. Experience of once-daily aminoglycoside dosing using a target area under the concentration-time curve. Aust NZ J Med 1995;25:230–235.

26. Gyselynek A, et al. Pharmacokinetics of gentamicin: distribution and plasma and renal clearance. J Infect Dis 1971;124(Suppl):70.

27. Christopher T, et al. Gentamicin pharmacokinetics during hemodialysis. Kidney Int 1974;6:38.

28. Danish M, et al. Pharmacokinetics of gentamicin and kanamycin during hemodialysis. Antimicrob Agents Chemother 1974;6:841.

29. Barza M, et al. Predictability of blood levels of gentamicin in man. J Infect Dis 1975;132:165.

30. Sawchuck R, Zaske, DE. Pharmacokinetics of dosing regimens which utilize multiple intravenous infusions: gentamicin in burn patients. J Pharmacokinet Biopharm 1976;4:183.

31. Regamey C, et al. Comparative pharmacokinetics of tobramycin and gentamicin. Clin Pharmacol Ther 1973;14:396.

32. Siber G, et al. Pharmacokinetics of gentamicin in children and adults. J Infect Dis 1975;132:637.

33. Hull J, Sarubbi, FA. Gentamicin serum concentrations: pharmacokinetic predictions. Ann Intern Med 1976;85:183.

34. Blouin R, et al. Tobramycin pharmacokinetics in morbidly obese patients. Clin Pharmacol Ther 1979;26:508.

35. Bauer L, et al. Amikacin pharmacokinetics in morbidly obese patients. Am J Hosp Pharm 1980;37:519.

36. Sampliner R, et al. Influence of ascites on tobramycin pharmacokinetics. J Clin Pharmacol 1984;24:43.

37. Hodgman T, et al. Tobramycin disposition into ascitic fluid. Clin Pharm 1984;3:203.

38. Esheverria P, et al. Age-dependent dose response to gentamicin. Pediatrics 1975;87:805.

39. Schentag J, et al. Tissue persistence of gentamicin in man. JAMA 1977;238:327.

40. Schentag J, Jusko WJ. Renal clearance and tissue accumulation of gentamicin. Clin Pharmacol Ther 1977;22:364.

41. Mendelson J, et al. Safety of bolus administration of gentamicin. Antimicrob Agents Chemother 1976;9:633.

42. Lynn K, et al. Gentamicin by intravenous bolus injections. NZ Med J 1977;80:442.

43. Demczar D, Nafziger AN, Bertino JS. Pharmacokinetics of gentamicin at traditional versus higher doses: implications for once-daily aminoglycoside dosing. Antimicrob Agents Chemother 1997;41:1115–1119.

44. Colburn W, et al. A model for the prospective identification of the prenephrotoxic state during gentamicin therapy. J Pharmacokinet Biopharm 1978;6:179.

45. Evans W, et al. A model for dosing gentamicin in children and adolescents that adjust for tissue accumulation with continuous dosing. Clin Pharmacokinet 1980;5:295.

46. Dionne R, et al. Estimating creatinine clearance in morbidly obese patients. Am J Hosp Pharm 1981;38:841–844.

47. Bauer L, et al. Influence of weight on aminoglycoside pharmacokinetics in normal weight and morbidly obese patients. Eur J Clin Pharmacol 1983;24:643–647.

48. Holt H, et al. Interactions between aminoglycoside antibiotics and carbenicillin or ticarcillin. Infection 1976;4:107.

49. Ervin F, et al. Inactivation of gentamicin by penicillins in patients with renal failure. Antimicrob Agents Chemother 1976;9:1004.

50. Weibert R, Keane, WF. Carbenicillin-gentamicin interaction in acute renal failure. Am J Hosp Pharm 1977;34:1137.

51. Riff L, Jackson, GG. Laboratory and clinical conditions for gentamicin inactivation by carbenicillin. Arch Intern Med 1972;130:887.

52. Konishi H, et al. Tobramycin inactivation by carbenicillin, ticarcillin, and piperacillin. Antimicrob Agents Chemother 1983;23:653.

53. Pickering L, Gerahart, P. Effect of time and concentration upon interaction between gentamicin, tobramycin, netilmicin, or amikacin, and carbenicillin or ticarcillin. Antimicrob Agents Chemother 1979;15:592.

54. Henderson J, et al. In vitro inactivation of tobramycin and netilmicin by carbenicillin, azlocillin, or mezlocillin. Am J Hosp Pharm 1981;38:1167.

55. Earp C, Barriere SL. The lack of inactivation of tobramycin by cefazolin, cefamandole, moxalactam in vitro. Drug Intell Clin Pharm 1985;19:677.

56. Kehoe W. Lack of effect of ceftizoxime on gentamicin serum level determinations. Hosp Pharm 1986;21:340.

57. Fischer J, et al. Pharmacokinetics and antibacterial activity of two gentamicin products given intramuscularly. Clin Pharm 1984;3:411.

58. Schultze R. Possible nephrotoxicity of gentamicin. J Infect Dis 1971;124(Suppl):145.

59. Kleinknecht D, et al. Acute renal failure after high doses of gentamicin and cephalothin. Lancet 1973;7812:1129.

60. Blieler R, Schedl, HP. Creatinine excretion: variability and relationships to diet and body size. J Lab Clin Med 1962;59:945.

61. Reiner N, et al. Nephrotoxicity of gentamicin and tobramycin in dogs on a continuous or once daily intravenous injection. Antimicrob Agents Chemother 1978;4(Suppl A):85.

62. Reguer L, et al. Pharmacokinetics of amikacin during hemodialysis and peritoneal dialysis. Antimicrob Agents Chemother 1977;11:214.

63. Christopher T, et al. Hemodialyzer clearance of gentamicin, kanamycin, tobramycin, amikacin, ethambutol, procainamide, and flucytosine with a technique for planning therapy. J Pharmacokinet Biopharm 1976;4:427.

64. Halprin B, et al. Clearance of gentamicin during hemodialysis: a comparison of four artificial kidneys. J Infect Dis 1976;133:627.

65. Gailiunas P, et al. Vestibular toxicity of gentamicin: incidence in patients receiving long-term hemodialysis therapy. Arch Intern Med 1978;138:1621.

66. Bauer L. Rebound gentamicin levels after hemodialysis. Ther Drug Monit 1982;4:99.

67. Gary N. Peritoneal clearance and removal of gentamicin. J Infect Dis 1971;124 (Suppl):96.

68. Lamiere N, et al. Peritoneal pharmacokinetics and pharmacological manipulation of peritoneal transport. In: Gokal R, ed. Continuous Ambulatory Peritoneal Dialysis. New York: Churchill Livingstone, 1986:56–93.

69. O'Brien M, Mason, NA. Systemic absorption of intra-peritoneal antimicrobials in continuous ambulatory peritoneal dialysis. Clin Pharm 1992; 11:246–54.

70. Horton M, et al. Treatment of peritonitis in patients undergoing continuous ambulatory peritoneal dialysis. Clin Pharm 1990;9:102–117.

71. Kaiser A. Aminoglycoside therapy of gram-negative bacillary meningitis. N Engl J Med 1975;293:1215.

72. Rahal J, et al. Combined intrathecal and intramuscular gentamicin for gram-negative meningitis. N Engl J Med 1974;290:1394.

73. Everett E, Stausbaugh, LJ. Antimicrobial agents and central nervous system. Neurosurgery 1980; 6:691.

74. Beringer PM, Vinks A, Jelliffe R, Shapiro B. Pharmacokinetics of tobramycin in adults with cystic fibrosis: implications for once-daily administration. Antimicrob Agents Chemother 2000;44:809–813.

2

CARBAMAZEPINE

Jeanne Hawkins Van Tyle and Michael E. Winter

Carbamazepine is an anticonvulsant compound that is structurally similar to the tricyclic antidepressant agents. It is the drug of choice for the treatment of trigeminal neuralgia[1] and is used in the treatment of seizures. It has FDA approval for generalized tonic–clonic (grand mal) and partial (psychomotor, temporal lobe) seizures as well as trigeminal neuralgia (tic douloureux) and glossopharyngeal neuralgia syndromes. It is used in a variety of other conditions including bipolar disorders,[2,3] pain syndromes,[1] migraine headaches,[4] neurologic disorders, and schizophrenia. Carbamazepine is most frequently prescribed for patients whose conditions have failed to respond to other anticonvulsant therapy or for those in whom significant side effects from other anticonvulsant agents have developed. The use of carbamazepine has increased in recent years in part due to its use in psychiatric illnesses. Carbamazepine is available in many dosage forms including oral suspension, chewable tablet, oral immediate-release tablet, extended-release tablet, and an extended-release capsule. It is available generically from several manufacturers. It is labeled for use in adults and children and is in pregnancy class D. Effective doses for seizure disorders are in the range of 15 to 25 mg/kg/day.

Carbamazepine is eliminated primarily by the metabolic route, with one of the metabolites (10,11-epoxide) having some anticonvulsant activity.[5,6] The ratios of carbamazepine-10,11-epoxide to carbamazepine are higher in infants and preschool children than in adults.[7] In addition, children have a higher carbamazepine clearance per kilogram of body weight than adults.[8] Carbamazepine is metabolized primarily by the P450 isozyme CYP3A4. Less than 2% of carbamazepine is excreted unchanged in the urine. Carbamazepine is bound to plasma albumin and α_1-acid glycoprotein to a significant extent.[9] The free fraction is approximately 0.2 to 0.3, indicating that alterations in serum protein concentration may affect the therapeutic range or the relationship between the measured carbamazepine concentration and its pharmacologic effect. Concomitant treatment with valproate sodium results in a higher free fraction of carbamazepine.

THERAPEUTIC AND TOXIC PLASMA CONCENTRATIONS

The range of therapeutic serum concentrations for carbamazepine[10] is commonly reported to be 4 to 12 mg/L. Many patients, however, will de-

KEY PARAMETERS: **Carbamazepine**	
Therapeutic Plasma Concentrations	4–12 mg/L
F	80%
S	1.0
V^a	1.4 L/kg
Cl^a	
Monotherapy[b]	0.064 L/kg/hr
Polytherapy[b]	0.1 L/kg/hr
Children (monotherapy)	0.11 L/kg/hr
α (free fraction)	0.2–0.3
$t\frac{1}{2}^b$	
Adult monotherapy	15 hr
Adult polytherapy	10 hr

[a]The values for volume of distribution and clearance are approximations based on oral administration data and an estimate of bioavailability.
[b]The clearance and half-life values represent adult values after induction has taken place. Polytherapy represents a patient receiving other enzyme-inducing anticonvulsants (e.g., phenobarbital, phenytoin).

velop symptoms of toxicity when plasma concentrations exceed 9 mg/L.[11] For this reason, many clinicians prefer to use a therapeutic range of approximately 4 to 8 mg/L.[12] The conversion of mass units to SI units is 1 µg/mL = 4.23 µmol/L. In the Advia Centaur assay, there is approximately a 7% cross-reactivity with the 10,11-epoxide which may cause a slight elevation in the reported carbamazepine concentrations. The clinician should be aware of conditions that can increase the formation of the 10,11-epoxide such as simultaneous administration of valproate sodium. In most patients, the ratio of carbamazepine to its major metabolite (10,11-epoxide) is relatively constant.[13] Carbamazepine has many drug interactions[14–19] resulting both from CYP3A4 inhibition[20] and CYP3A4 induction[21] which alter observed concentrations (Table 2.1). Under certain conditions, such as when felbamate[21] is added to a patient's carbamazepine regimen, the carbamazepine concentration is reduced and the 10,11-epoxide concentration is increased. This may explain the observation of central nervous system (CNS) side effects in some patients with relatively low carbamazepine concentrations.

TABLE 2.1 **Carbamazepine Drug Interactions**

Increased Plasma Carbamazepine	Decreased Plasma Carbamazepine
CYP 3A4 **inhibitors** that inhibit carbamazepine metabolism and increase plasma carbamazepine concentrations include:	CYP 3A4 **inducers** that induce the rate of carbamazepine metabolism and decrease plasma carbamazepine concentrations include:
Cimetidine	Carbamazepine[a]
Clarithromycin	Cisplatin
Diltiazem	Doxorubicin
Erythromycin	Felbamate
Fluoxetine	Phenobarbital
Isoniazid	Phenytoin
Itraconazole	Primidone
Loratadine	Rifampin
"Macrolides"	Theophylline
Niacinamide	
Propoxyphene	
Valproate	
Verapamil	

[a]Autoinduction.

Carbamazepine is associated with numerous adverse drug reactions. The most common adverse effects associated with carbamazepine involve the CNS: nystagmus, ataxia, blurred vision, and drowsiness[6]; however, carbamazepine is also associated with skin rashes, syndrome of inappropriate antidiuretic hormone (SIADH),[22] hyponatremia, and blood dyscrasias.[23] Carbamazepine is teratogenic[24,25] and has been associated with both hepatotoxicity[26] and interstitial nephritis.[27] There are a number of dermatologic and hematologic side effects that are not dose related, the most serious of which are rare but potentially fatal: aplastic anemia[23] and Stevens-Johnson syndrome.[22,28,29] A mild leukopenia occurs in approximately 10% of patients. The reaction is usually mild and transient, although a few cases of persistent neutropenia have been reported. Some clinicians recommend obtaining a baseline complete blood count (CBC) and liver function tests because carbamazepine is associated with blood dyscrasias and is highly metabolized.

BIOAVAILABILITY (F)

Carbamazepine is a lipid-soluble compound that is slowly and variably absorbed from the gastrointestinal tract. Peak plasma concentrations following immediate-release products occur approximately 6 hours (range: 2

to 24 hours) after oral ingestion.[5,6] Grapefruit juice[30] increases the bioavailability of carbamazepine by inhibiting CYP3A4. A high-fat meal diet[31] has been shown to increase the rate of absorption and elevate the peak concentration while not changing the extent as measured by the area under the curve (AUC). Although the bioavailability of carbamazepine has not been directly determined, it is estimated to be greater than 75%.[5,6] Because carbamazepine is slowly absorbed, changes in gastrointestinal function, especially those associated with rapid transit, could decrease its bioavailability and result in variable plasma concentrations of carbamazepine. For clinical purposes, the author assumes the bioavailability factor (F) to be approximately 0.8 for carbamazepine when administered as the oral tablet, chewable tablet, or suspension. The controlled release product (Tegretol-XR) is well absorbed, with bioavailability reported to be 89% of the suspension. Therefore, if the suspension is assumed to have a bioavailability of 80%, Tegretol-XR would have a corresponding oral bioavailability of approximately 70% (i.e., $0.71 = 0.89 \times 80$). The effects of gender and race on carbamazepine pharmacokinetics have not been systematically studied.

VOLUME OF DISTRIBUTION (V)

On average, the volume of distribution for carbamazepine is approximately 1.4 L/kg. Although there is a wide range of reported values (0.8 to 1.9 L/kg), this variability is probably due to alterations in plasma binding and calculation of the volume of distribution from oral administration data.[5,6] Carbamazepine, a neutral compound, is primarily bound to albumin[9] and α_1-acid glycoprotein[32] and has a free fraction (alpha) of approximately 0.2 to 0.3.[9] In uremic patients, significant increases in free carbamazepine concentrations are seen.[33,34] Although carbamazepine has significant binding to plasma proteins, there are very few clinical studies exploring alterations in plasma binding characteristics. This may be because carbamazepine is bound to multiple plasma proteins and with a free fraction of 0.2 to 0.3, fairly large changes in plasma binding to multiple plasma proteins would be required for the change in binding to become clinically significant.

CLEARANCE (Cl)

Carbamazepine is eliminated almost exclusively by the metabolic route, with less than 2% of an oral dose being excreted unchanged in the urine. Clearance values are difficult to estimate because bioavailability is uncertain. Nevertheless, the average clearance value appears to be approximately 0.064 L/kg/hr in adult patients who have received the drug chronically[35,36] and higher in children,[8] or about 0.11 L/kg/hr. In patients who are taking other enzyme-inducing antiepileptic drugs concurrently, the clearance is increased to approximately 0.1 L/kg/hr.[15,37] Single-dose studies suggest a clearance value that is one-half to one-third of the value observed in patients receiving chronic therapy.[38] The increase in clearance associated with chronic therapy is apparently due to autoinduction[39] of its metabolic enzymes. Therefore, the use of clearance values from single-dose studies is impractical in the calculation of a maintenance dose and may lead to errors.

The autoinduction[40,41] of carbamazepine metabolism has many clinical implications.[13,40] It is important to initiate patients with relatively low doses to avoid side effects early in therapy. The maintenance dose can be increased at 1-week to 2-week intervals. The autoinduction phenomenon also limits pharmacokinetic manipulation of carbamazepine dosing. For example, it is uncertain whether induction is an all-or-none or graded process that is dose related. Whereas most clinicians assume that induction is complete within 5 to 7 days, it is possible that the majority of induction occurs over the first 1 to 3 days. Finally, autoinduction of metabolism commonly causes changes in steady-state carbamazepine levels which are less than proportional to an increase in the maintenance dose.[40,41]

As with many of the anticonvulsant agents, carbamazepine has been associated with cross-induction (i.e., enhanced metabolism) of other anticonvulsants.[14,16,17,19] For this reason, whenever carbamazepine is added to an anticonvulsant regimen or other agents are added to a carbamazepine regimen, additional plasma level monitoring may be appropriate to ensure that the maintenance regimen continues to result in plasma levels that are optimal for therapeutic control.[42–44]

HALF-LIFE (t½)

Although single-dose studies predict a carbamazepine half-life of approximately 30 to 35 hours, steady-state data suggest a half-life of approximately 15 hours in adult patients receiving carbamazepine monotherapy, and approximately 10 hours in patients receiving other enzyme-inducing antiepileptic drugs (e.g., phenytoin, phenobarbital) concurrently. Children metabolize carbamazepine more rapidly than adults with reported steady-state half-lives of 4 to 12 hours.[8,13] Due to the autoinduction of carbamazepine, pharmacokinetic data derived from single-dose studies should not be used to calculate maintenance regimens.[38,45] Time to steady state is highly variable, with reports of 4 to 30 days even though the usual half-life would suggest achievement of steady-state within 1 week. Although not documented, part of this variability in time to steady state may be an interindividual inconsistency in the onset and extent of autoinduction.

TIME TO SAMPLE

Obtaining carbamazepine plasma samples within the first few weeks of therapy may be useful to establish a relationship between carbamazepine concentration and a patient's clinical response. However, these data should be interpreted cautiously if one is attempting to predict the long-term relationship between a carbamazepine dosing regimen and plasma levels. Once steady state has been achieved, the time of sampling within a dosing interval is somewhat arbitrary given the long half-life and relatively short dosing interval for carbamazepine. It is important to establish a fixed relationship between drug intake and blood sampling. The most sensible time to take routine samples is in the early morning before the first dose of medication is administered, or later in the day before the next dose. Such samples will reflect the trough concentration and are comparable from day to day. In addition, the clinician can monitor plasma drug levels without concern for artifactual errors, including the influence of diet and food intake on absorption of the drug from the gastrointestinal tract. Nevertheless, it is reasonable to obtain carbamazepine plasma samples at a consistent time within the dosing interval. As a general rule, samples should be obtained just before a dose (trough) unless this is significantly inconvenient for the patient. Inconvenience is most likely to be encountered in ambulatory patients who may be taking the drug on a schedule that is not consistent with their clinic appointments.

There are a number of reviews that provide additional information on the role of carbamazepine in the treatment of patients with seizure disorders.[15,46–53]

OXCARBAZEPINE (TRILEPTAL)

Carbamazepine has a number of limitations including autoinduction, many drug interactions, toxicities, and teratogenicity. Oxcarbazepine (Trileptal)[54–56] is chemically similar to carbamazepine and is reported to have an improved safety profile.[47] It is in pregnancy category C. Oxcarbazepine biotransformation does not involve epoxide metabolite formation. Although oxcarbazepine is an alternative, it is not commonly used in place of carbamazepine in most clinical settings.

Question #1. *N.S., a 36-year-old, 60-kg woman, is to be given carbamazepine as an anticonvulsant agent. Calculate a daily dose that will produce an average steady-state plasma concentration of approximately 6 mg/L.*

To calculate an average steady-state plasma concentration, the maintenance dose equation is used with an assumed bioavailability of 0.8 and an average clearance value of 3.84 L/hr (0.064 L/kg/hr × 60 kg). The fraction of the administered dose that is active drug (S) is 1.0.

$$\text{Maintenance Dose} = \frac{(Cl)(Css\ ave)(\tau)}{(S)(F)} \qquad \text{[Eq. 2.1]}$$

$$= \frac{(3.84 \text{ L/hr})(6 \text{ mg/L})(24 \text{ hr/1 day})}{(1)(0.8)}$$

$$= 691.2 \text{ mg/day}$$

This dose (approximately 700 mg/day) is that which would be required to achieve the steady-state level of 6 mg/L after autoinduction of carbamazepine metabolism had taken place. For this reason, N.S. should be started on a lower daily dose initially and increased at 1-week to 2-week intervals based on her clinical response. The usual initial daily dose for adult patients is 200 to 400 mg, with increases of approximately 200 mg every 7 to 14 days.

Question #2. *After 2 months, N.S.'s carbamazepine dose had been increased to 300 mg twice a day. With this regimen, she had some reduction in seizure frequency; however, seizure control was still considered unsatisfactory. The steady-state carbamazepine level at this time was reported to be 4 mg/L. What are possible explanations for this observed plasma level? What dose would be required to achieve a new steady-state carbamazepine level of 6 mg/L?*

Using the steady-state continuous infusion equation and a clearance of 3.84 L/hr, the anticipated carbamazepine level in N.S. for a dose of 600 mg/day would be approximately 5 mg/L. One should also consider whether to use literature values or patient observations when one has patient data that allow the calculation of clearance for the patient. Using the literature information:

$$\text{Css ave} = \frac{(S)(F)(\text{Dose}/\tau)}{Cl} \qquad \text{[Eq. 2.2]}$$

$$= \frac{(1)(0.8)(300 \text{ mg/12 hr})}{3.84 \text{ L/hr}}$$

$$= 5.2 \text{ mg/L}$$

The observed level of 4.0 mg/L is within the predicted range, considering the fact that both bioavailability and clearance values derived from average literature values may not be correct for N.S. At this point, it would be difficult to establish whether a slightly lower-than-expected bioavailability or a higher-than-average clearance was responsible for the observed level of 4.0 mg/L. As always, nonadherence to the prescribed dosing regimen should also be considered.

Because of carbamazepine's relatively slow absorption characteristics and long half-life, it is probable that the measured concentration of 4 mg/L represents an average steady-state value. At steady state, the average plasma concentration should be proportional to the daily dose. Therefore, to increase the plasma concentration from 4 to 6 mg/L, one would simply increase the carbamazepine dose by 50% (i.e., from 600 to 900 mg/day).

$$\text{New Maintenance Dose} = \left(\frac{\text{Css ave New}}{\text{Css ave Old}} \right) \text{Old Maintenance Dose} \qquad \text{[Eq. 2.3]}$$

$$= \left(\frac{6 \text{ mg/L}}{4 \text{ mg/L}} \right) 600 \text{ mg/day}$$

$$= 900 \text{ mg/day}$$

Another approach might be to calculate the apparent carbamazepine clearance for patient N.S. using a rearrangement of the maintenance dose Equation 2.1, the current maintenance dose of 300 mg/12 hr, and an assumed bioavailability of 0.8. In this case, patient observations are used rather that literature clearance:

$$\text{Cl} = \frac{\text{(S)(F)(Dose/}\tau\text{)}}{\text{Css ave}} \qquad \text{[Eq. 2.4]}$$

$$= \frac{(1)(0.8)(300 \text{ mg/12 hr})}{4 \text{ mg/L}}$$

$$= 5 \text{ L/hr}$$

This clearance value could then be used in the maintenance dose equation to calculate the maintenance dose as illustrated below. However, this time the clearance value that has been derived from the patient's specific data is used rather than an average value from the literature:

$$\text{Maintenance Dose} = \frac{\text{(Cl)(Css ave)(}\tau\text{)}}{\text{(S)(F)}}$$

$$= \frac{(5 \text{ L/hr})(6 \text{ mg/L})(24 \text{ hr/1 day})}{(1)(0.8)}$$

$$= 900 \text{ mg/day}$$

If N.S. were receiving other anticonvulsant agents, it would be appropriate to monitor their concentrations as well, because carbamazepine could induce their metabolism, thereby reducing their steady-state concentrations.

REFERENCES

1. Sindrup SH, Jensen TS. Pharmacotherapy of trigeminal neuralgia. Clin J Pain 2002; 18:22–27.
2. Goldberg JF. Treatment guidelines: current and future management of bipolar disorder. J Clin Psychiatr 2000;61(Suppl 13):12–18.
3. Griswold KS, Pessar LF. Management of bipolar disorder. Am Fam Physician 2000;62: 1343–1353.
4. Rozen TD. Antiepileptic drugs in the management of cluster headache and trigeminal neuralgia. Headache 2001;41:(suppl 1):S25–S32.
5. Bertilsson L. Clinical pharmacokinetics of carbamazepine. Clin Pharmacokinet 1978;3: 128–143.
6. Bertilsson L, Tomson T. Clinical pharmacokinetics and pharmacological effects of carbamazepine and carbamazepine-epoxide: an update. Clin Pharmacokinet 1986;11: 177–198
7. Iribarnegaray MFD, et al. Carbamazepine population pharmacokinetics in children: mixed-effect models. Ther Drug Monitor 1997;19:132–139.
8. Gray AL, Botha JH, Miller R. A model for the determination of carbamazepine clearance in children on mono- and polytherapy. Eur J Clin Pharmacol 1998;54:359–362.
9. Hooper WD, et al. Plasma protein binding of carbamazepine. Clin Pharmacol Ther 1975;17:433–440.
10. Mitchell PB. Therapeutic drug monitoring of psychotropic medications. Br J Clin Pharmacol 2001;52:45S–54S.
11. Bialer M, Levy RH, Perucca E. Does carbamazepine have a narrow therapeutic plasma concentration range? Ther Drug Monitor 1998;20:56–59.
12. Hoppener RJ, et al. Correlation between the daily fluctuations of carbamazepine serum levels and intermittent side effects. Epilepsia 1980;21:341–350.
13. Lanchote VL, et al. Factors influencing plasma concentrations of carbamazepine and carbamazepine-10,11-epoxide in epileptic children and adults. Ther Drug Monit 1995; 17:47–52.
14. Levy RH. Cytochrome P450 isozymes and antiepileptic drug interactions. Epilepsia 1995;36:(Suppl 5):S8–S13.
15. Levy RH, Kerr BN. Clinical pharmacokinetics of carbamazepine. J Clin Psychiatr 1988;49:(Suppl):58–62.
16. Patsalos PN, Duncan JS. Antiepileptic drugs: a review of clinically significant drug interactions. Drug Safety 1993;9:156–184.
17. Patsalos PN, Froscher W, Pisani F, van Rijn CM. The importance of drug interactions in epilepsy therapy. Epilepsia 2002;43:365–385.
18. Riva R, et al. Pharmacokinetic interactions between antiepileptic drugs. Clin Pharmacokinet 1996;31:470–493.
19. Spina E, Pisani F, Perucca E. Clinically significant pharmacokinetics drug interactions with carbamazepine: an update. Clin Pharmacokinet 1996;31:198–214.
20. Albani F, Riva R, Baruzzi A. Clarithromycin-carbamazepine interaction: a case report. Epilepsia 1993;34:161–162.
21. Albani F, Theodore WH, Washington P, et al. Effect of felbamate on plasma levels of carbamazepine and its metabolites. Epilepsia 1991;32:130–132.
22. Harden CL. Therapeutics safety monitoring: what to look for and when to look for it. Epilepsia 2000;41:(Suppl 8):S37–S44.
23. Blackburn SCF, Oliart AD, Rodriguez LAG, Gutthann SP. Antiepileptics and blood dyscrasias: a cohort study. Pharmacotherapy 1998;18:1277–1283.

24. Lewis DP, VanDyke DC, Stumbo PJ, Berg MJ. Drug and environmental factors associated with adverse pregnancy outcomes. Part I: Antiepileptic drugs, contraceptives, smoking and folate. Ann Pharmacother 1998;32:802–817.

25. Arpino C, et al. Teratogenic effects of antiepileptic drugs: use of an international database on malformations and drug exposure (MADRE). Epilepsia 2000; 41:1436–1443.

26. Morales-Diaz M, Pinilla-Roa E, Ruiz I. Suspected carbamazepine-induced hepatotoxicity. Pharmacotherapy 1999:19;252–255.

27. Mayan, Golubev N, Dinour D, Farfel Z. Lithium intoxication due to carbamazepine-induced renal failure. Ann Pharmacother 2001;35:560–562.

28. Rzany B, et al. Risk of Stevens-Johnson syndrome and toxic epidermal necrolysis during the first weeks of antiepileptic therapy: a case-controlled study. Lancet 1999;353:2190–2194.

29. Hebert AA, Ralston JP. Cutaneous reactions to anticonvulsant medications. J Clin Psychiatr 2001;62(Suppl 14):22–26.

30. Garg SK, Kumar N, Bhargava VK Prabhakar SK. Effect of grapefruit on carbamazepine bioavailability in patients with epilepsy. Clin Pharmacol Ther 1998;64:286–288.

31. McLean A, et al. The influence of food on the bioavailability of twice-daily controlled release carbamazepine formulation. J Clin Pharmacol 2001;41;183–186.

32. Baruzzi A, Contin M, Perucca E, Albani F, Riva R. Altered serum protein binding of carbamazepine in disease states associated with an increased alpha-1-acid glycoprotein concentration. Eur J Clin Pharmacol 1986;31:85–89.

33. Dasgupta A, Volk A.. Displacement of valproic acid and carbamazepine from protein binding in normal and uremic sera by tolmetin, ibuprofen and naproxen. Ther Drug Monit 1996;18:284–287.

34. Dasgupta A, Thompson WC. Carbamazepine-salicylate interaction in normal and uremic sera. Ther Drug Monit 1995:17;199–202.

35. Reith DM, Hooper WD, Parker J, Charles B. Population pharmacokinetic modeling of steady state carbamazepine clearance in children, adolescents, and adults. J Pharmacokinet Pharmacodyn 2001;28:79–92.

36. Graves NM, et al. Population pharmacokinetics of carbamazepine in adults with epilepsy. Pharmacotherapy 1998;19:273–281.

37. Eichelbaum M, Tomson T, Tybring G, Bertilsson L. Carbamazepine metabolism in man: induction and pharmacogenetic aspects. Clin Pharmacokinet 1985;10:80–90.

38. Arroyo S, Sander JWA. Carbamazepine in comparative trials: pharmacokinetic characteristics too often forgotten. Neurology 1999;53:1170–1174.

39. Kudriakova TB, et al. Autoinduction and steady-state pharmacokinetics of carbamazepine and its major metabolites. Br J Clin Pharmacol 1992;33:611–615.

40. Bernus I, et al. Early stage auto-induction of carbamazepine metabolism in humans. Eur J Clin Pharmacol 1994;47:355–360.

41. Bernus I, et al. Dose-dependent metabolism of carbamazepine in humans. Epilepsy Res 1996;24:163–172.

42. Cloyd JC, Remmel RP. Antiepileptic drug pharmacokinetics and interactions: impact on treatment of epilepsy. Pharmacotherapy 2000;20:(8 Pt 2):139S–151S.

43. Schoenenberger KA, Tanasjevic MJ, Jha A, Bates DW. Appropriateness of antiepileptic drug level monitoring. JAMA 1995;274:1622–1626.

44. Burstein AH, et al. Lack of effect of St. John's Wort on carbamazepine pharmacokinetics in healthy volunteers. Clin Pharmacol Ther 2000;68:605–612.

45. Westenberg HGM, et al. Kinetics of carbamazepine and carbamazepine-epoxide determined by use of plasma and saliva. Clin Pharmacol Ther 1978;23:320–328.

46. Bourgeois BFD. Important pharmacokinetics properties of antiepileptic frugs. Epilepsia 1995;36:(Suppl 5):S1–S7.

47. Bourgeois BFD. Pharmacokinetic properties of current antiepileptic drugs. What improvements are needed? Neurology 2000;55(11Suppl 3):S11–S16.

48. Browne TR. Pharmacokinetics of antiepileptic drugs. Neurology 1998;51 (5suppl4):S2–S7.

49. Browne TR, Holmes GL. Epilepsy (review). N Engl J Med 2001;344:1145–1151.

50. Eadie MJ. Therapeutic drug monitoring—antiepileptic drugs. Br J Clin Pharmacol 2001;52(1suppl1):1S–20S.

51. Eadie MJ. Plasma antiepileptic drug monitoring in a neurological practice: A 25-year experience. Ther Drug Monit 1994;16:458–468.

52. Faught E. Pharmacokinetic considerations in prescribing antiepileptic drugs. Epilepsia 2001;42(Suppl 4):19–23.

53. Mattson RH, Cramer JA, Collins JF. A comparison of valproate with carbamazepine for the treatment of complex partial deizures and secondarily generalized tonic-clonic seizures in adults. N Engl J Med 1992;327:765–771.

54. Tecoma ES. Oxcarbazepine. Epilepsia 1999;40(Suppl 5):S37–S46.

55. Glauser TA. Oxcarbazepine in the treatment of epilepsy. Pharmacotherapy 2001;21;904–919.

56. Baruzzi A, Albani F, Riva R. Oxcarbazepine: pharmacokinetic interactions and their clinical relevance. Epilepsia 1994;35(Suppl 3):S14–S19.

3

DIGOXIN

Michael E. Winter

Digoxin is an inotropic agent primarily used to treat congestive heart failure (CHF) and atrial fibrillation. It is incompletely absorbed and once absorbed, a substantial fraction is cleared by the kidneys. In the acute care setting, digoxin loading doses of $\approx$1 mg/70 kg (0.01 to 0.02 mg/kg) can be administered before the initiation of the usual maintenance dose of 0.125 to 0.25 mg/day. Because it has a relatively long elimination half-life in adults, digoxin is given once daily. Dosage adjustments can be important for patients who are being converted from parenteral to oral therapy or vice versa; patients with renal impairment, CHF, or thyroid abnormalities; or patients who take amiodarone concurrently.

THERAPEUTIC PLASMA CONCENTRATIONS

Although there is considerable variation between patients, plasma digoxin concentrations of $\approx$1 to 2 μg/L (ng/mL) are generally considered to be within the therapeutic range.[1,2] In recent years a therapeutic range of 0.5 to 1 μg/L for patients with CHF has been recognized by many clinicians. This lower target range is based on the fact that most patients with left ventricular dysfunction do not demonstrate additional therapeutic benefits from higher digoxin concentrations.[3-5] The use of pharmacokinetics to adjust the dosing regimen can reduce the incidence of digoxin toxicity.[2,6-8]

BIOAVAILABILITY (F)

The bioavailability of digoxin tablets ranges from 0.5 to greater than 0.9. Many clinicians use a bioavailability of 0.7 to 0.8. A bioavailability of 0.7 will be used in this text as an estimate of the average bioavailability figures reported in the literature.[9,10] The elixir appears to have a bioavailability of approximately 0.8, and soft gelatin capsules of digoxin appear to be completely absorbed.[11,12] The intravenous route of administration is also assumed to have 100% bioavailability.

St. John's wort has been reported to reduce the bioavailability of digoxin by approximately 25%. It has been postulated that the interaction is with p-glycoprotein; however, other mechanisms (such as an induction of hepatic metabolism) have also been proposed.[13-16] Similarly, various antibiotics have also been reported to alter the bioavailability of digoxin. In

KEY PARAMETERS: Digoxin

Therapeutic Range[a]	0.8–2 µg/L
F	
Tablets	0.7
Elixir	0.8
Soft gelatin capsule	1
S	1
V[b] (L)	(3.8)(Weight in kg) + (3.1)(Cl_{Cr} in mL/min)
Cl[b] (mL/min)	
Non-CHF patients	(0.8 mL/kg/min)(Weight in kg) + (Cl_{Cr} in mL/min)
Patients with CHF	(0.33 mL/kg/min)(Weight in kg) + (0.9)(Cl_{Cr} in mL/min)
$t\frac{1}{2}$[c]	2 days

[a]The therapeutic range in patients with CHF may be 0.5 to 1 µg/L; in some patients with atrial fibrillation, concentrations greater than 2 µg/L may be required to control ventricular rate adequately.
[b]See Table 3.1 for factors that alter V and Cl for digoxin.
[c]The t½ is longer in patients with renal failure and in patients receiving amiodarone.

most cases the antibiotics appear to increase the bioavailability, supposedly by suppressing bacteria in the gastrointestinal tract that metabolize digoxin. Other mechanisms such as metabolism or renal excretion may also play a role in how some of the antibiotics increase the plasma concentrations of digoxin. The most common class of antibiotics that have been reported to increase digoxin concentrations are macrolides, but others such as itraconazole are not a surprise.[17–21] Coadministration of cholestyramine has been reported to decrease the bioavailability of digoxin, and both cholestyramine and charcoal have been suggested as a treatment modality in patients who are digitalis toxic.[22,23]

VOLUME OF DISTRIBUTION (V)

The average volume of distribution for digoxin is ≈7.3 L/kg.[24] This V is decreased in patients with renal disease (see Question 4).

$$V_{Digoxin} \text{ (L/70 kg)} = 226 + \frac{(298)(Cl_{cr} \text{ in mL/min})}{29 + Cl_{cr} \text{ in mL/min}} \quad \text{[Eq. 3.1]}$$

$$V_{Digoxin} \text{ (L)} = (3.8 \text{ L/kg})(\text{Weight in kg}) + (3.1)(Cl_{cr} \text{ in mL/min}) \quad \text{[Eq. 3.2]}$$

In the above equations, the factors have been selected so that when creatinine clearance is in mL/min (Equations 3.1 and 3.2) and weight is in kilograms (Equation 3.2), the calculated volume of distribution units are L/70 kg (Equation 3.1) and L (Equation 3.2).

Digoxin V is also decreased in hypothyroid patients (see Question 12) and in patients who are taking quinidine (see Question 15). The volume of distribution is increased in hyperthyroid patients (see Question 12). In addition, the volume of distribution for digoxin in obese subjects appears to be more closely related to the non-obese or ideal body weight (IBW) than total body weight (TBW)[25] (Table 3.1).

TABLE 3.1 Factors That Alter Digoxin Volume of Distribution and Clearance

Factor[a]	
Volume of Distribution	
Creatinine clearance	See Equations 3.1 and 3.2
Obesity	IBW[b]
Quinidine	0.7
Thyroid	
Clinically hypothyroid	0.7
Clinically hyperthyroid	1.3
Clearance	
Creatinine clearance	See Equations 3.4 and 3.5
Congestive heart failure	See Equation 3.5
Obesity	IBW[b]
Amiodarone	0.5
Quinidine	0.5
Verapamil	0.75
Thyroid function	
Clinically hypothyroid	0.7
Clinically hyperthyroid	1.3

[a]Factor should be multiplied by calculated volume of distribution or clearance value. Multiple factors would increase the uncertainty of any volume or clearance prediction. Although not tested, one might anticipate the factors to be multiplicative.
[b]IBW = ideal body weight or "non-obese weight."

The manner in which digoxin is distributed in the body must be considered in the interpretation of plasma levels. The distribution of digoxin follows a two-compartment model (see Part I: Volume of Distribution: Two-Compartment Models). Digoxin first distributes into a small initial volume of distribution, Vi, consisting of plasma and other rapidly equilibrating tissues, and then distributes into a larger and more slowly equilibrating tissue compartment. The myocardium responds pharmacologically as though it were located in the larger more slowly equilibrating tissue compartment (Vt). Since plasma samples are obtained from Vi, plasma digoxin levels do not accurately reflect the drug's pharmacologic effects until the digoxin is completely distributed into both compartments. Serum concentrations of digoxin obtained before complete distribution are often misleading. Because the initial volume of distribution (Vi) of digoxin is relatively small ($\approx$1/10 Vt), high plasma concentrations are commonly reported immediately after a dose is administered. Because the heart behaves as though it were in the second or tissue compartment, the initial high serum concentrations that occur immediately after a dose are not reflective of either therapeutic or toxic potential of digoxin. Plasma concentrations are only meaningful when obtained after equilibration is complete (i.e., at least 4 hours after an intravenous dose[26] or 6 hours after an oral dose[27]). The clinical effects of a dose, however, may be observed much sooner than 4 to 6 hours because the distribution half-life α t$\frac{1}{2}$ is only about 35 minutes.[28] After approximately two α t$\frac{1}{2}$'s (i.e., 1 hour) the myocardium experiences the effects of 75% of an intravenous dose. However, a plasma sample taken at this time would be misleadingly high because the remaining 25% of the dose which is not yet distributed out of Vi would produce a plasma concentration that is high relative to that which would be observed once equilibrium between the two compartments is complete (Fig. 3.1).

CLEARANCE (Cl)

Digoxin clearance varies considerably among individuals and should be estimated for each patient. Total digoxin clearance (Cl$_t$) is the sum of its metabolic (Cl$_m$) and renal (Cl$_r$) clearances as illustrated by Equation 3.3:

$$Cl_t = Cl_m + Cl_r \qquad \text{[Eq. 3.3]}$$

In healthy individuals the metabolic clearance of digoxin is $\approx$0.57 to 0.86 mL/kg/min, and the renal clearance is about equal to or a little less than creatinine clearance. CHF reduces the metabolic clearance of digoxin to about one-half its usual value and may reduce the renal clearance slightly as well[10,29–31] [also see Part I: Clearance (Cl)].

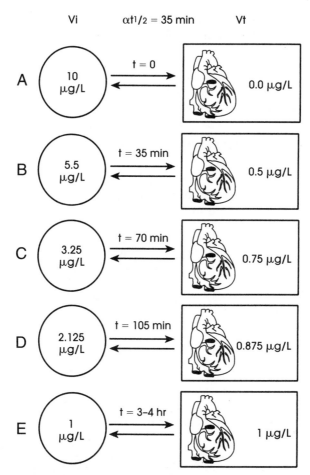

Vi $\alpha t^1/_2 = 35$ min   Vt

A — 10 µg/L — t = 0 → ← — 0.0 µg/L

B — 5.5 µg/L — t = 35 min → ← — 0.5 µg/L

C — 3.25 µg/L — t = 70 min → ← — 0.75 µg/L

D — 2.125 µg/L — t = 105 min → ← — 0.875 µg/L

E — 1 µg/L — t = 3–4 hr → ← — 1 µg/L

FIGURE 3.1. A theoretical two-compartment model for digoxin. The myocardium or target organ behaves as though it were in Vt and therefore responds to the theoretical digoxin concentration in Vt. Following complete distribution, the concentrations in Vi and Vt are assumed to be equal and the pharmacologic effect maximal. Note that the initial volume of distribution (Vi) is much smaller than the tissue volume of distribution (Vt); therefore, the digoxin concentrations are very high following an initial IV dose. Figure 3.1.A depicts digoxin concentration immediately following an IV bolus. All of the drug is in Vi and the plasma concentration is 10 µg/L, but no digoxin is in the tissue compartment Vt; therefore, no effect is present. Figure 3.1 E depicts complete digoxin distribution. Note that the two compartments are in equilibrium and that the digoxin concentration in both Vi and Vt is assumed to be equal (i.e., 1 µg/L). At this point, the plasma level accurately reflects the concentration in the tissue compartment and the potential for drug effect. Figures 3.1 B, 3.1.C, and 3.1 D depict the relative digoxin concentrations in Vi and Vt after one, two, and three distribution half-lives (α $t^1/_2$'s). After three α $t^1/_2$'s, 87.5% of the pharmacologic effect is achieved; however, it is still much too early to obtain a digoxin level, because the concentration in Vi is more than 100% higher than the final equilibrated concentration.

Using the data from Sheiner et al.,[29] the total digoxin clearance in mL/kg/min can be calculated in patients with and without CHF as follows:

$$\frac{\text{Total Cl}_{\text{Digoxin}} \text{ (mL/min)}}{\text{(Patients without CHF)}} = (0.8 \text{ mL/kg/min})(\text{Weight in kg}) + \text{Cl}_{\text{cr}} \text{ in mL/min} \qquad [\text{Eq. 3.4}]$$

$$\frac{\text{Total Cl}_{\text{Digoxin}} \text{ (mL/min)}}{\text{(Patients with CHF)}} = (0.33 \text{ mL/kg/min})(\text{Weight in kg}) + (0.9)(\text{Cl}_{\text{cr}} \text{ in mL/min}) \qquad [\text{Eq. 3.5}]$$

Creatinine clearance can be estimated from the patient's serum creatinine using Equations 3.6 and 3.7 below:

$$\frac{\text{Cl}_{\text{cr}} \text{ for males}}{\text{(mL/min)}} = \frac{(140 - \text{Age})(\text{Weight in kg})}{(72)(\text{SCr}_{\text{ss}})} \qquad [\text{Eq. 3.6}]$$

$$\frac{\text{Cl}_{\text{cr}} \text{ for females}}{\text{(mL/min)}} = (0.85)\frac{(140 - \text{Age})(\text{Weight in kg})}{(72)(\text{SCr}_{\text{ss}})} \qquad [\text{Eq. 3.7}]$$

Note that in the above equations the units do not cancel and the values of 140 in the numerator and 72 in the denominator result in a creatinine clearance that has a unit value of mL/min. Also, in obese subjects, creatinine clearance is normally calculated using ideal body weight (IBW). The most common method of estimating IBW is as follows:

Ideal body weight for males in kg = 50 + (2.3)(Height in Inches > 60)   [Eq. 3.8]

Ideal body weight for females in kg = 45 + (2.3)(Height in Inches > 60)   [Eq. 3.9]

Similarly, IBW should also be used to estimate digoxin clearance (renal and metabolic) in obese patients. These and other methods for estimating digoxin clearance are illustrated in the questions later in this chapter. See Table 3.1 for common factors that alter digoxin clearance.

HALF-LIFE (t½)

The half-life for digoxin is approximately 2 days in patients with normal renal function. In anephric patients, the half-life increases to approximately 4 to 6 days. This increase in the digoxin half-life is less than might be expected based on the reduction in clearance because the volume of distribution is also decreased in patients with diminished renal function (see Question 4 and Equations 3.1, 3.2, and 3.17).

TIME TO SAMPLE

Plasma samples for routine digoxin level monitoring are ideally obtained 7 to 14 days after a maintenance regimen is initiated or changed. This delay in obtaining digoxin samples helps to ensure that steady state has been attained on the current dosing regimen. Samples may be obtained before steady state is achieved, but caution should be used in assessing the relationship between the current dosing regimen and the eventual steady-state concentration. In addition, in patients with end-stage renal disease it may take 15 to 20 days to achieve steady state because of the prolonged half-life.

Plasma samples obtained within 24 hours of an initial loading dose may help confirm the relationship between the digoxin plasma concentration and pharmacologic response or establish the apparent volume of distribution. When plasma samples are obtained this early, however, they are of little value in evaluating the maintenance regimen.

Once steady state has been achieved, routine plasma samples for digoxin monitoring should be drawn just before the next dose (trough levels); however, any sampling time that avoids the distribution phase (at least 4 hours following an intravenous dose or 6 hours following an oral dose) is acceptable.

Patients taking digoxin who are to be given amiodarone are likely to require digoxin plasma level monitoring to determine the extent to which the digoxin pharmacokinetics are altered[32-34] (see Question 14). If quinidine is being used as the antiarrhythmic, there is the possibility that digoxin concentrations will fluctuate within a quinidine dosing interval. Consequently, in patients taking quinidine and digoxin, samples should be obtained at a time that corresponds to the trough of the quinidine dosing interval and that also avoids the distribution phase for digoxin.

The time course for the expected change in digoxin concentrations will depend on whether the drug interaction alters digoxin volume of distribution or clearance or both. In addition, the time required for the interacting drug to accumulate and effect a change in the digoxin's pharmacokinetic parameter(s) should also be considered. When drugs are added to a patient's therapy that can alter the disposition of digoxin, the nature of the drug interaction and expected change in half-life should provide some clues as to the time course and extent of the expected change in the digoxin concentration.

Question #1. *Estimate a digoxin loading dose that will produce a plasma concentration of 1 μg/L for a 70-kg patient being treated for CHF.*

Estimating a loading dose requires knowledge of the volume of distribution of the drug. In this case, the average literature value for the V of digoxin (7.3 L/kg) will be used. If one knew the renal function, a volume of distribution based on renal function would be calculated instead (see

Question 4 and Equations 3.1 and 3.2).[24] Using Equation 3.10, the loading dose can be calculated as follows:

$$\text{Loading Dose} = \frac{(V)(C)}{(S)(F)} \qquad [\text{Eq. 3.10}]$$

$$= \frac{(7.3 \text{ L/kg})(70 \text{ kg})(1 \text{ } \mu g/L)}{(1)(0.7)}$$

$$= \frac{(511 \text{ L})(1 \text{ } \mu g/L)}{0.7}$$

$$= \frac{511 \text{ } \mu g}{0.7}$$

$$= 730 \text{ } \mu g \text{ or } \approx 750 \text{ } \mu g$$

In this case, it was assumed that the loading dose was to be given orally as tablets; therefore, a bioavailability (F) of 0.7 was used.[9] If the loading dose was to have been given intravenously, F would have been 1 and the calculated loading dose would have been 511 μg (≈500 μg). In both cases, S is 1 because digoxin is not administered as a salt.

Loading doses of digoxin are not usually given to patients with CHF in the ambulatory care setting. Loading doses are used in the acute care setting. The difference may be the level of acuity, the ability to closely monitor the patient during the loading process, and perhaps the economic pressures that force clinicians to achieve therapeutic goals as quickly as possible.

Question #2. *How should this loading dose be divided, and what would be an appropriate interval between doses?*

Loading doses of digoxin are almost always administered in divided doses so that the patient can be evaluated for toxicity and efficacy in the course of receiving the total loading dose. If the patient appears to develop toxicity or is therapeutically controlled, the remainder of the calculated loading dose is withheld. The usual procedure is to give one-half of the calculated loading dose initially, followed by one-fourth in 6 hours; the remaining fourth is administered 6 hours after the second dose.

Six hours is the usual interval between doses because it is the approximate time to ensure that the oral dose of digoxin has been absorbed and distributed into the myocardium.[27] Even following an intravenous (IV) injection, 2 to 4 hours are required for a single dose of digoxin to exhibit its full effect.[26] In an emergency, when it is important to rapidly achieve pharmacologic effects, clinical decisions about efficacy/toxicity can be made 1 to 2 hours following an IV dose. This is because the majority of digoxin will have been distributed into the tissue compartment and ≈75% to 90% of the pharmacologic effect can be evaluated at this time. It would still be too soon, however, to evaluate plasma concentrations due to the distribution phase (see Fig. 3.1 and Part I: Loading Dose).

Question #3. *Assume the patient in Question 1 is R.J., a 50-year-old man with a serum creatinine of 1 mg/dL. Calculate a maintenance dose that will achieve an average plasma digoxin concentration of 1 μg/L.*

Since the objective is to achieve an average digoxin concentration of 1 μg/L at steady state (Css ave), Equation 3.11 can be used to calculate the maintenance dose:

$$\text{Maintenance Dose} = \frac{(Cl)(Css\ ave)(\tau)}{(S)(F)} \qquad \text{[Eq. 3.11]}$$

When using Equation 3.11, it is important to ensure that the units will cancel properly and are easy to use. In the case of digoxin, the concentrations are usually reported as μg/L, and therefore, the digoxin dose should be expressed as μg. Given that the dosing interval (τ) is usually expressed in days, the clearance should be expressed as L/day. If the dosing interval is thought of as hours (e.g., 24 hours), then clearance would be in the units of L/hr. Therefore, assuming the dosing interval (τ) to be 1 day, the bioavailability (F) 0.7 for oral tablets, and the fraction of the dose that is digoxin (S) to be 1, the digoxin clearance (Cl) is the only remaining parameter to be calculated.

The digoxin clearance for R.J. can be determined by use of Equation 3.5:

$$\begin{array}{l}\text{Total } Cl_{\text{Digoxin}}\text{ (mL/min)} \\ \text{(Patients with CHF)}\end{array} = (0.33\text{ mL/kg/min})(\text{Weight in kg}) + (0.9)(Cl_{cr}\text{ in mL/min})$$

Although the creatinine clearance (Cl_{cr}) for R.J. is unknown, it can be estimated easily from his serum creatinine by use of Equation 3.6, assuming all the criteria for the use of this formula are met (i.e., serum creatinine is at steady state, and R.J.'s muscle mass is average for a 50-year-old man):

$$\begin{aligned}Cl_{cr}\text{ for males} &= \frac{(140 - \text{Age})(\text{Weight in kg})}{(72)(SCr_{ss})} \\ &= \frac{(140 - 50\text{ yrs})(70\text{ kg})}{(72)(1\text{ mg/dL})} \\ &= 87.5\text{ mL/min}\end{aligned}$$

This creatinine clearance can now be used in Equation 3.5 to estimate R.J.'s total digoxin clearance:

$$\begin{aligned}
\text{Total Cl}_{\text{Digoxin}} \text{ (mL/min)} &= (0.33 \text{ mL/kg/min})(\text{Weight in kg}) + \\
\text{(Patients with CHF)} &\quad (0.9)(\text{Cl}_{\text{cr}} \text{ in mL/min}) \\
&= (0.33 \text{ mL/kg/min})(70 \text{ kg}) + \\
&\quad (0.9)(87.5 \text{ mL/min}) \\
&= 23.1 \text{ mL/min} + 78.8 \text{ mL/min} \\
&= 101.9 \text{ mL/min}
\end{aligned}$$

The digoxin clearance can be used to calculate the maintenance dose in ng/min, but a maintenance dose stated in μg/day is more practical. The clearance in mL/min can be converted to L/day by multiplying the value by the number of minutes per day (1440 min/day) and dividing by the number of milliliters per liter (1000 mL/L) as shown below:

$$\text{Cl (L/day)} = \text{(Cl as mL/min)}\left(\frac{1440 \text{ min/day}}{1000 \text{ mL/L}}\right) \qquad \text{[Eq. 3.12]}$$

$$\begin{aligned}
&= (101.9 \text{ mL/min})\left(\frac{1440 \text{ min/day}}{1000 \text{ mL/L}}\right) \\
&= 146.7 \text{ L/day}
\end{aligned}$$

The maintenance dose can now be calculated using Equation 3.11:

$$\begin{aligned}
\text{Maintenance Dose} &= \frac{(\text{Cl})(\text{Css ave})(\tau)}{(\text{S})(\text{F})} \\
&= \frac{(146.7 \text{ L/day})(1 \text{ μg/L})(1 \text{ day})}{(1)(0.7)} \\
&= \frac{146.7 \text{ μg}}{0.7} \\
&= 210 \text{ μg} \\
&= 0.210 \text{ mg}
\end{aligned}$$

One could elect to give either 0.125 or 0.25 mg/day since these are the most convenient oral dosage forms. Another solution is to give 0.125 and 0.25 mg on alternate days for an average dose of 0.1875 mg/day. Given that the 0.210 mg/day dosing rate is only an estimate, most clinicians would probably give 0.25 mg/day unless there was reason to believe that R.J is at undue risk for digitalis toxicity; if R.J. is being treated for CHF, a lower digoxin concentration might be desirable.

Question #4. *If the patient in Question 1 had a serum creatinine of 5 mg/dL, would the estimated loading dose have been different?*

For a number of years it was assumed that renal function influenced only the clearance of digoxin. A number of studies have indicated, however, that patients with decreased creatinine clearance also have a decreased volume of distribution for digoxin.[24,29,35]

The relationship between volume of distribution (V), plasma concentration (C), and amount of drug in the body is described by Equation 3.13 below:

$$V = \frac{\text{Amount of drug in the body}}{C} \qquad \text{[Eq. 3.13]}$$

In uremic patients, it is assumed that digoxin is displaced from the tissue compartment. As a result, C is higher and V is smaller.

$$\downarrow V = \frac{\text{Amount of drug in the body}}{\uparrow C}$$

There is some controversy about the significance of this tissue displacement of digoxin. Myocardial digoxin concentrations at any given plasma digoxin level are lower relative to their non-uremic counterparts.[36] Consequently, some have suggested that no change in the loading dose is necessary.[37] Almost all clinicians today assume that the higher the digoxin concentrations the greater the drug effect, both therapeutic and toxic. Therefore, they generally target digoxin concentrations, in renal failure patients, that are similar to or lower than the concentrations for patients with normal renal function. Many clinicians, however, do not recognize that the volume of distribution is likely to be reduced in patients with significant renal dysfunction and therefore do not always make the appropriate initial reduction in digoxin loading doses.

Because very little digoxin is bound to plasma proteins ($\approx 30\%$), a change in the desired therapeutic plasma concentration is unlikely to result from plasma protein displacement[38] [see Part I: Desired Plasma Concentration (C): Protein Binding].

There are a number of ways to estimate the volume of distribution for digoxin in a patient with decreased renal function; Equations 3.1:

$$V_{\text{Digoxin}} \ (\text{L/70 kg}) = 226 + \frac{(298)(Cl_{cr} \text{ in mL/min})}{29 + Cl_{cr} \text{ in mL/min}}$$

and 3.2 are the most commonly used.

$$V_{\text{Digoxin}} \ (\text{L}) = (3.8 \text{ L/kg})(\text{Weight in kg}) + (3.1)(Cl_{cr} \text{ in mL/min})$$

Equation 3.1 is adjusted for a 70 kg person and, therefore, requires that the creatinine clearance (Cl_{Cr}) be expressed as mL/min/70 kg. If the patient is smaller or larger than 70 kg, the volume of distribution can be adjusted in proportion to the patient's body size. The second equation is for a specific patient; therefore, the estimated Cl_{Cr} should be expressed in mL/min for that patient. The volume of distribution for digoxin in uremic patients can vary considerably. For this reason, the values obtained from these equations and the calculated loading dose should be considered only rough estimates.

Using Equation 3.6, the patient's creatinine clearance is determined to be approximately 20 mL/min. Note that we are assuming the patient is not receiving any type of dialysis, as dialysis invalidates Equations 3.6 and 3.7.

$$Cl_{Cr} \text{ for males} = \frac{(140 - \text{Age})(\text{Weight in kg})}{(72)(SCr_{ss})}$$

$$= \frac{(140 - 50 \text{ yrs})(70 \text{ kg})}{(72)(5 \text{ mg/dL})}$$

$$= 17.5 \text{ mL/min or} \approx 20 \text{ mL/min}$$

Using this value in Equations 3.1 and 3.2, the estimated volumes of distribution would be 347.6 L and 328 L, respectively:

$$V_{Digoxin} \text{ (L/70 kg)} = 226 + \frac{(298)(Cl_{Cr} \text{ in mL/min})}{29 + Cl_{Cr} \text{ in mL/min}}$$

$$= 226 + \frac{(298)(20 \text{ mL/min})}{29 + 20 \text{ mL/min}}$$

$$= 226 + \frac{5960}{49}$$

$$= 347.6 \text{ L}$$

Since this patient weighs 70 kg, the Cl_{Cr} calculated from Equation 3.1 can be used directly. If the patient had not been 70 kg, the Cl_{Cr} would need to be adjusted to what it would have been if the patient were 70 kg. The V then generated from Equation 3.1 would represent that expected for a 70 kg person and would have to be adjusted for the patient's actual weight. Equation 3.2 takes into account the patient's actual weight:

$$V_{Digoxin} \text{ (L)} = (3.8 \text{ L/kg})(\text{Weight in kg}) + (3.1)(Cl_{Cr} \text{ in mL/min})$$

$$= (3.8 \text{ L/kg})(70 \text{ kg}) + (3.1)(20 \text{ mL/min})$$

$$= (266 \text{ L}) + (62)$$

$$= 328 \text{ L}$$

Since both of these approaches give similar estimates, either could be used. However, it is the author's opinion that Equation 3.2 appears to be useful over a wider range of creatinine clearance values, especially in young adults with good renal function.[39]

If the volume of distribution is assumed to be approximately 330 L (as calculated from Equation 3.2), the estimated oral loading dose using Equation 3.10 would be approximately 500 µg:

$$\text{Loading Dose} = \frac{(V)(C)}{(S)(F)}$$

$$= \frac{(330 \text{ L})(1 \text{ } \mu g/L)}{(1)(0.7)}$$

$$= \frac{330 \text{ } \mu g}{0.7}$$

$$= 471 \text{ } \mu g \text{ or } \approx 500 \text{ } \mu g$$

Again, as in Question 1, S and F are assumed to be 1 and 0.7, respectively. The total loading dose should be divided and administered as described in Question 2. Again, the loading dose is divided so that the patient's response can be evaluated between each of the partial loading doses. This is to guard against the possibility that the patient's volume of distribution is smaller than anticipated or that the patient is more sensitive to the pharmacologic effects than expected. One should also consider the possibility that the volume of distribution may be much larger than expected and additional doses may have to be administered to achieve the desired plasma concentration or pharmacologic effect.

It should be pointed out that dosing to a therapeutic endpoint is common in patients with atrial fibrillation in whom the therapeutic endpoint is increased atrial-ventricular nodal blockade and a decrease in ventricular rate. Patients with CHF, however, are more difficult to evaluate, and it is much less common to increase the loading dose beyond the initial targeted amount. Of course, in either atrial fibrillation or CHF, if toxicity is observed, the process of administering the loading dose would be stopped.

Question #5. *Estimate the daily dose that would maintain the average digoxin concentration at 1 µg/L in this same 70-kg, 50-year-old patient with a serum creatinine of 5 mg/dL.*

As in Question 3, Equation 3.11 would be used to estimate the maintenance dose:

$$\text{Maintenance Dose} = \frac{(Cl)(Css \text{ ave})(\tau)}{(S)(F)}$$

Using the creatinine clearance estimate of 20 mL/min (see Question 4), the digoxin clearance can be estimated using Equation 3.5 (for CHF):

$$\text{Total Cl}_{\text{Digoxin}} \text{ (mL/min)} \atop \text{(Patients with CHF)} = \text{(0.33 mL/kg/min)(Weight in kg)} + \text{(0.9)(Cl}_{\text{cr}} \text{ in mL/min)}$$

$$= \text{(0.33 mL/kg/min)(70 kg)} + \text{(0.9)(20 mL/min)}$$

$$= 23.1 \text{ mL/min} + 18 \text{ mL/min}$$

$$= 41.1 \text{ mL/min}$$

The digoxin clearance can be converted from mL/min to L/day as described in Question 3 using Equation 3.12:

$$\text{Cl (L/day)} = \frac{\text{(Cl as mL/min)(1440 min/day)}}{1000 \text{ mL/L}}$$

$$= \frac{\text{(41.1 mL/min)(1440 min/day)}}{1000 \text{ mL/L}}$$

$$= 59.2 \text{ L/day}$$

Again, assuming S to be 1 and F to be 0.7 for digoxin tablets, the approximate daily dose (calculated using Equation 3.11) would be 85 µg/day or 0.085 mg/day:

$$\text{Maintenance Dose} = \frac{\text{(Cl)(Css ave)(}\tau\text{)}}{\text{(S)(F)}}$$

$$= \frac{\text{(59.2 L/day)(1 µg/L)(1 day)}}{\text{(1)(0.7)}}$$

$$= \frac{59.2 \text{ µg}}{0.7}$$

$$= 84.6 \text{ µg of digoxin each day}$$

Again this dose is not convenient, and most clinicians would probably administer 0.125 mg/day as digoxin comes in 0.125 mg tablets and this is a reasonably standard dose for many patients with significantly diminished renal function. Given that the 0.125 mg/day dose is almost 50% higher than our estimated dose, one could consider 0.125 mg every other day or possibly alternating between 0.0625 mg (half of a 0.125 mg tablet) and 0.125 mg every other day. This second possibility would give an average administration rate of 93.75 µg/day, which is only slightly higher than our initial estimates but is more complicated and therefore less desirable.

Question #6. *Assume that the patient described above can take nothing by mouth and must be converted to daily intravenous doses* *of digoxin. Assume he was taking one 0.125-mg tablet each day. Calculate an equivalent intravenous dose.*

If the bioavailability of digoxin is assumed to be 0.7, the equivalent intravenous dose would be 0.0875 or 0.09 mg/day as calculated from Equations 3.14 and 3.15:

$$\text{Amount of Drug Absorbed or Reaching the Systemic Circulation} = \text{(F)(Dose)} \qquad [\text{Eq. 3.14}]$$

$$= (0.7)(0.125 \text{ mg})$$

$$= 0.0875 \text{ mg}$$

$$\frac{\text{Dose of New Dosage Form}}{} = \frac{\text{Amount of Drug Absorbed From Current Dosage Form}}{\text{F of New Dosage Form}} \qquad [\text{Eq. 3.15}]$$

$$= \frac{0.0875 \text{ mg}}{1}$$

$$= 0.0875 \text{ mg or} \approx 0.09 \text{ mg}$$

If the dose is not adjusted to account for the increased bioavailability of the intravenous dose, higher steady-state digoxin concentrations would eventually be achieved [see Part I: Elimination Rate Constant (K) and Half-Life (t½) and Figure 16].

Question #7. *B.G., a 62-year-old, 50-kg woman, was admitted to the hospital for possible digoxin toxicity. Her serum creatinine was 3 mg/dL, and her dosing regimen at home had been 0.25 mg of digoxin daily for many months. The digoxin plasma concentration on admission was 4 μg/L. How long will it take for the digoxin concentration to fall from 4 to 2 μg/L?*

The answer to this question requires knowledge of the digoxin half-life (t½) or the elimination rate constant (K), both of which are dependent on the clearance and volume of distribution for digoxin in B.G. The relationship between these parameters is described by Equations 3.16 and 3.17:

$$K = \frac{Cl}{V} \qquad [\text{Eq. 3.16}]$$

$$t½ = \frac{(0.693)(V)}{Cl} \qquad [\text{Eq. 3.17}]$$

Three basic steps are required to solve this problem: 1) estimate digoxin clearance, 2) estimate the V for digoxin, and 3) calculate the half-life.

Step 1. Estimate Clearance. We can estimate digoxin clearance as illustrated in previous questions by first determining B.G.'s creatinine clearance through the use of Equation 3.7 for women:

$$\text{Cl}_{cr} \text{ for females} = (0.85)\frac{(140 - \text{Age})(\text{Weight in kg})}{(72)(\text{SCr}_{ss})}$$

$$= (0.85)\frac{(140 - 62 \text{ yrs})(50 \text{ kg})}{(72)(3 \text{ mg/dL})}$$

$$= 15.3 \text{ mL/min}$$

This estimation of Cl_{cr} then can be used to determine the digoxin clearance by use of Equation 3.5 (for CHF):

$$\begin{array}{l}\text{Total Cl}_{\text{Digoxin}} \text{ (mL/min)} \\ \text{(Patients with CHF)}\end{array} = (0.33 \text{ mL/kg/min})(\text{Weight in kg}) + (0.9)(\text{Cl}_{cr} \text{ in mL/min})$$

$$= (0.33 \text{ mL/kg/min})(50 \text{ kg}) + (0.9)(15.3 \text{ mL/min})$$

$$= 16.5 \text{ mL/min} + 13.8 \text{ mL/min}$$

$$= 30.3 \text{ mL/min}$$

Converted to L/day by Equation 3.12, the digoxin clearance would be 43.6 L/day.

$$\text{Cl (L/day)} = \frac{(\text{Cl as mL/min})(1440 \text{ min/day})}{1000 \text{ mL/L}}$$

$$= \frac{(30.3 \text{ mL/min})(1440 \text{ min/day})}{1000 \text{ mL/L}}$$

$$= 43.6 \text{ L/day}$$

A more patient-specific approach would be to use the patient's dosing history and the observed digoxin concentrations to derive a patient-specific digoxin clearance. If one assumes that the digoxin half-life is significantly longer than the dosing interval, the observed digoxin plasma concentration should closely reflect the average concentration at steady state; from this the digoxin clearance can be calculated [i.e., this level is relatively independent of the volume of distribution; see Part I: Elimination Rate Constant (K) and Half-Life ($t\frac{1}{2}$): Dosing Interval (τ)].

Therefore, the observed digoxin concentration can be used in Equation 3.18 to estimate B.G.'s clearance:

$$Cl = \frac{(S)(F)(Dose/\tau)}{Css\ ave} \qquad \text{[Eq. 3.18]}$$

$$= \frac{(1)(0.7)(250\ \mu g/day)}{4\ \mu g/L}$$

$$= \frac{175\ \mu g/day}{4\ \mu g/L}$$

$$= 43.75\ L/day$$

This lower than average digoxin clearance of 43.75 L/day calculated from B.G.'s dosing history and observed plasma level is very close to what we calculated using literature estimates for a 50-kg, 62-year-old woman with a serum creatinine of 3 mg/dL. In most cases, our estimates and the actual values are not this close. Given the usual uncertainty in predicting clearance, we would expect most of our patients to have an observed clearance that is between ½ to 2 times the predicted value. Actual clearance values outside of this range should be evaluated carefully to determine if the patient is substantially different from the assumed pharmacokinetic population. In most cases, it is more likely that we have made an error in our calculations or in our assumptions (see Question 3.9).

Step 2. Calculate B.G.'s digoxin volume of distribution. Because our only digoxin plasma concentration represents something approaching Css ave, we cannot derive a patient-specific volume and will have to rely on a literature estimate that we can calculate using Equation 3.2.

$$V_{Digoxin}\ (L) = (3.8\ L/kg)(Weight\ in\ kg) + (3.1)(Cl_{cr}\ in\ mL/min)$$

$$= (3.8\ L/kg)(50\ kg) + (3.1)(15.3\ mL/min)$$

$$= (190\ L) + (47)$$

$$= 237\ L$$

Step 3. The digoxin elimination rate constant and half-life for B.G. can now be estimated from Equations 3.16 and 3.17 using our patient-specific digoxin clearance and the literature estimate of volume of digoxin:

$$K = \frac{Cl}{V}$$

$$= \frac{43.75 \text{ L/day}}{237 \text{ L}}$$

$$= 0.184 \text{ day}^{-1}$$

$$t\tfrac{1}{2} = \frac{(0.693)(V)}{Cl}$$

$$= \frac{(0.693)(237 \text{ L})}{43.75 \text{ L/day}}$$

$$= 3.8 \text{ days}$$

We now have the data necessary to answer the original question. The time required for B.G.'s plasma concentration of digoxin to fall from 4 to 2 µg/L (one-half the original level) is one half-life, or 3.8 days.

In most situations the calculations are not this easy (i.e., one $t\tfrac{1}{2}$). When the time of decay is not obvious, the time required for the plasma concentration to fall to a predetermined level can be calculated using Equation 3.19:

$$t = \frac{\ln\left(\dfrac{C_1}{C_2}\right)}{K} \qquad \text{[Eq. 3.19]}$$

In the above equation t represents the time required for C_1, the initial higher concentration, to decay to C_2, the lower concentration, for any given elimination rate constant K. Of course the equation assumes a first-order decay process (i.e., Cl and V are constant) and that no drug is administered or absorbed between the concentrations C_1 and C_2 [see Part I: Elimination Rate Constant (K) and Half-Life ($t\tfrac{1}{2}$): Elimination Rate Constant (K)].

$$t = \frac{\ln\left(\dfrac{C_1}{C_2}\right)}{K}$$

$$t = \frac{\ln\left(\dfrac{4\ \mu g/L}{2\ \mu g/L}\right)}{0.184\ \text{days}^{-1}}$$

$$= \frac{\ln(2)}{0.184\ \text{days}^{-1}}$$

$$= \frac{0.693}{0.184\ \text{days}^{-1}}$$

$$= 3.8\ \text{days}$$

Question #8. *Calculate a daily dose that will maintain B.G.'s average digoxin plasma concentration at 2 μg/L.*

Using the clearance value of 43.75 L/day calculated from B.G.'s data, and assuming S, F, and τ to be 1, 0.7, and 1 day, respectively, the new maintenance dose can be estimated using Equation 3.11.

$$\text{Maintenance Dose} = \frac{(Cl)(Css\ ave)(\tau)}{(S)(F)}$$

$$= \frac{(43.75\ \text{L/day})(2\ \mu g/L)(1\ \text{day})}{(1)(0.7)}$$

$$= \frac{87.5\ \mu g}{0.7}$$

$$= 125\ \mu g$$

or 0.125 mg digoxin daily

Alternatively, the previous maintenance dose could be adjusted proportionately to the desired change in steady-state plasma level because clearance and other factors were assumed to be constant. Therefore, if the new steady-state level is to be one-half of the previous value, the new maintenance dose should be one-half the previous maintenance dose.

Question #9. *R.N., a female who has been taking the same dose of digoxin for 15 days, is seen in the clinic and is found to be doing well clinically. A digoxin plasma level drawn on the morning of her visit is 3.4 μg/L. What are the possible explanations for this elevated serum digoxin concentration?*

Because this serum digoxin concentration theoretically represents an average steady-state concentration (Css ave), one must evaluate each of the factors that could alter steady state. The relationship of each of these factors to the average steady-state concentration may be seen by studying Equation 3.20:

$$\text{Css ave} = \frac{(S)(F)(Dose/\tau)}{Cl} \qquad \text{[Eq. 3.20]}$$

a) (S)(F). R.N. may be absorbing more than 70% (average bioavailability) from the oral dosage form. Since there are no salt forms of digoxin, S should be 1. Whereas an increase in F could account for some of the elevated digoxin concentration, F alone could only increase the digoxin by a factor of 1.4 (i.e., 1/0.7)

b) Dose. R.N. may be taking more than the prescribed dose, although taking less than the prescribed dose is more common.[7,40] Of course each tablet may not contain the labeled amount, but given current manufacturing standards this is not high on the list of possibilities.

c) τ. R.N. may be taking the proper dose more often than prescribed.

d) Cl. R.N.'s clearance or ability to eliminate the drug may be less than we estimated. We expect most patients to be within the range of ½ to 2 times the expected clearance values (i.e., 2 times to ½ the expected Css ave).

e) Css ave. The assay could be in error. Interfering substances may be present or the plasma level may have been drawn during the distribution phase of the drug.

Plasma levels obtained during the distribution phase of digoxin are higher than anticipated because digoxin is absorbed from the gastrointestinal tract into the plasma and Vi faster than it is distributed into the tissues or Vt. Since the myocardium responds to digoxin as though it were in the tissue compartment (Vt), plasma levels obtained before distribution is complete do not correlate with pharmacologic effects of the drug.[7,27] Digoxin plasma levels should be obtained just before the next dose is given, or at least 6 hours after the oral digoxin dose[27] (see the discussion on Digoxin Volume of Distribution and Time to Sample).

Question #10. *Outline a reasonable plan to determine the cause of R.N.'s higher than predicted digoxin level.*

a) Ask R.N. when that day's digoxin dose was taken relative to when the blood sample was obtained.

b) Determine R.N.'s adherence to the digoxin regimen. This is difficult but must be attempted through a history or pill count.

c) Determine whether any drugs interfered with the digoxin assay. Literature reports of interference by drugs having a steroid nucleus are applicable only to the antibody assay used in the particular report and to the assay techniques and may not apply to the assay used to determine R.N.'s digoxin plasma level. Therefore, the laboratory measuring the serum level would have to be contacted about the possibility of assay interference.[31,41–44] While falsely elevated digoxin concentrations are most commonly reported and should be considered in R.N.'s case, interfering substances may also result in a falsely decreased assay measurement.[44]

Patients with poor renal function and newborn infants accumulate an endogenous digoxin-like compound that can produce a falsely elevated or false-positive digoxin assay result. The usual range of the false-positive reaction is from 0.1 to > 1 μg/L,[45–47] with an average of ≈0.1 to 0.4 μg/L. This interference does not appear to represent a cross-reactivity with digoxin metabolites, since it has been observed in patients who have never received digoxin. The assay interference in these patients with apparent renal dysfunction is assay-specific and is much more significant for some assays than for others.[46,48]

d) Reschedule a second digoxin plasma level, but be certain that it is drawn at least 6 hours after a dose. Preferably, obtain the sample in the morning before the daily dose is taken.

e) Evaluating R.N.'s Cl and F is difficult and costly because such evaluation would require hospitalization. Furthermore, it would only result in the obvious conclusion that the dose should be reduced if, in fact, the dosage level was too high. This approach would only be used under the most unusual circumstances. In addition, F could only increase from the assumed 0.7 to a maximum of 1 and could not, by itself, account for the observed elevation in Css ave.

Question #11. *T.S., a female receiving digoxin 0.375 mg/day for several months, has a reported digoxin plasma concentration of 0.3 μg/L. Her CHF is poorly controlled. What is the most probable explanation?*

The answer to this question is essentially the same as that to Question 9; the same factors should be considered. T.S. should be asked if she is receiving the same brand or dosage form of digoxin because bioavailability may vary between products. T.S. also could be one of the very rare patients who has a large metabolic and renal clearance for digoxin.[49] As indicated in Question 10, there are some drugs that result in a falsely decreased digoxin assay result and that possibility should also be considered.[44] The most likely explanation for the subtherapeutic digoxin concentrations is noncompliance with the prescribed regimen.[40]

Question #12. *In 1966, Doherty and Perkins[50] evaluated the pharmacokinetics of digoxin in hyperthyroid, hypothyroid, and euthyroid patients. Figure 3.2 is a representation of one of the graphs from this study. Using the graph, discuss the implications of thyroid disease on the loading dose, maintenance dose, and the time required to reach steady state relative to the euthyroid state. Assume that the same Css ave is desired in all patients.*

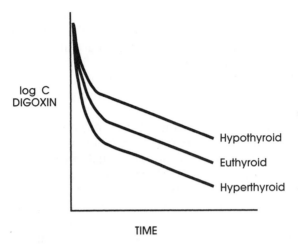

TIME

FIGURE 3.2. Digoxin and thyroid function. Note the distribution and elimination of digoxin when administered by the intravenous route to hypothyroid, hyperthyroid, and euthyroid patients.[50]

Loading Dose. Since hypothyroid patients have higher plasma levels following a single loading dose, they must have a decreased apparent volume of distribution. Therefore, a decrease in the loading dose may be appropriate. Hyperthyroid patients have lower plasma levels and would be expected to require larger loading doses because of a larger volume of distribution. In addition, atrial fibrillation is one of the common cardiac arrhythmias in hyperthyroid patients. In these patients, higher than average digoxin concentrations are often necessary to achieve adequate AV nodal blockade and ventricular rate control.

Time To Reach Steady State. The slope of all the decay curves is the same. Therefore, the half-lives and elimination rate constants are equal, and the time required to reach steady state will be the same for hyperthyroid, hypothyroid, and euthyroid patients receiving digoxin.

Maintenance Dose. Since K is the same in all patients, the clearance and volume of distribution must both be changed by the same proportion and in the same direction. See Equation 3.16 below.

$$K = \frac{Cl}{V}$$

$$K \text{ (Same in All Patients Studied)} = \frac{Cl \text{ (Variable)}}{V \text{ (Variable)}}$$

Hypothyroid patients must have a decreased clearance, since the volume of distribution is decreased. This reduction in Cl would necessitate a reduction in maintenance doses. Similarly, the larger V in the hyperthyroid patients is consistent with an increased clearance; therefore, an increase in maintenance dose would be indicated if Css ave is to remain the same as that used for euthyroid patients.

It is important to reemphasize, however, that although K and V were used to estimate clearance, V is an independent variable, which, like Clearance, is affected by thyroid disease. As both Cl and V were affected in the same direction and to the same degree, the half-life (and K) did not change (see Table 3.1).

Two other studies[51,52] have examined the pharmacokinetics of digoxin in patients with thyroid disease. Both of these suggest that the changes in the digoxin clearance result from an increased glomerular filtration rate associated with hyperthyroidism. If this increased renal function is the primary factor responsible for the altered digoxin clearance observed in hyperthyroid patients, it would be possible to encounter such patients with decreased digoxin clearance if they also had intrinsic renal dysfunction.

Question #13. *Do patients receiving hemodialysis require additional digoxin following dialysis?*

No. Whereas digoxin has a molecular weight of about 500 daltons and will pass through the dialysis membrane, most of the digoxin is in the deeper, more slowly equilibrating tissue compartment and is difficult to remove by any intermittent hemofiltration process. The dialysis clearance for digoxin is only 10 mL/min using dialysis membranes having a molecular weight cutoff of about 1000 daltons. Therefore, < 3% of the total amount of drug in the body is removed during hemodialysis.[53] This dialysis clearance of 10 mL/min may seem significant when compared with the metabolic clearance of 23 mL/min/70 kg for patients with CHF,[29] but the dialysis takes place for only 3 to 4 hours every few days, while the metabolic clearance is continuous. High-efficiency or high-flux membranes with a molecular weight cutoff in the range of 10,000 to 20,000 will have higher digoxin clearance values and be more efficient in clearing plasma digoxin, but the digoxin in the deep compartment is slowly equilibrating and unlikely to be effectively eliminated in the usual 3- or 4-hour dialysis run. Continuous renal replacement therapy (CRRT) may be more effective over several days in removing digoxin because it is continuous. However, given the long $t_{1/2}$ of digoxin, even with the increased clearance, changes in concentration are likely to be over several days and any necessary dose adjustments can be made as needed.[54]

Dialysis, however, can induce digitalis toxicity by altering serum electrolyte concentrations and acid–base balance. For example, a decrease in serum potassium or other electrolytes may occur during dialysis and result in digoxin toxicity during or just following dialysis. If digoxin plasma samples are to be obtained around the time of dialysis, it would be wise to sample before dialysis is started or to wait at least 4 hours following the end of dialysis to ensure that the vascular and deep tissue concentrations of digoxin have had sufficient time to re-equilibrate.

Question #14. *C.B is a patient with atrial fibrillation who was given digoxin for ventricular rate control. He is taking a maintenance dose of 0.25 mg/day of digoxin. Now, however, amiodarone will be added to C.B.'s drug regimen in an attempt to further control his ventricular response and, it is hoped, to convert him to normal sinus rhythm. What are the pharmacokinetic considerations with regard to the amiodarone-digoxin drug interaction?*

Amiodarone is well recognized to decrease both the metabolic and renal clearance of digoxin. Although estimates vary, most patients have about a 50% reduction in digoxin clearance when amiodarone is added to their regimen.[32–34,55] While the digoxin volume of distribution may also decrease slightly, the change is small.[32,33] In addition, amiodarone has a very long $t\frac{1}{2}$ of approximately 40 days and accumulates slowly in the body.[56] As a result, following the initiation of amiodarone, digoxin concentrations rise slowly over a 1- to 2-week period (Fig. 3.3, Line C).

Given that the change in digoxin disposition is primarily a 50% reduction in clearance, we would expect to reduce the patient's digoxin maintenance dose by 50% if our goal was to maintain the same steady-state digoxin concentration after the initiation of amiodarone. Although the change in digoxin occurs slowly, most clinicians reduce the digoxin maintenance dose at the time of starting amiodarone to ensure that the change in the digoxin regimen is not forgotten. If the digoxin steady-state concentration was very low at the time of initiating amiodarone, no change in digoxin may be necessary if the goal was to approximately double the digoxin concentration.

Although not related to the question at hand, many if not most patients with atrial fibrillation are receiving warfarin. Amiodarone also reduces the clearance of warfarin and as a result the INR increases. If the patient's INRs are not closely monitored and the warfarin doses adjusted, the patient's INR will almost certainly increase significantly. It would not be good pharmaceutical care to prevent a digitalis intoxication only to have the patient develop a major bleeding episode.

Question #15. *What if patient C.B. above was to be given quinidine? Are the considerations the same as for amiodarone?*

Although quinidine is no longer one of the more common antiarrhythmic agents, it is still used on occasion. Understanding how quinidine alters the disposition of digoxin helps to explain the differences in how the interaction is managed. Patients receiving digoxin have a rapid and sustained rise in the serum digoxin concentration following the addition of quinidine[57–59] (see Fig. 3.3, line B). This rapid rise in digoxin within the first 24 hours apparently results from the displacement of digoxin by quinidine from tissue sites. The increased digoxin concentration reflects a decrease in digoxin's volume of distribution to 70% of the original value. The initial rise in digoxin concentrations to approximately 1.5 times the original concentration is followed by a relatively slow accumulation over the next week to a steady-state digoxin concentration that is approximately double the original value.[57,60] Many patients develop signs of digitalis toxicity (primarily gastrointestinal in nature) which subside when the dose and plasma concentrations of digoxin are adjusted.[57] However, it should be recognized that while gastrointestinal side effects are the most common for digitalis, side effects do not occur in a progressive order from least to most toxic or dangerous. The first sign of digoxin toxicity could be a life-threatening cardiac arrhythmia.

The rapid and sustained changes in digoxin concentrations (see Fig. 3.3) suggest that the initial change in digoxin concentration is due to a decline in the volume of distribution, which is slightly smaller than the decline in the clearance. This is illustrated by the initial rapid increase in serum digoxin concentration followed by a gradual increase in the serum concentration to the final steady-state value.

Given the initial rapid rise in digoxin concentration (decrease in V) and the eventual doubling of the steady-state concentration (decrease in Cl), the usual approach is to hold one daily dose of digoxin in an attempt to blunt the initial rapid rise in digoxin, and then reinitiate the digoxin maintenance dose at half the previous rate.[61-65] Again this approach assumes that the goal is to maintain the same digoxin concentration following the initiation of quinidine therapy.[66-68]

The patient's digoxin concentration at the time of adding quinidine should be considered carefully. For example, adding quinidine to a patient with a digoxin level of 0.5 μg/L may require no digoxin dose adjustment. A patient with a level of ≈1 μg/L may have one dose withheld

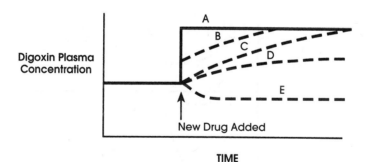

TIME

FIGURE 3.3. Digoxin. Figure 3.3 represents the anticipated changes in digoxin concentration following the initiation of an interacting agent (↑). The solid line A represents the effect of a drug that changes the volume of distribution in proportion to the decrease in the digoxin clearance. Broken line B represents the effect of a drug that produces a decrease in volume of distribution that is less than proportional to the decrease in digoxin clearance (e.g., quinidine). Line C represents the effect of a drug that decreases the digoxin clearance to approximately the same extent as quinidine, but produces no apparent change in the volume of distribution (e.g., amiodarone). Line D represents the effect of a drug that decreases digoxin clearance to a lesser extent than that observed with quinidine (e.g., verapamil). Line E represents a drug that decreases bioavailability or increases clearance or both and hence the decline in digoxin concentrations (e.g., St. John's wort).

and the maintenance dose halved. In a patient with a digoxin concentration of 2 μg/L or higher, it may not be appropriate to add quinidine, given the expected increase in digoxin concentrations and the potential risk of toxicity.

In addition, digoxin concentrations also may vary within a quinidine dosing interval because of varying degrees of tissue displacement. This has been demonstrated at relatively low quinidine concentrations and should be considered when obtaining digoxin plasma levels. For this reason it is generally advisable to obtain plasma digoxin concentrations just before a quinidine dose so that the digoxin plasma levels will be reasonably reproducible. Any change in digoxin concentration sampled in this way should represent actual changes in digoxin disposition rather than transient changes within a quinidine dosing interval[62] (Fig. 3.4).

In the case of both amiodarone[55] and verapamil, if a reduction in digoxin dose is contemplated, it is not necessary to skip a daily dose. Instead, the maintenance regimen should be reduced by the appropriate amount at about the time the amiodarone or verapamil therapy is instituted.

Procainamide does not appear to interact with digoxin and might be considered as an alternative to quinidine. This choice might be most rational when patients require relatively high digoxin concentrations.

Question #16. *What other drugs commonly used in patients receiving digoxin are likely to cause a significant change in its disposition?*

Amiodarone is probably the most significant and common drug that interacts with digoxin. However, other compounds, such as propafenone

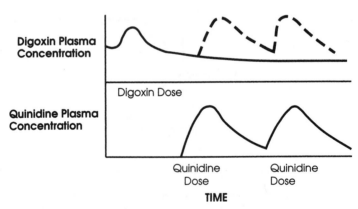

FIGURE 3.4. **Displacement of digoxin by quinidine.** The digoxin plasma concentration with no quinidine (——) and following the administration of two quinidine doses (- - -). Note that as the quinidine plasma concentrations rise and then fall, the digoxin levels also rise and then fall. The elevation of digoxin levels appears to be minimal at quinidine concentrations below 1 mg/L.[62]

and verapamil, also reduce digoxin clearance.[65,69–72] The decrease in digoxin clearance with the addition of propafenone ranges from less than 25% to more than 50%. Most of the change appears to be associated with the metabolic route of digoxin elimination. In addition, the decrease in metabolism appears to increase as the concentration of propafenone increases. Monitoring digoxin plasma levels may be helpful in evaluating the extent of the propafenone-digoxin interaction. Careful consideration should be given to those patients with renal dysfunction or who are to be given large doses of propafenone.

Although the change in clearance for verapamil is not remarkable, approximately a 25% reduction, there may be individual patients in whom a modest reduction in the digoxin maintenance dose is warranted. Broken line D in Figure 3.3 depicts the anticipated rise in digoxin concentration following the institution of verapamil therapy. Note that the slow rise in digoxin concentration suggests that the volume of distribution for digoxin is not altered. The clearance, while reduced, is not reduced to the same extent as that associated with concomitant amiodarone or quinidine therapy; this is consistent with the smaller increase in steady-state digoxin concentrations associated with verapamil. Nifedipine and diltiazem appear to have relatively little influence on digoxin disposition; verapamil has modest effects.

St. John's wort can reduce digoxin concentrations by approximately 25%.[13–16] The most common explanation is a reduced bioavailability, but hepatic enzyme induction and an increase in clearance has also been proposed as a possible mechanism.[15,16] Note in Figure 3.3, Line E, that the digoxin concentration decreases with the addition of an agent that either reduces bioavailability or increases clearance.

Question #17. *A.P., a 75-year-old, 60-kg man, was admitted with complaints of increased shortness of breath (SOB) and yellow sputum production. He has a medical history of chronic obstructive pulmonary disease (COPD) and CHF. During his hospital stay, he developed atrial fibrillation and was given digoxin to slow his ventricular rate. He received 250 µg IV every 3 hours × 3 doses (starting at 9:00 p.m., day 1) and was given a maintenance dose of 250-µg tablets each morning (starting at 9:00 a.m., day 2). His serum creatinine is stable at 1.5 mg/dL. A digoxin level obtained at 9:00 a.m. on the morning of day 4 (2.5 days after the loading dose) was reported to be 1.5 µg/L. A.P. had, therefore, received his initial IV loading dose and two oral maintenance doses when a plasma sample was drawn on the morning of day 4. What would you expect his digoxin concentration to be?*

To calculate the expected concentration, just before the third maintenance dose, one would first need to calculate A.P.'s expected digoxin pharmacokinetic parameters. Using Equation 3.6 for Cl_{cr}, an estimate of 36.1 mL/min is calculated:

$$Cl_{cr} \text{ for males} = \frac{(140 - Age)(Weight \text{ in kg})}{(72)(SCr_{ss})}$$

$$= \frac{(140 - 75 \text{ yrs})(60 \text{ kg})}{(72)(1.5 \text{ mg/dL})}$$

$$= 36.1 \text{ mL/min}$$

Then using Equation 3.2 for digoxin V and Equation 3.5 for the digoxin clearance in patients with CHF, the corresponding values can be obtained.

$$V_{Digoxin} \text{ (L)} = (3.8 \text{ L/kg})(Weight \text{ in kg}) + (3.1)(Cl_{cr} \text{ in mL/min})$$

$$= (3.8 \text{ L/kg})(60 \text{ kg}) + (3.1)(36.1 \text{ mL/min})$$

$$= (228 \text{ L}) + (111.9)$$

$$= 339.9 \text{ L}$$

$$\frac{Total \; Cl_{Digoxin} \text{ (mL/min)}}{\text{(Patients with CHF)}} = (0.33 \text{ mL/kg/min})(Weight \text{ in kg}) + (0.9)(Cl_{cr} \text{ in mL/min})$$

$$= (0.33 \text{ mL/kg/min})(60 \text{ kg}) + (0.9)(36.1 \text{ mL/min})$$

$$= 19.8 \text{ mL/min} + 32.5 \text{ mL/min}$$

$$= 52.3 \text{ mL/min}$$

The $Cl_{Digoxin}$ in mL/min can be converted to the more convenient units of L/day using Equation 3.12:

$$Cl \text{ (L/day)} = \frac{(Cl \text{ as mL/min})(1440 \text{ min/day})}{1000 \text{ mL/L}}$$

$$= \frac{(52.3 \text{ mL/min})(1440 \text{ min/day})}{1000 \text{ mL/L}}$$

$$= 75.3 \text{ L/day}$$

Using the calculated volume of distribution of approximately 340 L and clearance of approximately 75 L/day, Equation 3.16 estimates an elimination rate constant of 0.22 days^{-1}.

$$K = \frac{Cl}{V}$$

$$= \frac{75 \text{ L/day}}{340 \text{ L}}$$

$$= 0.22 \text{ day}^{-1}$$

Equation 3.17 estimates a half-life of approximately 3 days.

$$t\frac{1}{2} = \frac{(0.693)(V)}{Cl}$$

$$= \frac{(0.693)(340\ L)}{75\ L/day}$$

$$= 3.15\ days$$

To calculate A.P.'s digoxin plasma concentration, one needs to consider the loading dose plus the two maintenance doses. To model this series of doses, refer to Part I, Selecting the Appropriate Equation: Series of Individual Doses, Figure 27, in which the loading dose plus the two maintenance doses are depicted as D_1, D_2, and D_3. Because his loading dose of 750 µg (250 µg × 3 doses) was given over a total of 6 hours and A.P.'s expected digoxin half-life is 3.15 days, one can group the entire loading dose together as though it were administered as a single dose, all administered when the first 250-µg dose was given [i.e., time from start to end of loading (tin) is ≤ 1/6 t½].

$$C_{(Sum)} = \frac{(S)(F)(D_1)}{V}(e^{-Kt_1}) + \frac{(S)(F)(D_2)}{V}(e^{-Kt_2}) + \frac{(S)(F)(D_3)}{V}(e^{-Kt_3})\cdots \quad [Eq.\ 3.21]$$

$$= \frac{(1)(1)(750\ \mu g)}{340\ L}(e^{-(0.22\ day^{-1})(2.5\ days)}) + \frac{(1)(0.7)(250\ \mu g)}{340\ L}(e^{-(0.22\ day^{-1})(2\ days)})$$

$$+ \frac{(1)(0.7)(250\ \mu g)}{340\ L}(e^{-(0.22\ day^{-1})(1\ day)})$$

$$= (2.2\ \mu g/L)(0.58) + (0.51\ \mu g/L)(0.64) + (0.51\ \mu g/L)(0.8)$$

$$= 1.3\ \mu g/L + 0.33\ \mu g/L + 0.41\ \mu g/L$$

$$= 2\ \mu g/L$$

Note that the predicted digoxin concentration of 2 µg/L is greater than the observed value of 1.5 µg/L. Unfortunately, revision of pharmacokinetic parameters at this point would be difficult. After only 2.5 days and with a half-life of 3 days, it is relatively easy to see that we have gone beyond one-third of the half-life since the loading dose was administered. Generally, to accurately estimate volume of distribution following a loading dose, we would want a plasma sample within one-third of a half-life. Furthermore, A.P.'s maintenance dose has not been administered longer than two half-lives, which limits our ability to extract information about clearance. The observed plasma concentration may reflect a larger-than-expected V, a higher-than-expected Cl, or some combination of both of these factors. To more accurately determine A.P.'s digoxin clearance, it will be necessary to wait several more days to obtain a plasma concentration that might reasonably be expected to yield information about clearance. Given his expected half-life of approximately 3 days and the probability that his half-life is less than expected, an additional 2 or 3 days would probably be sufficient to begin to get at least some information that will help to predict A.P.'s final steady-state concentration.

Question #18. *C.A. is a 60-year-old, 65-kg man with a serum creatinine of 1.3 mg/dL. He had been taking 0.25 mg of digoxin at 9:00 a.m. orally for his CHF. On the day of admission, a digoxin level of 0.8 µg/L was measured. His outpatient maintenance dose was continued. On the fifth day, just before his morning dose (four doses of digoxin having been administered each day at 9:00 a.m.), a second digoxin sample was obtained. Using the expected pharmacokinetic parameters, calculate C.A.'s digoxin concentration on the morning of the fifth day.*

Again, to calculate the expected plasma concentration, one would first have to estimate C.A.'s creatinine clearance and then use the appropriate equations to calculate his volume of distribution, clearance, elimination rate constant, and half-life.

Using Equation 3.6, we calculate a creatinine clearance of 55.6 mL/min.

$$Cl_{cr} \text{ for males} = \frac{(140 - \text{Age})(\text{Weight in kg})}{(72)(SCr_{ss})}$$

$$= \frac{(140 - 60 \text{ yrs})(65 \text{ kg})}{(72)(1.3 \text{ mg/dL})}$$

$$= 55.6 \text{ mL/min}$$

Then using Equation 3.2 for digoxin V, and Equation 3.5 for the digoxin clearance in patients with CHF, the corresponding values can be obtained.

$$V_{Digoxin} \text{ (L)} = (3.8 \text{ L/kg})(\text{Weight in kg}) + (3.1)(Cl_{cr} \text{ in mL/min})$$

$$= (3.8 \text{ L/kg})(65 \text{ kg}) + (3.1)(55.6 \text{ mL/min})$$

$$= (247 \text{ L}) + (172.4)$$

$$= 419.4 \text{ L}$$

$$\text{Total } Cl_{Digoxin} \text{ (mL/min)} \atop \text{(Patients with CHF)} = (0.33 \text{ mL/kg/min})(\text{Weight in kg}) + (0.9)(Cl_{cr} \text{ in mL/min})$$

$$= (0.33 \text{ mL/kg/min})(65 \text{ kg}) + (0.9)(55.6 \text{ mL/min})$$

$$= 21.5 \text{ mL/min} + 50 \text{ mL/min}$$

$$= 71.5 \text{ mL/min}$$

The $Cl_{Digoxin}$ in mL/min can be converted to the units of L/day using Equation 3.12

$$Cl \ (L/day) = \frac{(Cl \ as \ mL/min)(1440 \ min/day)}{1000 \ mL/L}$$

$$= \frac{(71.5 \ mL/min)(1440 \ min/day)}{1000 \ mL/L}$$

$$= 103 \ L/day$$

Using the calculated volume of distribution and clearance, Equation 3.16 estimates an elimination rate constant of 0.25 days^{-1}.

$$K = \frac{Cl}{V}$$

$$K = \frac{103 \ L/day}{419 \ L}$$

$$= 0.25 \ day^{-1}$$

Equation 3.17 estimates a half-life of approximately 3 days.

$$t\frac{1}{2} = \frac{(0.693)(V)}{Cl}$$

$$= \frac{(0.693)(419 \ L)}{103 \ L/day}$$

$$= 2.8 \ days$$

To model the initial digoxin concentration decay and the four subsequent doses, several approaches could be used. One approach is to use Equation 3.22 to model the initial digoxin concentration and subsequent decay:

$$C_{(Sum)} = C_1(e^{-Kt_1}) + \frac{(S)(F)(D_1)}{V}(e^{-Kt_1}) + \frac{(S)(F)(D_2)}{V}(e^{-Kt_2}) + \frac{(S)(F)(D_3)}{V}(e^{-Kt_3})\cdots$$ [Eq. 3.22]

In the above equation, the digoxin concentration of 0.8 would be C_1, the first t_1 the time from that concentration to the time of sampling (4 days), D_1 the initial dose of 250 μg, and the second t_1 the time from that dose to the time of the sample (again 4 days). D_2 is the second dose, t_2

the second time interval (3 days), etc. The calculations would then be as follows:

$$C_{(Sum)} = (0.8\ \mu g/L)(e^{-(0.25\ day^{-1})(4\ days)}) + \frac{(1)(0.7)(250\ \mu g)}{419\ L}(e^{-(0.25\ day^{-1})(4\ days)})$$

$$+ \frac{(1)(0.7)(250\ \mu g)}{419\ L}(e^{-(0.25\ day^{-1})(3\ days)})$$

$$+ \frac{(1)(0.7)(250\ \mu g)}{419\ L}(e^{-(0.25\ day^{-1})(2\ days)})$$

$$+ \frac{(1)(0.7)(250\ \mu g)}{419\ L}(e^{-(0.25\ day^{-1})(1\ day)})$$

Note that because S and F as well as each of the digoxin doses were the same, the above equation can be factored to the following:

$$C_{(Sum)} = (0.8\ \mu g/L)(e^{-(0.25\ day^{-1})(4\ days)})$$

$$+ \frac{(1)(0.7)(250\ \mu g)}{419\ L}\left[\begin{array}{l}(e^{-(0.25\ day^{-1})(4\ days)}) + (e^{-(0.25\ day^{-1})(3\ days)})\\ + (e^{-(0.25\ day^{-1})(2\ days)}) + (e^{-(0.25\ day^{-1})(1\ day)})\end{array}\right]$$

$$C_{(Sum)} = (0.8\ \mu g/L)(0.37) + 0.42\ \mu g/L\ [(0.37) + (0.47) + (0.61) + (0.78)]$$

$$= (0.3\ \mu g/L) + 0.42\ \mu g/L\ [2.23]$$

$$= (0.3\ \mu g/L) + 0.94\ \mu g/L$$

$$= 1.24\ \mu g/L$$

An alternative approach is to use a model that takes advantage of digoxin's long half-life relative to the dosing interval (see Part I: Selecting the Appropriate Equation, Figure 25). In this model, one could choose to decay the initial digoxin plasma concentration and then add the four subsequent doses by treating them as a continuous infusion as depicted in Equation 3.23 below:

$$C_t = (C_1)(e^{-Kt_1}) + \frac{(S)(F)(Dose/\tau)}{Cl}(1 - e^{-Kt_1}) \qquad \text{[Eq. 3.23]}$$

Note that, in the infusion part of the nonsteady-state equation, Dose/τ is the rate of drug administration and t_1 is the duration of drug administration. Therefore, Dose/τ × t_1 should equal the total amount of drug administered. In this case, there were four doses administered for 1000 μg. Given that the rate of administration is 250 μg/day, t_1 would be 4 days.

Using the appropriate doses, times, and pharmacokinetic parameters, a digoxin concentration of 1.37 $\mu g/L$ is calculated.

$$C_t = (0.8\ \mu g/L)(e^{-(0.25\ \text{day}^{-1})(4\ \text{days})}) + \frac{(1)(0.7)(250\ \mu g/day)}{103\ L/day}(1 - e^{-(0.25\ \text{day}^{-1})(4\ \text{days})})$$

$$= (0.8\ \mu g/L)(0.37) + (1.7\ \mu g/L)(1 - 0.37)$$

$$= (0.3\ \mu g/L) + (1.07\ \mu g/L)$$

$$= 1.37\ \mu g/L$$

The concentration predicted by the first method (individual bolus doses) and the second method (digoxin given as an infusion) are similar, indicating that either method is a reasonable way to predict C.A.'s digoxin concentration on the morning of the fifth day. Also note that the predicted steady-state concentration produced by a maintenance dose of 0.25 mg/day (250 μg/day) would be ≈1.7 μg/L. See above part of Equation 3.22 that represents Css ave or Equation 3.20 below.

$$\text{Css ave} = \frac{(S)(F)(Dose/\tau)}{Cl}$$

$$= \frac{(1)(0.7)(250\ \mu g/day)}{103\ L/day}$$

$$= 1.7\ \mu g/L$$

Question #19. *C.A.'s digoxin level reported from the laboratory was 1.6 μg/L. Since the observed digoxin concentration is greater than the predicted level (1.24 to 1.37 μg/L), what would one expect C.A.'s digoxin clearance and subsequent steady-state digoxin concentration to be on his current regimen of 0.25 mg/day?*

Either of the two approaches in the previous question can be used to resolve this problem. Clearance could be calculated by first assuming C.A.'s digoxin volume of distribution to be 419 L. Then, using a trial and error method or iterative search, one could substitute various clearance values and the corresponding elimination rate constant values until the equation predicted the observed digoxin concentration of 1.6 μg/L. Since this process could be laborious, an alternative approach is to use the mass balance technique and solve directly for C.A.'s clearance. See Part I: Interpretation of Plasma Drug Concentrations: Nonsteady-State Revision of Clearance (Mass Balance). The expected steady-state digoxin concentration for C.A. could then be more easily calculated.

$$Cl = \frac{(S)(F)(Dose/\tau) - \dfrac{(C_2 - C_1)V}{t}}{C\ \text{ave}} \qquad \text{[Eq. 3.24]}$$

In this equation t is the time interval between C_1 and C_2 and therefore is 4 days, since this is the interval between C_1 (0.8 µg/L) and C_2 (1.6 µg/L). C ave is calculated as the arithmetic mean of the two plasma concentrations.

$$C\ ave = \frac{C_1 + C_2}{2} \qquad \text{[Eq. 3.25]}$$

$$= \frac{0.8\ µg/L + 1.6\ µg/L}{2}$$

$$= 1.2\ µg/L$$

Substituting the appropriate values in Equation 3.24, a digoxin clearance of 76 L/day can be calculated.

$$Cl = \frac{(S)(F)(Dose/\tau) - \dfrac{(C_2 - C_1)V}{t}}{C\ ave}$$

$$= \frac{(1)(0.7)(250\ µg/day) - \dfrac{(1.6\ µg/L - 0.8\ µg/L)(419\ L)}{4\ days}}{1.2\ µg/L}$$

$$= \frac{(91.2\ µg/day)}{1.2\ µg/L}$$

$$= 76\ L/day$$

Note that this calculated digoxin clearance and our assumed volume of distribution of 419 L is consistent with an expected half-life of approximately 3.8 days (Equation 3.17).

$$t\frac{1}{2} = \frac{(0.693)(V)}{Cl}$$

$$= \frac{(0.693)(419\ L)}{76\ L/day}$$

$$= 3.8\ days$$

Evaluating the revised half-life is an important step in our assessment of the clearance prediction of 76 L/day. As mentioned in Part I, there are three key issues or rules to be considered when using the mass balance approach when solving for clearance, using nonsteady-state data:

1) t or time interval between C_1 and C_2 should be at least one half-life but not more than two half-lives. If t is very short, relative to the drug half-life, small differences in C_1 and C_2 can result in widely varying estimates

of drug accumulation or drug loss. If t is much more than two half-lives, the second concentration would be approaching steady-state and our C ave would be an underestimate of the average concentration within the time interval t. Hence, the rule that t should be at least one but not more than two half-lives.

2) The plasma concentration values should be reasonably close to one another, therefore: $C_2/C_1 \leq 2$ if the concentration is increasing and $C_2/C_1 \geq 0.5$ if the concentration is decreasing. If there is a large difference between C_1 and C_2, it means that relatively little of the dose administered between C_1 and C_2 has been eliminated. In this situation, volume of distribution and the total dose administered are the critical factors and the drug concentrations contain very little information about clearance. If the concentration has declined more than one $t\frac{1}{2}$, i.e., $C_2/C_1 \geq 0.5$, there will be a significant curve in the decay line and the arithmetic mean of C_1 and C_2 (i.e., $(C_1 + C_2)/2$) will not be a good estimate of the average drug concentration over the time interval t. Ideally C_1 and C_2 would be very close together and the net drug accumulation or loss would be approaching zero, suggesting near steady-state conditions and therefore ideal conditions for estimating clearance.

3) The rate of drug administration $[(S)(F)(Dose/\tau)]$ should be regular and result in a reasonably smooth progression from C_1 to C_2. If the doses are very irregular because either the interval is not consistent or the dose is changing, the accumulation pattern will not be a smooth transition from C_1 to C_2. Therefore, the C ave as calculated from the arithmetic mean of C_1 and C_2 (i.e., $(C_1 + C_2)/2$) will not accurately represent the true C ave between C_1 and C_2. Another potential problem with the mass balance approach is when the dosing interval is longer than the drug half-life. Under these conditions there will be significant increases and decreases in the drug concentration within each dosing interval. The progression from C_1 to C_2 will not be smooth and result in the arithmetic mean $((C_1 + C_2)/2)$ being a poor estimate of the true average concentration.

Assuming we have met all three rules above and are using the revised clearance value and Equation 3.20, the expected steady-state digoxin concentration of approximately 2.3 μg/L can be calculated.

$$Css\ ave = \frac{(S)(F)(Dose/\tau)}{Cl}$$

$$= \frac{(1)(0.7)(250\ \mu g/day)}{76\ L/day}$$

$$= 2.3\ \mu g/L$$

Because this value is somewhat above the upper limit of the usually accepted therapeutic range, one might choose to reduce the digoxin maintenance dose at this time. This is especially true given that most patients with CHF do well clinically with digoxin concentrations in the range of 0.5 to 1 μg/L. An alternative approach would be to obtain another digoxin sample after approximately one additional half-life (3 to 4 days) to determine if the digoxin concentration is accumulating as anticipated. In one half-life, the digoxin concentration should accumulate to a concentration of approximately 2 μg/L, or half-way between the present concentration of 1.6 μg/L and the expected steady-state value of 2.3 μg/L. The time interval of one half-life was chosen for two reasons. First, a significant time interval is required, usually at least one half-life, to distinguish true drug accumulation from assay variability. Second, it is desirable to detect accumulation early enough to avoid unnecessary toxicity risks. In this case, the time interval chosen has placed C.A.'s digoxin concentration at the upper end of the therapeutic range.

REFERENCES

1. Smith TW. Digitalis toxicity: epidemiology and clinical use of serum concentration measurements. Am J Med 1975;58:470.
2. Smith TW, Haber. E. Digoxin intoxication: the relationship of clinical presentation to serum digoxin concentration. J Clin Invest 1970;49:2377.
3. HFSA Guidelines for management of patients with heart failure caused by left ventricular systolic dysfunction-pharmacologic approaches. J Cardiac Failure 1999;5:357–382.
4. Sameri RM, Soberman JE, Finch CK, Self TH. Lower serum digoxin concentrations in heart failure and reassessment of laboratory report forms. Am J Med Sci 2002;324:10–13.
5. Adams KF Jr, et al. Clinical benefits of low serum digoxin concentrations in heart failure. J Am Coll Cardiol 2002;39:946–953.
6. Kock-Weser J, et al. Influence of serum digoxin concentration measurements on frequency of digitoxicity. Clin Pharmacol Ther 1974;16:284.
7. Sheiner LB, et al. Instructional goals for physicians in the use of blood level data and the contribution of computers. Clin Pharmacol Ther 1974;16:260.
8. Ogilvie RI, Ruedy J. An educational program in digitalis therapy. JAMA 1972;222:50.
9. Huffman DH, et al. Absorption of digoxin from different oral preparations in normal subjects during steady state. Clin Pharmacol Ther 1974;16:310.
10. Lisalo E. Clinical pharmacokinetics of digoxin. Clin Pharmacokinet 1977;2:1.
11. Mallis GI, et al. Superior bioavailability of digoxin solution in capsules. Clin Pharmacol Ther 1975;18:761.
12. Marcus FI, et al. Digoxin bioavailability: formulations and rates of infusions. Clin Pharmacol Ther 1976;20:253.
13. Johne A, et al. Pharmacokinetic interaction of digoxin with an herbal extract from St John's wort (Hypericum perforatum). Clin Pharmacol Ther 1999;66:338–345.
14. Izzo AA, Ernst E. Interactions between herbal medicines and prescribed drugs: a systematic review. Drugs 2001;61:2163–2175.
15. Durr D, et al. St John's wort induces intestinal P-glycoprotein/MDR1 and intestinal and hepatic CYP3A4. Clin Pharmacol Ther 2000;68:598–604.
16. Henderson L, et al. St John's wort (Hypericum perforatum): drug interactions and clinical outcomes. Br J Clin Pharmacol 2002;54:349–356.

17. Bizjak ED, Mauro VF. Digoxin-macrolide drug interaction. Ann Pharmacother 1997;31:1077–1079.

18. Gooderham MJ, Bolli P, Fernandez PG. Concomitant digoxin toxicity and warfarin interaction in a patient receiving clarithromycin. Ann Pharmacother 1999;33:796–799.

19. Wakasugi H, et al. Effect of clarithromycin on renal excretion of digoxin: interaction with P-glycoprotein. Clin Pharmacol Ther 1988;64:123–128.

20. Lindenbaum J, et al. Inactivation of digoxin by the gut flora: reversal by antibiotic therapy. N Engl J Med 1981;305:789–794.

21. Partanen J, Jalava KM, Neuvonen PJ. Itraconazole increases serum digoxin concentration. Pharmacol Toxicol 1996;79:274–276.

22. Henderson RP, Solomon CP. Use of cholestyramine in the treatment of digoxin intoxication. Arch Intern Med 1988;148:745–746.

23. Neuvonen PJ, Kivisto K, Hirvisalo EL. Effects of resin and activated charcoal on the absorption of digoxin, carbamazepine and frusemide. Br J Pharmacol 1988;25:229–233.

24. Reuning RH, et al. Role of pharmacokinetics in drug dosage adjustment: I. Pharmacologic effect kinetics and apparent volume of distribution of digoxin. J Clin Pharmacol 1973;13:127.

25. Abernethy DR, et al. Digoxin disposition in obesity: Clinical pharmacokinetic investigation. Am Heart J 1981;102:740–744.

26. Shapiro W, et al. Relationship of plasma digitoxin and digoxin to cardiac response following intravenous digitalization in man. Circulation 1970;42:1065.

27. Walsh FM, et al. Significance of non-steady state serum digoxin concentrations. Am J Clin Pathol 1975;63:446.

28. Kramer WG, et al. Pharmacokinetics of digoxin: comparison of a two and a three compartment model in man. J Pharmacokinet Biopharm 1974;2:299.

29. Sheiner LB, et al. Estimation of population characteristics of pharmacokinetic parameters from routine clinical data. J Pharmacokinet Biopharm1977;5:445.

30. Sheiner LB, et al. Modeling of individual pharmacokinetics for computer-aided drug dosage. Comput Biomed Res 1972;5:441.

31. Smith TW, et al. Clinical value of the radioimmunoassay of the digitalis glycosides. Pharmacol Rev 1973;25:219.

32. Fenster PE, White NW Jr, Hanson CD. Pharmacokinetic evaluation of the digoxin-amiodarone interaction. J Am Coll Cardiol 1985;5:108–112.

33. Nademanee K, et al. Amiodarone-digoxin interaction: clinical significance, time course of development, potential pharmacokinetic mechanisms and therapeutic implications. J Am Coll Cardiol 1984;4:111–116.

34. Trujillo TC, Nolan PE. Antiarrhythmic agents: drug interactions of clinical significance. Drug Saf 2000;23:509–532.

35. Jusko WH, et al. Pharmacokinetic design of digoxin dosage regimens in relation to renal function. J Clin Pharmacol 1974;14:525.

36. Jusko WJ, Wintraub M. Myocardial distribution of digoxin and renal function. Clin Pharmacol Ther 1974;16:449.

37. Wagner JG. Loading and maintenance doses of digoxin in patients with normal renal function and those with severely impaired renal function. J Clin Pharmacol 1974;14:329.

38. Ohnhaus EE, et al. Protein binding of digoxin in human serum. Eur J Clin Pharmacol 1972;5:34.

39. Koup JR, et al. Pharmacokinetics of digoxin in normal subjects after intravenous bolus and infusion doses. J Pharmacokinet Biopharm 1975;3:181.

40. Wintraub M, et al. Compliance as a determinant of serum digoxin concentration. JAMA 1973;224:481.

41. Lader S, et al. The measurement of plasma digoxin concentrations: a comparison of two methods. Eur J Clin Pharmacol 1972;5:22.

42. Silber B, et al. Associated digoxin radioimmunoassay interference. Clin Chem 1979;25:48.

43. Dasgupta A. Endogenous and exogenous digoxin-like immunoreactive substances: impact on the therapeutic drug monitoring of digoxin. Am J Clin Pathol 2002;118:132–140.

44. Steimer W, Muller C, Eber B. Digoxin assays: frequent, substantial and potentially dangerous interference by spironolactone, canrenone, and other steroids. Clin Chem 2002;48:507–516.

45. Graves SW, et al. An endogenous digoxin-like substance in patients with renal impairment. Ann Intern Med 1983;99:604.

46. Pudek MR, et al. Seven different digoxin immunoassay kits compared with respect to interference by a digoxin-1ike immunoreactive substance in serum from premature and full-term infants. Clin Chem 1983;29:1972.

47. Yatscoff RW, et al. Digoxin-1ike immunoreactivity in the serum of neonates and uremic patients, as measured in the Abbott TDX (Letter). Clin Chem 1984;30:588.

48. Avendano C, et al. Interference of digoxin-like immunoreactive substances with TDx Digoxin II assay in different patients. Ther Drug Monit 1991;13:523–527.

49. Luchi RJ, Gruber JW. Unusually large digitalis requirements. Am J Med 1968;45:322.

50. Doherty JE, Perkins WH. Digoxin metabolism in hypo-and hyperthyroidism. Ann Intern Med 1966;64:489.

51. Lawrence JR. Digoxin kinetics in patients with thyroid dysfunction. Clin Pharmacol Ther 1977;22:7.

52. Croxson MS, Ibbertson HK. Serum digoxin in patients with thyroid disease. Br Med J 1985;3:566.

53. Ackerman GL, et al. Peritoneal and hemodialysis of tritiated digoxin. Ann Intern Med 1967;67:4:718.

54. Reetze-Bonorden P, Bohler J, Keller E. Drug dosage in patients during continuous renal replacement therapy. Clin Pharmacokinet 1993;24:362–379.

55. Lesko LJ. Pharmacokinetic drug interactions with amiodarone. Clin Pharmacokinet 1989;17:130–140.

56. Hardman JG, Limbird LE, Gilman AG, eds. The Pharmacological Basis of Therapeutics. 10th Ed. New York: McGraw Hill, 2001.

57. Ejvinsson G. Effect of quinidine of plasma concentrations of digoxin. Br Med J 1978;279.

58. Leahey EB Jr, et al. Interactions between quinidine and digoxin. JAMA 1978;240:533.

59. Bauer LA, Horn JR, Pettit H. Mixed-effect modeling for detection and evaluation of drug interactions: digoxin-quinidine and digoxin-verapamil combinations. Ther Drug Monit 1996;18:46–52.

60. Leahey EB, et al. Quinidine-digoxin interaction: time course and pharmacokinetics. Am J Cardiol 1981;48:1141.

61. Hager DW, et al. Digoxin-quinidine interaction. N Engl J Med 1979;300:1238.

62. Powell JR, et al. Quinidine-digoxin interaction. N Engl J Med 1980;302:176.

63. Doering W. Quinidine-digoxin interaction. N Engl J Med 1979;301:400.

64. Fichtl B, Doering W. The quinidine-digoxin interaction in perspective. Clin Pharmacokinet 1983;8:137.

65. Bussey HI. The influence of quinidine and other agents on digitalis glycosides. Am Heart J 1982;104:289.

66. Steiness E, et al. Reduction of digoxin-induced inotropism during quinidine administration. Clin Pharmacol Ther 1980;27:791.

67. Schenck-Gustafsson K, et al. Cardiac effects of treatment with quinidine and digoxin, alone and in combination. Am J Cardiol 1983;51:777.

68. Belz GB, et al. Quinidine-digoxin interaction; cardiac efficacy of elevated serum digoxin concentration. Clin Pharmacol Ther 1982;31:548.

69. Nolan PE Jr, et al. Effects of coadministration of propafenone on the pharmacokinetics of digoxin in healthy volunteer subjects. J Clin Pharmacol 1989;29:46–52.

70. Bigot MC, et al. Serum digoxin levels related to plasma propafenone levels during concomitant treatment. J Clin Pharmacol 1991;31:521–526.

71. Belz GG, Doering W, Munkes R, Matthews J. Interactions between digoxin and calcium antagonists and antiarrhythmic drugs. Clin Pharmacol Ther 1983;33:410–417.

72. Pedersen KE, et al. Verapamil-induced changes in digoxin kinetics and intraerythrocytic sodium concentration. Clin Pharmacol Ther 1983;34:8.

4

ETHOSUXIMIDE

Melissa M.L. Choy and Michael E. Winter

Ethosuximide is an anticonvulsant which has been used primarily for the treatment of uncomplicated absence seizures.[1] It is available as 250 mg capsules and as a solution containing 250 mg of ethosuximide per 5 mL. Ethosuximide is eliminated primarily by metabolism to an inactive hydroxyethyl metabolite which is excreted in the urine as the glucuronide. Approximately 20% of unchanged ethosuximide is excreted in the urine. The usual dosage range is 15 to 30 mg/kg/day. Children 3 to 6 years of age usually receive a single daily dose of ≈250 mg. Some pediatric clinicians, however, prefer administering a maintenance dose of 15 to 40 mg/kg/day (usually not to exceed 1500 mg/day), divided into two daily doses given every 12 hours. Older children and adults generally receive their daily regimen in two divided doses, although some older patients appear to do well on once-daily dosing.

THERAPEUTIC AND TOXIC PLASMA CONCENTRATIONS

The range of therapeutic plasma concentrations for ethosuximide (measured just before the next dose) is 40 to 100 mg/L. Most patients with plasma concentrations in this range respond with a significant or complete reduction in seizure activity; patients with plasma concentrations less than 40 mg/L are less likely to have well-controlled seizure activity.[2,3] The incidence of adverse effects associated with ethosuximide therapy is relatively low and does not correlate well with plasma concentrations. Whereas side effects associated with ethosuximide are uncommon, those most usually encountered are related to the gastrointestinal tract and include abdominal discomfort, nausea and vomiting, and anorexia. Drowsiness, dizziness, fatigue, and headaches are also observed occasionally. Many patients with plasma concentrations in excess of 100 mg/L experience no side effects.[4] Plasma levels are, therefore, primarily used to evaluate a patient's potential for clinical response and compliance. Alterations in plasma concentrations due to plasma protein binding changes are not a consideration for ethosuximide because very little is protein bound.[5]

KEY PARAMETERS: Ethosuximide

Therapeutic Plasma Concentrations	40–100 mg/L
F	100%
S	1.0
V	0.7 L/kg
Cl	
Child	0.39 L/kg/day
Adult	0.23 L/kg/day
$t\frac{1}{2}$	
Child	30 hr
Adult	50 hr

BIOAVAILABILITY (F)

Ethosuximide appears to be well absorbed following oral administration, with peak levels occurring within 2 to 4 hours after administration of a dose. Available data suggest that the bioavailability approaches 100%.[6,7] The salt factor (S) for ethosuximide is 1.

VOLUME OF DISTRIBUTION (V)

The volume of distribution for ethosuximide appears to be ≈0.7 L/kg.[7] There is an insignificant amount of plasma and tissue protein binding.[5,8]

CLEARANCE (Cl)

Ethosuximide is eliminated from the body primarily by metabolism, with a relatively small percentage of drug being excreted unchanged. Children have an average clearance value of ≈0.39 L/kg/day, and adults have a lower clearance value of ≈0.23 L/kg/day .[6,7] These clearance values vary considerably from patient to patient, making plasma level monitoring useful in designing dosing regimens.

Because the primary route of ethosuximide elimination is hepatic metabolism, anticonvulsant inducers (such as phenytoin, phenobarbital, primidone, and carbamazepine) may increase the clearance of ethosuximide.[9] For patients receiving these drugs concomitantly, higher dosages of ethosuximide may be needed to achieve therapeutic drug concentrations and plasma levels of the administered anticonvulsants should be monitored. Conversely, valproic acid may increase,[10] decrease,[11] or may not change[12] ethosuximide plasma levels. Thus, careful monitoring of plasma concentrations of both drugs are recommended.

Based on ethosuximide's relatively small molecular weight (141 daltons), small volume of distribution, and negligible plasma protein binding, one would predict significant removal by hemodialysis. Data indicate that ≈50% of ethosuximide is removed during a standard hemodialysis run.[13] One would also predict significant elimination of ethosuximide by continuous renal replacement therapies (e.g., CVVH, CVVHD). This is based on the parameters above (molecular weight, volume of distribution, protein binding) and an extracorporeal clearance that is expected to be significant relative to a patient's residual renal and nonrenal clearance.[14]

HALF-LIFE (t½)

The elimination half-life of ethosuximide is ≈30 hours in children and ≈50 hours in adults. Due to the wide variation in clearance values, the half-life can be less than one-half or greater than twice these average values.[6,7] The long half-life of ethosuximide suggests that once-daily dosing regimens would be appropriate; however, in some cases gastrointestinal side effects may require dividing the dose to twice daily.[15]

TIME TO SAMPLE

The timing of the ethosuximide sample within a dosing interval is not critical because of its long elimination half-life. Although trough levels are recommended for the sake of consistency, obtaining trough concentrations should not be considered crucial if it is inconvenient. Ethosuximide concentrations require approximately 4 to 7 days to reach steady state in children. An even longer period will be required in adults. For this reason, early plasma level monitoring may cause confusion about the final steady-state concentration and should be avoided.

Question #1. *C.A., an 8-year-old, 25-kg male, is receiving 250 mg ethosuximide BID for treatment of absence seizures. Predict C.A.'s trough plasma concentration of ethosuximide at steady state.*

To calculate the anticipated trough concentration of ethosuximide, the expected volume of distribution and elimination rate constant would have to be calculated and the appropriate values placed in Equation 4.1 below:

$$Css\ min = \frac{\frac{(S)(F)(Dose)}{V}}{(1 - e^{-K\tau})}(e^{-K\tau}) \qquad [Eq.\ 4.1]$$

In this case, however, it is important to recognize that the difference between the trough and average concentrations will be relatively small because the dosing interval of 12 hours is short compared to the anticipated half-life of ≈30 hours. For this reason, an average plasma concentration of ethosuximide could be calculated by using Equation 4.2 and the estimated clearance value of 0.39 L/kg/day or 9.75 L/day (0.39 L/kg/day × 25 kg).

$$Css\ ave = \frac{(S)(F)(Dose/\tau)}{Cl} \qquad [Eq.\ 4.2]$$

$$= \frac{(1)(1)(250\ mg/0.5\ days)}{9.75\ L/day}$$

$$= 51.3\ mg/L$$

This average concentration of ≈50 mg/L could then be used as an approximation of the anticipated trough concentration.

Question #2. *Because C.A.'s seizure control has been poor, an ethosuximide level is ordered and reported as 35 mg/L. How would one interpret this ethosuximide concentration? What would be an appropriate course of action?*

The measured ethosuximide concentration of 35 mg/L is below the usual therapeutic range; therefore, it might be assumed that increasing the plasma concentration into the therapeutic range would result in better seizure control. Before a dose is adjusted, however, C.A. or his family should be questioned carefully to ascertain whether the low ethosuximide concentration is the result of increased metabolism (clearance) or nonadherence to the prescribed regimen. If it can be determined that C.A. has been compliant, then the dosing regimen should be adjusted.

Because ethosuximide concentrations should not change much during a dosing regimen, the plasma concentration of 35 mg/L probably represents an average plasma concentration. The average steady-state plasma concentration is proportional to the dosing rate; therefore, a change in the maintenance regimen should result in a proportional change in the steady-state plasma concentration. For example, using Equation 4.3, if the daily dose was increased from 500 mg to 750 mg, the plasma concentration should increase by 50% (i.e., from 35 mg/L to $\approx$52 mg/L):

$$\text{Css ave (new)} = [\text{Css ave (old)}]\left[\frac{\text{Maintenance Dose (new)}}{\text{Maintenance Dose (old)}}\right] \qquad \text{[Eq. 4.3]}$$

$$= [35 \text{ mg/L}]\left[\frac{750 \text{ mg/day}}{500 \text{ mg/day}}\right]$$

$$= [35 \text{ mg/L}][1.5]$$

$$= 52.5 \text{ mg/L}$$

An alternate approach would be to use the steady-state level of 35 mg/L to calculate C.A.'s apparent ethosuximide clearance. This could be accomplished by using the maintenance regimen of 250 mg every 12 hours (250 mg/0.5 days) and Equation 4.4:

$$Cl = \frac{(S)(F)(Dose/\tau)}{(Css \text{ ave})} \qquad \text{[Eq. 4.4]}$$

$$= \frac{(1)(1)(250 \text{ mg/0.5 days})}{(35 \text{ mg/L})}$$

$$= 14.3 \text{ L/day}$$

This clearance of 14.3 L/ day could then be used in Equation 4.5, below, to calculate the dose that would be required to maintain any desired steady-state ethosuximide level. For example, if an average plasma concentration of 50 mg/L were inserted in this equation, the calculated maintenance dose would be 715 mg/day:

$$\text{Maintenance Dose} = \frac{(Cl)(Css \text{ ave})(\tau)}{(S)(F)} \qquad \text{[Eq. 4.5]}$$

$$= \frac{(14.3 \text{ L/day})(50 \text{ mg/L})(1 \text{ day})}{(1)(1)}$$

$$= 715 \text{ mg}$$

Ethosuximide is available in 250 mg capsules; an appropriate dose would be 250 mg every 8 hours or 250 mg given once daily and 500 mg given 12 hours later. Once-daily therapy would not be advisable because the estimated half-life for C.A. is $\approx$20 hours, as shown below using Equation 4.6.

$$t\frac{1}{2} = \frac{(0.693)(V)}{Cl} \qquad \text{[Eq. 4.6]}$$

$$= \frac{(0.693)(0.7 \text{ L/kg})(25 \text{ kg})}{14.3 \text{ L/day}}$$

$$= \frac{(0.693)(17.5 \text{ L})}{14.3 \text{ L/day}}$$

$$= 0.848 \text{ days}$$

or

$$= 0.848 \text{ days } (24 \text{ hr/day})$$

$$= 20.4 \text{ hr}$$

REFERENCES

1. Brodie MJ, Dichter MA. Antiepileptic drugs. N Engl J Med 1996;334:168–175.
2. Browne TR, Dreifuss FE. Ethosuximide in the treatment of absence seizures. Neurology 1975;25:515–24.
3. Sherwin AL, Robb JP. Ethosuximide: relation of plasma levels to clinical control. In: Woodbury DM, et al., eds. Anti-Epileptic Drugs. New York: Raven Press, 1972:443–448.
4. Sherwin AL, et al. Plasma ethosuximide levels: a new aid in the management of epilepsy. Ann R Coll Surg Can 1971;4:48.
5. Johannessen SI. Antiepileptic drugs: pharmacokinetic and clinical aspects. Ther Drug Monit 1981;2:17–37.
6. Buchanan RA, et al. Absorption and elimination of ethosuximide in children. J Clin Pharmacol 1969;9:393–8.
7. Buchanan RA, et al. The absorption and excretion of ethosuximide. Int J Clin Pharmacol Res 1973;7:213–218.
8. Chang T, et al. Ethosuximide: absorption, distribution and excretion. In: Woodbury DM, et al., eds. Anti-Epileptic Drugs. New York: Raven Press, 1972:417–423.
9. Riva R, et al. Pharmacokinetic interactions between antiepileptic drugs: clinical considerations. Clin Pharmacokinet 1996;31:470–493.
10. Mattson RH, et al. Valproic acid and ethosuximide interaction. Ann Neurol 1980;7:583–584.
11. Battino D, et al. Ethosuximide plasma concentrations: influence of age and associated concomitant therapy. Clin Pharmacokinet 1982;7:176–180.
12. Bauer LA, et al. Ethosuximide kinetics: possible interaction with valproic acid. Clin Pharmacol Ther 1982;31:741–745.
13. Marbury TC, et al. Hemodialysis clearance of ethosuximide in patients with chronic renal failure. Am J Hosp Pharm 1981;38:1757–1760.
14. Reetze-Bonorden P, et al. Drug dosage in patients during continuous renal replacement therapy: pharmacokinetic and therapeutic considerations. Clin Pharmacokinet 1993;24:362–379.
15. Dooley JM, et al. Once-daily ethosuximide in the treatment of absence epilepsy. Pediatr Neurol 1990;6:38–39.

5

IMMUNOSUPPRESSANTS: CYCLOSPORINE, TACROLIMUS, AND SIROLIMUS

David J. Quan and Michael E. Winter

Immunosuppression plays a vital role in preventing and treating allograft rejection in the transplant recipient and in the treatment of various autoimmune disorders.

Many of the immunosuppressive drugs have a narrow therapeutic window, such that the concentration range between subtherapeutic and toxic is small. In addition, many of these drugs exhibit pharmacokinetic variability. There can be large fluctuations in the observed blood levels between patients receiving the same dose normalized for weight (interpatient variability) and within the same patient receiving the same dose (intrapatient variability). Subtherapeutic levels and wide fluctuations in drug levels are risk factors for allograft rejection and decreased graft survival. Therapeutic drug monitoring is essential in optimizing the patient's immunosuppressive drug regimen to minimize the risk of allograft rejection and dose-related adverse effects.

Immunosuppressive drug therapy is usually individualized to the patient and may be specific to the organ(s) transplanted, time after transplant, indication for transplantation, and transplant-center–specific immunosuppression protocols. Although there are many immunosuppressive drugs available, this chapter focuses on the three drugs that routinely undergo therapeutic drug monitoring in the setting of organ transplantation: cyclosporine, tacrolimus, and sirolimus.

CYCLOSPORINE

Cyclosporine is a cyclical peptide used in clinical practice since 1978 for the prevention of allograft rejection in solid organ transplant recipients, for the prevention of graft-versus-host disease in bone marrow transplant recipients, and for the management of various autoimmune disorders. The primary immunosuppressive effects of cyclosporine are to inhibit the production and secretion of interleukin-2 (IL-2) and other cellular growth factors by inhibiting the enzyme, calcineurin. IL-2 plays a vital role in the rejection process by signaling for cytotoxic T lymphocyte activation and

KEY PARAMETERS: Cyclosporine[a]

Therapeutic Concentration	See Table 5.2
F[b]	30% (range: 8–60%)
V[c]	4–5 L/kg
Cl[d]	5–10 mL/kg/min
$t^1/_2$	6–12 hours
Free Fraction (α)[e]	<10%

[a]As with the therapeutic range, pharmacokinetic parameters will vary, depending on the biologic fluid and assay procedure used.
[b]Bioavailability is both inter- and intraindividually variable.
[c]Cyclosporine is distributed into multiple compartments; however, toxicity is not known to be associated with drug concentrations in the distribution phase.
[d]Clearance is primarily by hepatic metabolism.
[e]Cyclosporine is extensively bound to many blood elements and, in plasma, it is extensively bound to lipoproteins.

proliferation. Cyclosporine is used to prevent acute allograft rejection, not to treat rejection. Cyclosporine is usually given in combination with a corticosteroid and an antiproliferative agent such as azathioprine or mycophenolate mofetil as part of an immunosuppression regimen.

Cyclosporine is available in several different formulations; the reader should refer to Table 5.1 for the various immunosuppressive drug formulations. The original formulation of cyclosporine, Sandimmune, is formulated in olive oil. Absorption of the oil-based formulation is dependent on bile for emulsification. External bile drainage, cholestasis, or diarrhea may reduce the amount of bile for emulsification and impair cyclosporine absorption. In addition to poor and erratic absorption of cyclosporine, there is substantial intrapatient and interpatient pharmacokinetic variability. The newer formulation, Neoral, a microemulsion of cyclosporine, and other bioequivalent preparations (cyclosporine modified) are readily absorbed in the absence of bile. The newer formulations will be collectively referred to as cyclosporine modified, and the Sandimmune formulation as cyclosporine. The cyclosporine modified formulations compared to the cyclosporine formulation are absorbed faster (shorter tmax), to a greater extent (greater area-under-the-concentration-time-curve and larger Cmax), and more consistently (decreased intrapatient and interpatient variability).[1] Figure 5.1 compares the typical concentration time curves of cyclosporine and cyclosporine modified after an oral dose. Because cyclosporine and cyclosporine modified are absorbed differently, they are

TABLE 5.1 **Immunosuppressive Drug Formulations**

Drug	Formulations
Cyclosporine	
Sandimmune	25, 100 mg capsules
	100 mg/mL oral solution
	50 mg/5 mL ampules for intravenous infusion
Cyclosporine modified	
Neoral, Gengraf, and others	25, 100 mg capsules
	100 mg/mL oral solution
Tacrolimus	
Prograf	0.5, 1, 5 mg capsules
	5 mg/mL ampules for intravenous infusion
Sirolimus	
Rapamune	1, 2 mg tablets
	1 mg/mL oral solution

not considered bioequivalent formulations and therefore should not be used interchangeably. Because of the pharmacokinetic limitations, the original cyclosporine formulation is no longer commonly used. Patients may be receiving Sandimmune brand if they are on a stable regimen and wish to continue with this particular formulation. Most patients who are newly initiated on a cyclosporine-based immunosuppression regimen are started with a cyclosporine modified formulation.

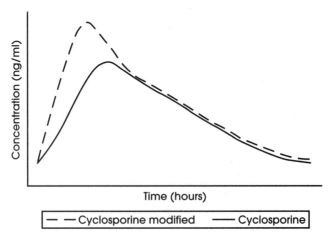

FIGURE 5.1. The typical concentration time curves of cyclosporine and cyclosporine modified after an oral dose.

The typical starting dose of cyclosporine or cyclosporine modified to prevent allograft rejection is approximately 5 to 10 mg/kg/day given as a divided dose twice a day (e.g., 2.5 to 5 mg/kg given every 12 hours). Target cyclosporine blood trough concentrations will vary according to the organ(s) transplanted, time after transplant, and transplant-center–specific immunosuppression protocols. For the treatment of rheumatoid arthritis or psoriasis, the starting dose is 2.5 mg/kg/day given as a divided dose twice a day.

Cyclosporine and cyclosporine modified are available in oral liquid formulations for those unable to swallow the capsules. The oral syringe enclosed with the cyclosporine solution should be used to measure the dose. The cyclosporine modified solution should be diluted with orange juice or apple juice in a glass container, stirred, and ingested immediately. The container should be rinsed with more diluent and should be consumed to ensure delivery of the entire dose. Grapefruit juice should be avoided because it can inhibit the metabolism of cyclosporine.[2]

Cyclosporine preparations exhibit a narrow therapeutic window. The concentration range between subtherapeutic levels, at which patients are at risk of developing acute rejection, and toxic levels, at which the patient is at risk of developing adverse effects, is narrow. Regular therapeutic drug monitoring is essential in maintaining cyclosporine levels within a target blood concentration range to maximize immunosuppression and minimize dose-related adverse effects.

Therapeutic and Toxic Concentrations (Blood)

Cyclosporine is a lipid-soluble compound that is approximately 20% bound to leukocytes and 40% bound to erythrocytes; 40% remains in the plasma fraction of blood where it is highly bound to lipoproteins which comprise a relatively small fraction of the plasma proteins.[3,4] Cyclosporine binding to these different blood elements is temperature dependent. Thus, assays performed on a sample other than whole blood must be done at 37°C. Otherwise, the therapeutic range needs to be temperature corrected for changes in protein binding. For this reason, whole blood is the preferred matrix for measurement.[5] Whereas cyclosporine is available in several different formulations, with different absorption characteristics it is the parent compound, cyclosporine, that is measured in the blood.

As can be seen from Table 5.2, nonspecific assays measure not only cyclosporine but its metabolites as well. Polyclonal and monoclonal fluorescence polarization immunoassays are most commonly used in clinical practice. Because the polyclonal assay also detects cyclosporine metabolites, the therapeutic range is substantially higher than that for the more specific monoclonal methods. As a general rule, high performance liquid chromatography (HPLC) assay results have the same range as monoclonal methods. While requiring more technical support, many institutions prefer the HPLC methods as they are less expensive than the monoclonal assays and it is easier to discern assay interference and to detect metabolites.

TABLE 5.2 **Cyclosporine Assay Methods and Therapeutic Range**

Assay	Serum/Plasma[a] (μg/L or ng/mL)	Whole Blood[a] (μg/L or ng/mL)
Monoclonal radioimmunoassay (RIA)	50–125	150–400
Fluorescence polarization immunoassay (FPIA)		
Polyclonal	150–400	200–800
Monoclonal	50–125	150–400
High-performance liquid chromatography (HPLC)	50–125	150–400

[a]Therapeutic range is variable and will depend on dosing interval (τ), time of sampling, assay technique, and temperature.

Clearly, clinicians must be aware of the assay procedure and biologic fluids used at their institution to ensure appropriate interpretation of cyclosporine concentrations. The lack of a single standard assay method has made it difficult to establish therapeutic ranges. When concentrations in whole blood are measured, most clinicians accept trough levels of 150 to 400 μg/L (ng/mL) as the target range, where allograft rejection and adverse effects are minimal. This range however, may be different depending on the type of transplant, time after transplant, and the use of other concomitant immunosuppressive drugs.

The goal of monitoring cyclosporine concentrations is to maximize the benefit to risk ratio so that the patient has an optimal chance of achieving a positive therapeutic outcome with minimal toxicity. Thus, low-risk patients (e.g., recipients of HLA-identical grafts or patients receiving other concurrent immunosuppressive therapy) might be acceptably controlled with lower-than-usual cyclosporine concentrations. Conversely, high-risk groups (including those with poorly HLA-matched grafts) might require higher cyclosporine concentrations to prevent allograft rejection.

Adverse Effects

The most common adverse effect associated with cyclosporine is renal dysfunction, which usually improves when the dose is decreased or the drug discontinued. Although the mechanism for nephrotoxicity is unclear, it may be related to cyclosporine-induced renal vasoconstriction. Because irreversible renal failure develops in some patients, the cyclosporine doses and target concentrations are often lowered in patients who show early signs of nephrotoxicity. Other dose-related adverse effects include neurotoxicity (headache, tremors, paresthesias, seizures) and hypertension.[6] Some other adverse effects associated with cyclosporine include hirsutism, gingival hyperplasia, nausea, opportunistic infections, and malignancies.

Bioavailability (F)

Cyclosporine is a highly lipophilic compound with limited and highly variable bioavailability. Cyclosporine undergoes pre-systemic metabolism via gut cytochrome P450 or more specifically CYP 3A4. In addition, cyclosporine is a substrate for P-glycoprotein, the drug efflux pump. These factors contribute in part to the incomplete and variable absorption. A low or variable bioavailability is a risk factor for allograft rejection.[7,8] The bioavailability of the oil-based formulation, Sandimmune, is approximately 30%. Peak concentrations occur in about 4 to 6 hours for the cyclosporine formulation and 1 to 2 hours after an oral dose for the cyclosporine modified formulations. Rapid gastrointestinal transit may also reduce the bioavailability and should be considered in a patient with diarrhea who is receiving oral cyclosporine.[9] One issue that is unique to liver transplant recipients during the immediate postoperative period is the lack of a sufficient amount of bile salts that are necessary for the adequate absorption of cyclosporine due to cholestasis or external biliary drainage. This problem can be overcome by administering the drug intravenously or by refeeding bile with the dose of cyclosporine to enhance solubility and absorption.[10] Bioavailability of cyclosporine modified is assumed to be approximately 30% but is probably more consistently absorbed than the original product. In addition, cyclosporine modified formulations do not require bile for emulsification and are absorbed in a similar fashion, even in the setting of external biliary drainage.[11]

Volume of Distribution (V)

The volume of distribution of cyclosporine is approximately 4 to 5 L/kg. This relatively large V is consistent with the observation that cyclosporine is significantly bound to plasma and blood elements, that the unbound portion in the plasma is less than 10%, and that it is probably extensively bound to tissues outside the vascular space.[12–14] Part of the variability in reported V can be attributed to the fact that cyclosporine exhibits two-compartment modeling with a substantial alpha or distribution phase.[12] The assay method and the type of biologic fluid assayed will influence the measured concentration and, therefore, the derived pharmacokinetic parameters. The uncertainty surrounding cyclosporine's volume of distribution does not influence its clinical use to a large degree because loading doses are seldom administered (see Clinical Application of Cyclosporine Pharmacokinetics).

Clearance (Cl)

Cyclosporine undergoes extensive metabolism via CYP 3A4 in the liver and gut to multiple metabolites. These metabolites are generally thought to be less active than the parent compound. The whole blood clearance by cyclosporine is approximately 5 to 10 mL/kg/min in adult patients, indicating that it is probably a drug with a low extraction ratio. In other words, its elimination is influenced primarily by the unbound cyclosporine concentration.[14,15] These clearance values are based on whole blood determinations and are lower than would be estimated using room temperature serum or plasma concentration data or those derived from nonspecific assay methods. There are a number of drugs that have been reported to influence the metabolism and clearance of cyclosporine (Table 5.3).

Half-Life (t½)

The average half-life calculated from the values indicated in the preceding sections and Equation 5.1 would suggest a value of approximately 7 hours.

TABLE 5.3   Immunosuppressive Drug-Drug Interactions

Drugs that inhibit cytochrome P450 (CYP 3A4) and P-glycoprotein[a] (and *increase* cyclosporine/tacrolimus/sirolimus concentrations)	
Calcium channel blockers	*Antifungal agents*
Diltiazem	Fluconazole
Nicardipine	Itraconazole
Verapamil	Ketoconacole
	Voriconazole
Antibiotics	*HIV protease inhibitors*
Clarithromycin	Indinavir
Erythromycin	Ritonavir
Others	
Danazol	
Grapefruits and grapefruit juice	
Nefazodone	
Drugs that induce cytochrome P450 (CYP 3A4) and P-glycoprotein[a] (and *decrease* cyclosporine/tacrolimus/sirolimus concentrations)	
Antibiotics	*Anticonvulsants*
Rifabutin	Carbamazepine
Rifampin	Phenobarbital
	Phenytoin
	Primidone
Others	
St. John's wort *(hypericum perforatum)*	

[a]This is a partial list of drugs that can interact with cyclosporine, tacrolimus, or sirolimus.

$$t_{1/2} = \frac{(0.693)(V)}{Cl} \qquad \text{[Eq. 5.1]}$$

$$= \frac{(0.693)(4.5 \text{ L/kg})}{(7.5 \text{ mL/kg/min})\left(\dfrac{60 \text{ min/hr}}{1000 \text{ mL/L}}\right)}$$

$$= 6.93 \text{ hr}$$

This half-life is variable, however, due to the uncertainty associated with the volume of distribution and clearance estimates for cyclosporine. The multi-compartmental nature of cyclosporine also may result in an underestimation of the terminal half-life and associated pharmacokinetic parameters. The most commonly reported values for cyclosporine half-life are in the range of 6 to 12 hours.

Time to Sample

Although there are a number of ways of monitoring cyclosporine therapy, the most widely used method is to sample the trough (just before the dose) concentration. However, this approach does not always correlate well with clinical outcomes. Cyclosporine exposure as represented by the area-under-the-concentration time curve (AUC_{0-12}) is a more sensitive method for predicting clinical outcomes. To determine the AUC_{0-12}, multiple blood samples over the 12-hour dosing interval are necessary. The added cost and inconvenience of multiple blood samples limits the widespread use of the AUC_{0-12} method. There is a poor correlation between trough levels and AUC with the cyclosporine formulation. Cyclosporine modified formulations show a stronger correlation between trough levels and AUC.[16] The improved predictability of cyclosporine exposure makes the trough level a more reliable aid for therapeutic drug monitoring in a clinical setting. Abbreviated AUC (or sparse-sampling) algorithms utilize a limited number of sampling points to estimate the AUC. Most of the variability in absorption occurs within the first 4 hours after administration of cyclosporine modified. The AUC_{0-4} is a very sensitive predictor for acute rejection.[17] The cyclosporine concentration at 2 hours after administration of Neoral (C_2) is the most accurate single-sample marker for AUC_{0-4}.[18] There is a 15-minute period before and after the 2-hour time point, during which the C_2 sample can be taken to remain within an acceptable margin of error. The precise timing of the sample dictates that this method of monitoring should be performed in a controlled environment, such as a hospital or clinic. Although not the most sensitive predictor for outcomes, the trough concentration is still the most commonly used method to monitor cyclosporine therapy.

Clinical Application of Cyclosporine Pharmacokinetics

Complex computer programs or relatively straightforward approaches can be used to evaluate a patient's pharmacokinetic parameters; however, in most cases the clinical result is essentially the same. When the cyclosporine concentration is low, the dose is increased; when the concentration is high, the dose is decreased. If the cyclosporine concentration is low, it is appropriate to evaluate patient adherence to the prescribed regimen and determine if any drugs have been added which might alter cyclosporine absorption or metabolism. If there are no easily correctable problems, most clinicians would increase the dose modestly, recognizing that the change in concentration should be approximately proportional to the change in the maintenance dose. If the cyclosporine concentration is high, it is important to first determine if the sample has been obtained at the appropriate time. In addition, patient adherence should be assessed as well as the potential for any drug–drug interactions that might account for the increased cyclosporine concentration. If the sample is valid, many clinicians will hold a dose and then restart on a proportionally lower maintenance dose, or simply lower the dose to bring the cyclosporine concentration into the desired range. Occasionally, patients have an isolated elevated or decreased cyclosporine concentration for which no logical explanation can be found. The patient should be assessed to determine if he or she is clinically stable, and the clinician should then recheck the cyclosporine concentration as soon as reasonably possible.

Question #1. *R.I., a 39-year-old, 51-kg woman, received an unrelated renal transplant 1 year ago. Following transplantation, her serum creatinine stabilized in the range of 1.4 to 1.7 mg/dL. She has been receiving cyclosporine modified orally, 125 mg BID over the past 6 months. Cyclosporine concentrations have been 85 to 110 μg/L (whole blood HPLC assay). Her last clinic appointment was 3 weeks ago. Other immunosuppressive medications included prednisone 10 mg/day and mycophenolate mofetil 1000 mg BID. She returned to the clinic yesterday complaining of increasing fatigue since her last clinic appointment. Blood and urine cultures were taken, and she was admitted to the hospital with a serum creatinine of 2.8 mg/dL. How would you adjust R.I.'s cyclosporine modified dose to increase the cyclosporine concentration to approximately 200 μg/L?*

First, it is important to determine whether the rise in serum creatinine is due to graft rejection or cyclosporine toxicity. If the increase in serum creatinine is presumed to be a sign of allograft rejection, the patient would probably also receive additional acute immunosuppressant therapy including methylprednisolone and antithymocyte globulin (ATG) or muromonab (OKT3). A kidney biopsy will usually be obtained to definitively diagnose allograft rejection. Using approach number three as outlined in Part I: Interpretation of Drug Concentrations: Choosing a Model to Revise or Estimate a Patient's Clearance at Steady State, a revised set of pharmacokinetic parameters can be calculated:

First, we would start by estimating a revised elimination rate constant.

$$K_{Revised} = \frac{\ln\left(\dfrac{Css\ min + \dfrac{(S)(F)(Dose)}{V}}{Css\ min}\right)}{\tau} \qquad \text{[Eq. 5.2]}$$

The average cyclosporine concentration of approximately 100 µg/L would be used as the Css min, F would be 0.3, and the dose would be expressed as 125,000 µg. The V would have to be estimated (4.5 L/kg), and τ would be 12 hours. Using these values, the revised elimination rate constant is approximately 0.0807 hr^{-1}.

$$= \ln\left(\frac{100\ \mu g/L + \dfrac{(1)(0.3)(125{,}000\ \mu g)}{(4.5\ L/kg)(51\ kg)}}{100\ \mu g/L}\right) \Big/ 12\ hr$$

$$= \frac{\ln\left(\dfrac{263.4\ \mu g/L}{100\ \mu g/L}\right)}{12}$$

$$= 0.0807\ hr^{-1}$$

This $K_{Revised}$ would correspond to a clearance of 18.5 L/hr:

$$Cl = (K_{Revised})(V) \qquad \text{[Eq. 5.3]}$$

$$= (0.0807\ hr^{-1})(4.5\ L/kg)(51\ kg)$$

$$= (0.0807\ hr^{-1})(229.5\ L)$$

$$= 18.5\ L/hr$$

and a half-life of approximately 8 or 9 hours.

$$t\tfrac{1}{2} = \frac{0.693}{K} \qquad \text{[Eq. 5.4]}$$

$$= \frac{0.693}{0.0807\ hr^{-1}}$$

$$= 8.6\ hr$$

Using the revised pharmacokinetic parameters, a new dose can be calculated by rearranging Equation 5.5 to solve for dose.

$$\text{Css min} = \frac{\dfrac{(S)(F)(Dose)}{V}}{(1 - e^{-K\tau})}(e^{-K\tau}) \qquad \text{[Eq. 5.5]}$$

$$\text{Dose} = \frac{(Css\ min)(V)(1 - e^{-K\tau})}{(S)(F)(e^{-K\tau})} \qquad \text{[Eq. 5.6]}$$

Making the appropriate substitutions for Css min, V, S, F, K, and τ, a dose of approximately 250 mg can be calculated.

$$= \frac{(200\ \mu g/L)(4.5\ L/kg)(51\ kg)(1 - e^{-(0.0807)(12)})}{(1)(0.3)(e^{-(0.0807)(12)})}$$

$$= \frac{(200\ \mu g/L)(229.5\ L)(1 - 0.38)}{(1)(0.3)(0.38)}$$

$$= 249{,}631\ \mu g\ or \approx 250\ mg\ Q12h$$

Note that this dose adjustment to 250 mg every 12 hours is double the original dose of 125 mg every 12 hours and should result in a proportional change in the steady-state trough concentration. This method of using the desired change in the plasma concentration as the same ratio change for maintenance dose is useful as long as the dosing interval is not altered. Because the dosing interval remains the same, this is the most common method of adjusting the cyclosporine dose. Most clinicians do not calculate the elimination rate constant or clearance values associated with steady-state trough concentrations of cyclosporine. They simply make a proportional or clinically reasonable change.

Question #2. *E.R., a 48-year-old, 59-kg male patient, received a living-related renal transplant 1.5 years ago. He is currently receiving Sandimmune 300 mg orally as the solution BID and, in addition, prednisone 5 mg/day and azathioprine 75 mg/day. E.R.'s current serum creatinine is 2.1 mg/dL and his steady-state cyclosporine trough concentration is 590 μg/L. The physician has ruled out the possibility of rejection and believes that the recent rise in serum creatinine is due to cyclosporine toxicity. What questions would one ask E.R. and how would one adjust his cyclosporine regimen to achieve a new steady-state cyclosporine concentration of approximately 200 μg/L?*

First, confirm that E.R. has been taking his Sandimmune 300 mg BID as prescribed and determine if any new medications have been added to his regimen or if he has consumed grapefruits or grapefruit juice. Also verify the time of sampling relative to when he took his last dose to ensure that the level is in fact a trough and not a peak concentration. If there are no easily correctable reasons for the elevated cyclosporine level, at least one cyclosporine dose should be held and then E.R. should be restarted on a new regimen. The dose decrease should approximate the proportionate decrease in cyclosporine concentration that is desired:

$$\text{Desired Dose} = \frac{\text{Css Desired}}{\text{Css Current}} \times \text{Current Dose} \qquad \text{[Eq. 5.7]}$$

Using the current steady-state cyclosporine concentration of 590 μg/L and the new target concentration of 200 μg/L, the new cyclosporine dose is approximately 100 mg.

$$\text{Desired Dose} = \frac{200 \ \mu g/L}{590 \ \mu g/L} \times 300 \text{ mg}$$

$$= 0.339 \times 300 \text{ mg}$$

$$= 101.7 \text{ mg or} \approx 100 \text{ mg}$$

This new dose assumes that the bioavailability remains the same and that the drug will be administered at the same interval of 12 hours. It is unclear why E.R. requires a lower than average cyclosporine dose (200 mg/day or ≈3.4 mg/kg/day). He may be absorbing more than the usual 30%, his hepatic metabolism may be unusually low, or a combination of both factors may be contributing.

Question #3. *M.J., a 78-kg liver transplant patient, is receiving 200 mg/day of cyclosporine as a continuous IV infusion. Currently, his hepatic function tests appear to be stable, and for the past 3 days he has been improving clinically with steady-state cyclosporine concentrations of approximately 220 μg/L. What would be an appropriate oral cyclosporine dose for M.J.?*

Because the usual bioavailability for cyclosporine is approximately 30%, most clinicians give an oral dose that is 3 times the parenteral dose. In this case, it would be approximately 600 mg/day, or 300 mg every 12 hours. Some clinicians prefer dividing the dose to reduce the volume of cyclosporine liquid or the number of capsules per dose. Dividing the daily dose should maintain the same steady-state average concentration but increase the trough and decrease the peak concentrations. This is because when the same rate of drug administration is given as smaller doses more often, a constant infusion model is more closely approximated and the peak and trough concentrations are moving toward the steady state average (see Part I: Interpretation of Plasma Drug Concentrations: Revising Pharmacokinetic Parameters: Clearance, Figure 31). Again, pharmacokinetic calculations could have been performed; however, the outcome would have been essentially the same as adjusting the dose in proportion to the desired change in steady-state plasma concentration.

In this case we have the additional factor of a change in route and, therefore, bioavailability to consider:

$$\text{New Dose} = \frac{\text{Css Desired}}{\text{Css Current}} \times \frac{\text{F Current}}{\text{F New Dosage Form}} \times \text{Current Dose} \qquad \text{[Eq. 5.8]}$$

Assuming the reported cyclosporine concentration of 220 µg/L is acceptable, the new dose will be approximately 600 mg/day.

$$= \frac{220 \ \mu g/L}{220 \ \mu g/L} \times \frac{1.0}{0.3} \times 200 \ mg$$

$$= 1 \times 3.33 \times 200 \ mg$$

$$= 666 \ mg \approx 600 \ mg$$

Again, if the dose is divided and given as 300 mg every 12 hours, trough levels will be somewhat higher than those produced by single daily doses. However, the bioavailability will probably be a more important influence on the trough cyclosporine concentration.

Question #4. *A.H. is a 63-year-old woman who received a liver transplant 10 years ago. She was taking a stable regimen of Sandimmune 150 mg PO BID and prednisone 5 mg PO QD, with a cyclosporine level 150 ng/mL 1 month ago. Since then, she had a surgical procedure to relieve a bile duct obstruction. As a result of the procedure, A.H. received a T-tube drain (a tube that will drain the bile into an external bag). Her cyclosporine level in the clinic yesterday was 25 ng/mL. A.H. states that she is compliant with her medication regimen and has not taken any new medications or changed the way that she takes her medications. What would account for A.H.'s low cyclosporine concentration?*

Cyclosporine (Sandimmune) is an oil-based formulation that requires bile for absorption. Since A.H. received a T-tube that will drain the bile externally, there is insufficient bile in her gastrointestinal tract for emulsification of cyclosporine for absorption. A.H. could be re-fed her bile along with her cyclosporine dose or be changed to a cyclosporine modified product. For patients who are being switched from the Sandimmune formulation to one of the cyclosporine modified formulations, the same daily dose that was previously used for Sandimmune can be used (1:1 dose conversion). In patients who have poor or erratic absorption, the conversion from Sandimmune to cyclosporine modified may result in increased cyclosporine blood trough concentrations as the result of increased absorption with the cyclosporine modified formulation. The dose of cyclosporine modified should be adjusted to obtain the desired cyclosporine blood trough concentration. The cyclosporine blood trough concentration should be monitored closely until a stable target level is achieved. For many patients, the dose required for cyclosporine modified will be somewhat less than the dose that was being given as Sandimmune.

TACROLIMUS

Tacrolimus is a macrolide antibiotic with immunosuppressive effects that is used to prevent allograft rejection. Whereas tacrolimus has a chemical structure similar to sirolimus, its mechanism of action is like that of cyclosporine. Tacrolimus, like cyclosporine, inhibits the activity of calcineurin, leading to a decrease in the production and release of IL-2. Tacrolimus is used as part of an immunosuppressive drug regimen to prevent allograft rejection.

KEY PARAMETERS: **Tacrolimus**	
Therapeutic Concentration[a]	5–20 ng/mL
F	25% (range: 4–93%)
V[b]	1 L/kg (range: 0.85–1.94 L/kg)
Cl[b]	0.04–0.083 L/kg/hr
$t^{1}/_{2}$	8–12 hours (range: 4–41 hours)
Free Fraction (α)[c]	1%

[a]Whole blood trough concentration. Target concentrations may vary with the organ(s) transplanted and transplant-center–specific immunosuppression protocols.
[b]Based on blood concentrations.
[c]The blood to plasma ratio is approximately 35 (range: 12–67), indicating extensive partitioning into blood cells. Tacrolimus is bound mainly to albumin and alpha-1 acid glycoprotein.

Tacrolimus is available as 0.5, 1, and 5 mg capsules and a solution for intravenous administration. The recommended initial oral dose of tacrolimus is approximately 0.2 mg/kg/day in kidney transplant recipients, 0.1 to 0.15 mg/kg/day in liver transplant recipients, and 0.15 to 0.2 mg/kg/day in pediatric liver transplant recipients. The oral doses are usually given as divided doses every 12 hours. The intravenous formulation must be diluted in 5% dextrose or 0.9% normal saline to a concentration of 0.004 to 0.02 mg/ml and given as a continuous infusion. The diluted infusion must not be stored in PVC containers or infused through PVC containing infusion sets, to minimize extraction of phthalates and adsorption onto the tubing. Intravenous tacrolimus is not commonly used because most patients can take it orally immediately after transplant, and it has an increased incidence of adverse effects compared to oral administration.

Tacrolimus, like cyclosporine and sirolimus, has a narrow therapeutic window and exhibits variability in its pharmacokinetic parameters. In addition, tacrolimus is also a substrate for CYP 3A4 and P-glycoprotein. There are many drugs known to be inhibitors or inducers of CYP 3A4 and P-glycoprotein. Table 5.3 lists commonly used drugs that can interact with tacrolimus. Like cyclosporine, therapeutic drug monitoring of tacrolimus is essential in optimizing immunosuppression and minimizing dose-related toxicity.

Therapeutic and Toxic Concentrations (Blood)

The therapeutic range of tacrolimus is 5 to 20 μg/L (ng/mL). Subtherapeutic tacrolimus concentrations are associated with an increased risk for allograft rejection, and levels above the therapeutic range are associated with increased risk for toxic effects (such as renal dysfunction, neurotoxicity, and hypertension).[19] There is considerable overlap between subtherapeutic levels and toxic levels. Patients may experience rejection and/or exhibit signs of toxicity even within the therapeutic range. The target blood concentrations of tacrolimus will vary according to the organ(s) transplanted, time after transplant, and transplant-center–specific immunosuppression protocols.

Adverse Effects

Tacrolimus is associated with a wide range of adverse effects. The most significant dose-related adverse effects include nephrotoxicity, post-transplant diabetes mellitus, neurotoxicity (headache, tremor, paresthesia, seizures), and hypertension. Other adverse effects include hyperkalemia, nausea, diarrhea, myocardial hypertrophy, opportunistic infections, and malignancies. The intravenous formulation contains castor oil, which can cause anaphylactic reactions.

Bioavailability (F)

The oral bioavailability of tacrolimus is poor. The bioavailability is approximately 25% (range: 4% to 93%).[20] The low bioavailability in part may be the result of pre-systemic metabolism in the gut wall by intestinal CYP 3A4 and the activity of the drug efflux pump, P-glycoprotein.[21,22] Tacrolimus is a lipophilic compound whose absorption is dissolution rate-limited. There may be delayed absorption in patients with impaired gut motility. Food decreases the rate and extent of tacrolimus absorption.[23] When tacrolimus is given with meals or after meals, the tmax increases 5- to 7-fold, the Cmax decreases by 39% to 77%, and the AUC decreases by 27% to 37%. To minimize variability of absorption, tacrolimus should be given consistently with or without food, preferably on an empty stomach to maximize absorption. Tacrolimus is rapidly absorbed, with peak concentrations being reached in approximately 0.5 to 2 hours after oral administration.

Volume of Distribution (V)

The volume of distribution of tacrolimus is greater than 20 L/kg when based on plasma concentration.[20] This indicates extensive distribution outside the plasma compartment. The blood to plasma ratio of 35 (range: 12 to 67) is consistent with extensive distribution into red blood cells. The volume of distribution is approximately 1 L/kg when based on blood concentration. The plasma protein binding of tacrolimus is approximately 99%. Tacrolimus is bound mainly to albumin and alpha-1-acid glycoprotein.

Clearance (Cl)

Tacrolimus is extensively metabolized in the liver and gut via CYP 3A4 to several hydroxylated and demethylated metabolites. Several of the metabolites have immunosuppressive activity.[24] The presence of active metabolites should be taken into consideration when using a tacrolimus assay that measures both the parent compound and its metabolites, such as the microparticulate enzyme immunoassay (MEIA) and enzyme-linked immunosorbent assay (ELISA) methods.

The systemic clearance of tacrolimus in plasma is very high, ranging from 0.6 to 5.4 L/kg/hr. However, the extensive distribution of tacrolimus into red blood cells limits its clearance from blood. Systemic clearance of tacrolimus in blood ranges from 0.04 to 0.083 L/kg/hr. Clearance decreases as hepatic function progressively declines. The clearance of tacrolimus is higher in children compared with adults.[25] Children require higher doses of tacrolimus to achieve similar target concentrations.[26]

Half-Life (t½)

The elimination half-life of tacrolimus is approximately 8 to 12 hours (range: 4 to 41 hours) and is prolonged in patients with impaired hepatic function.

Time to Sample

Tacrolimus blood levels are usually drawn just before the dose (trough). Given the elimination half-life of about 8 to 12 hours, it is reasonable to wait 24 to 36 hours after initiating or altering therapy before checking tacrolimus blood levels.

Question #5. *C.F. is a 55-year-old man who just received a liver transplant. His current immunosuppression regimen is intravenous methylprednisolone 160 mg/day and mycophenolate mofetil 1000 mg PO BID. His weight is 80 kg, and his serum creatinine is 1.1 mg/dL. What dose of tacrolimus would you recommend?*

The recommended starting dose is approximately 0.1 mg/kg/day given as 0.05 mg/kg every 12 hours.

$$\text{Daily Dose} = 80 \text{ kg} \times 0.1 \text{ mg/kg/day} = 8 \text{ mg/day}$$

$$\text{Administered Dose} = 4 \text{ mg PO every 12 hours}$$

Many clinicians will initiate therapy at lower doses and increase the dose over the next few days to determine if the patient will tolerate tacrolimus. Typical starting doses range from 1 to 2 mg PO every 12 hours and would be increased over the next few days to a target dose of 4 mg PO every 12 hours if tolerated.

Given the elimination half-life of approximately 8 to 12 hours, it is necessary to wait 24 to 36 hours (approximately 3.3 half-lives) to reach steady state after initiating or altering therapy. It would be reasonable to wait 2 days before checking tacrolimus blood levels. Tacrolimus concentrations are usually drawn as trough levels (just before the dose).

Clinically, tacrolimus blood levels are monitored on a daily basis during the immediate post-transplant period. The frequency of tacrolimus level monitoring decreases as the patient's condition becomes more stable.

Question #6. *L.J. is a 45-year-old woman who had a liver transplant. She is receiving a stable regimen of tacrolimus 4mg PO every 12 hours and prednisone 5 mg PO QD. Two weeks ago her tacrolimus level on this regimen was 12 ng/mL. She was prescribed diltiazem XR 300mg PO QD for hypertension 1 week ago, and now presents with headaches and tremors. Her serum creatinine is 1.4 mg/dL (baseline 1.1 mg/dL), and her tacrolimus level is 26 ng/mL. How can you account for the elevated tacrolimus level? How would you manage her tacrolimus dose to achieve a tacrolimus concentration of 10 to 15 ng/mL?*

L.J. is experiencing adverse effects as a result of elevated tacrolimus blood levels. Nephrotoxicity and neurotoxicity are related to tacrolimus concentration. In assessing the elevated tacrolimus level, one should determine if the tacrolimus blood level was drawn at the appropriate time relative to when the last dose was taken. Levels drawn too early may not represent trough levels. In addition, patient adherence should be assessed, and it should be determined if the patient is taking any medications or foods that may interact with tacrolimus.

Tacrolimus is primarily metabolized by CYP 3A4 in the liver and the gut, which accounts for a significant first-pass metabolism. In addition to being a substrate for CYP 3A4, tacrolimus is also a substrate for P-glycoprotein, the drug efflux pump in the gut. P-glycoprotein is a membrane-localized drug transporter found on the luminal face of enterocytes that pumps drug from the cells back into the lumen of the gut. Diltiazem is an inhibitor of both CYP 3A4 and P-glycoprotein. The net effect is increased absorption (from decreased gut wall metabolism) and decreased drug efflux. L.J. can be managed by either discontinuing diltiazem and choosing another antihypertensive agent that does not inhibit CYP 3A4 or by decreasing the dose of tacrolimus. The pharmacokinetics of tacrolimus are highly variable within an individual patient and between patients. It is reasonable to decrease the tacrolimus dose by one-half and to target a tacrolimus concentration range of 10 to 15 ng/ml using Equation 5.7.

$$\text{Desired Dose} = \frac{\text{Css Desired}}{\text{Css Current}} \times \text{Current Dose}$$

$$= \left(\frac{12 \text{ ng/mL}}{26 \text{ ng/mL}} \right) 8 \text{ mg/day}$$

$$= (0.461)8 \text{ mg/day}$$

$$= 3.7 \text{ mg/day} \approx 4 \text{ mg/day}$$

or

$$2 \text{ mg Q12h}$$

SIROLIMUS

Sirolimus is a macrolide antibiotic that has a chemical structure similar to tacrolimus. Although sirolimus and tacrolimus are structurally related,

KEY PARAMETERS: Sirolimus	
Therapeutic Concentration[a]	5–15 ng/mL
F[b]	
Liquid formulation	14%
Tablet formulation	18%
V[c]	12 L/kg
Cl[c,d]	139–221 ml/kg/hr
$t^1/_2$	62 hours
Fraction free (α)[e]	2–8%

[a]Trough blood concentration. Target concentrations may vary with the organ(s) transplanted and transplant-center–specific immunosuppression protocols.
[b]High-fat meals will increase the bioavailability of sirolimus by 23% to 35% (tablets and liquid, respectively).
[c]Volume of distribution and clearance are calculated as V/F and Cl/F, respectively. Therefore, true values are lower than those reported (see Sirolimus Volume of Distribution and Clearance).
[d]Sirolimus is extensively metabolized in the liver and is a substrate of CYP 3A4 and P-glycoprotein.
[e]In the plasma fraction, approximately 40% is associated with lipoproteins.

they have different mechanisms of action. Tacrolimus blocks the production of IL-2 by inhibiting calcineurin, whereas sirolimus prevents the IL-2 driven cell cycle progression. Sirolimus is usually used in combination with a calcineurin inhibitor, such as cyclosporine and prednisone, to prevent allograft rejection.

Sirolimus, like cyclosporine and tacrolimus, has a narrow therapeutic window and exhibits variability in its pharmacokinetic parameters. Sirolimus is also a substrate for CYP 3A4 and P-glycoprotein. There are many drugs known to interact with sirolimus. Table 5.3 lists commonly used drugs that can interact with sirolimus.

The typical loading dose of sirolimus is 6 to 15 mg (3 times the maintenance dose). The normal maintenance dose is 2 to 5 mg/day.

Sirolimus is available as 1 and 2 mg tablets and an oil-based oral solution (1 mg/ml). The solution should be mixed with at least 60 to 120 ml (2 to 4 ounces) of water or orange juice in a glass or plastic container. After drinking the mixture, the container should be rinsed with a similar volume of water or orange juice and consumed to maximize delivery of the dose.

Therapeutic and Toxic Concentrations (Blood)

The therapeutic range of sirolimus is 5 to 15 ng/mL. Concentrations less than 5 ng/mL are associated with an increased risk of rejection, and concentrations greater than 15 ng/mL are associated with an increased risk of adverse effects. The target concentration will vary according to the organ(s) transplanted and transplant-center–specific immunosuppression protocols. Results from assays may differ depending on methodology. Chromatographic methods such as high-performance liquid chromatography with ultraviolet detection (HPLC UV) or high-performance liquid chromatography with tandem mass-spectrometric detection (HPLC/MS/MS) will be approximately 20% lower than immunoassay techniques for whole blood concentrations.[27] Adjustments for the target levels should be made based on the assay used.

Adverse Effects

The most common adverse effects associated with sirolimus are dose-dependent hypertriglyceridemia, hypercholesterolemia, thrombocytopenia, and leukopenia. Other adverse effects include anemia, hypokalemia, impaired wound healing, formation of lymphoceles, rash, and increased risk of hepatic artery thrombosis in liver transplant recipients. While sirolimus has a chemical structure similar to tacrolimus, sirolimus is devoid of any nephrotoxic effects, commonly seen with tacrolimus.[28]

Bioavailability (F)

Sirolimus is a lipophilic compound with limited oral absorption. The systemic bioavailability of the liquid formulation is approximately 14%. When sirolimus is given with a high-fat meal, the area-under-the-concentration-time-curve (AUC) is increased by approximately 35%. To minimize variability, sirolimus should be taken consistently with or without food. The bioavailability of the tablets is about 27% higher relative to the solution, that is, the tablets are approximately 18% absorbed (F ≈ 0.18). Whereas the tablets are not bioequivalent to the liquid formulation, the 2 mg dose is clinically equivalent, and no dose adjustment is clinically necessary.

Volume of Distribution (V)

The volume of distribution of sirolimus is approximately 12 L/kg. This large volume of distribution was calculated from oral dosing. The reported value is V/F, indicating that the actual volume of distribution is in the range of one-tenth (assuming an oral bioavailability of 10%) to one-fifth (assuming an oral bioavailability of 20%) the reported value. Sirolimus extensively distributes in tissues. The blood-to-plasma ratio of sirolimus is about 36, indicating that sirolimus partitions extensively into blood cells. Sirolimus in the plasma is also extensively protein bound (approximately 92%) to albumin, alpha-1-acid glycoprotein, and lipoproteins.[29] Although sirolimus bioavailability is low, peak concentrations occur approximately 1 to 2 hours after an oral dose.

Clearance (Cl)

Sirolimus undergoes extensive metabolism. The clearance of sirolimus is approximately 139 to 221 mL/kg/hr. Like volume of distribution, the reported clearance values were determined following oral doses without taking into account the limited bioavailability (i.e., the clearance value is Cl/F). Therefore, the actual clearance of sirolimus is probably in the range of one-tenth to one-fifth the reported value, assuming an oral bioavailability of 10% to 20%. Sirolimus, like cyclosporine and tacrolimus, is a substrate for CYP 3A4 and P-glycoprotein. Drugs that inhibit CYP 3A4, such as the fluconazole, erythromycin, and diltiazem, can decrease the clearance of sirolimus and result in increased blood concentrations. Grapefruits and grapefruit juice can also inhibit CYP 3A4 and P-glycoprotein and should be avoided.

Half-Life (t½)

The elimination half-life of sirolimus is approximately 62 hours.[29]

Time to Sample

Because sirolimus has a relatively long half-life (approximately 62 hours), it is reasonable to wait at least 1 week (approximately 3 half-lives to achieve steady state) before drawing a whole blood concentration when initiating or changing therapy. Because the trough concentrations correlate well with the AUC, trough levels are most commonly used when monitoring sirolimus drug concentrations.

Question #7. *A.B. just received a cadaveric renal transplant. It is determined that A.B. will receive an immunosuppression regimen that utilizes sirolimus, cyclosporine modified, and prednisone. What dose of sirolimus should A.B. receive?*

Because sirolimus has a relatively long half-life, a loading dose is commonly used to achieve therapeutic concentrations in a timely fashion. The usual daily maintenance dose of sirolimus is 2 mg. The loading dose is typically 3 times the maintenance dose; in this case, 6 mg. A.B. should receive 6 mg of sirolimus as a loading dose immediately, then begin a maintenance dose of 2 mg per day starting the next day.

Question #8. *A.B. is to begin an immunosuppression regimen consisting of cyclosporine modified 300 mg PO BID, sirolimus 2 mg PO QD, and prednisone taper. Does it matter when A.B. takes his sirolimus?*

Sirolimus is typically given in combination with other immunosuppressive drugs (e.g., cyclosporine and prednisone). When sirolimus is administered simultaneously with cyclosporine-modified capsules, the Cmax and AUC of sirolimus are increased by 116 and 230%, respectively. When sirolimus is administered 4 hours after cyclosporine capsules modified, the Cmax and AUC are increased by 37% and 80%, respectively. It is recommended by the manufacturer to administer sirolimus 4 hours after cyclosporine modified. The Cmax and AUC of cyclosporine did not change when sirolimus was administered simultaneously or 4 hours after cyclosporine modified. Clinically, the most important factor is for the patient to consistently take their medications at the same time of the day to minimize variations. Some patients may find it easier to take their dose of sirolimus with their dose of cyclosporine modified. While this will result in an increased exposure (AUC) to sirolimus, the most important factor is for the patient to do this consistently, so that the blood concentrations can be interpreted appropriately and the dosage regimen adjusted if necessary.[29,30]

Question #9. *A.B. is being given sirolimus in a liquid formulation during his hospital stay. He mixes his daily dose with orange juice but does not like the taste. Can A.B. be switched to the tablet formulation?*

Sirolimus is available in a liquid and tablet formulation. The liquid formulation must be mixed with water or orange juice. Other liquids for dilution are not to be used. Many patients complain of an unpleasant taste. The tablet formulation may be more convenient in an outpatient setting, since it does not need to be refrigerated or diluted with water or orange juice. A.B. can be switched from the liquid to the tablet formulation at the same dose of 2 mg/day.

Question #10. *C.G. was taking a stable regimen of cyclosporine modified 200 mg PO BID, sirolimus 2 mg PO QD, and prednisone*

10 mg PO QD. Her cyclosporine concentration was 200 ng/mL (via HPLC assay) and sirolimus level was 9 ng/mL on this regimen. C.G. was started on itraconazole 200 mg PO QD to treat a fungal infection. Two weeks later, her platelet count decreased from 200K to 75K, and her WBC decreased from 7K to 2.5K. Her latest cyclosporine blood level was 470 ng/mL and sirolimus level was 22 ng/mL. What could account for her thrombocytopenia and leukopenia and elevated cyclosporine and sirolimus levels?

Patient adherence should always be assessed. In addition, it should be determined if there have been any changes to C.G.'s medication regimen and how C.G. takes her sirolimus. It appears that C.G. was on a stable immunosuppression regimen, with therapeutic cyclosporine and sirolimus blood levels. She was recently started on itraconazole. Itraconazole is a potent inhibitor of CYP 3A4 and P-glycoprotein. Sirolimus is a substrate for both CYP 3A4 and P-glycoprotein. Itraconazole will decrease the metabolism of sirolimus and cyclosporine and result in increased blood levels of both. The elevated blood levels of sirolimus could account for her thrombocytopenia and leukopenia. Since C.G. is manifesting toxicity (leukopenia, thrombocytopenia) from a supratherapeutic level of sirolimus, a lower dose of sirolimus would be warranted. The blood concentration of sirolimus is dose proportional over a wide range. If her dose of sirolimus was lowered to 1 mg/day, her sirolimus dose would be estimated to be approximately 11 ng/mL. Alternatively, she could be given another appropriate antifungal regimen that did not inhibit CYP 3A4 and be maintained on her current immunosuppression regimen.

REFERENCES

1. Wahlberg J, et al. Consistent absorption of cyclosporine from a microemulsion formulation assessed in stable renal transplant recipients over a one-year study period. Transplantation 1995;60:648–652.
2. Yee GC, et al. Effect of grapefruit juice on blood cyclosporine concentration. Lancet 1995;345:955–956.
3. LeMarie M, Tillement JP. Role of lipoproteins and erythrocytes in the in vivo binding and distribution of cyclosporin A in the blood. J Pharm Pharmacol 1982;34:715–718.
4. Niederberger W, et al. Distribution and binding of cyclosporine in blood and tissue. Transplant Proc 1983;15:2419–2421.
5. Oellerich M, et al. Lake Louise Consensus Conference on Cyclosporin Monitoring in Organ Transplantation: report of the consensus panel. Ther Drug Monit 1995;17: 642–654.
6. De Groen PC, et al. Central nervous system toxicity after liver transplantation: the role of cyclosporine and cholesterol. N Engl J Med 1987;317:861–866.
7. Kahan BD, et al. Variable absorption of cyclosporine: a biopharmaceutical risk factor for chronic renal allograft rejection. Transplantation 1996;62:599–606.
8. Lindholm A, Kahan BD. Influence of cyclosporine pharmacokinetics trough concentrations, and AUC monitoring on outcomes after kidney transplantation. Clin Pharmacol Ther 1993;54:205–218.

9. Atkinson K, et al. Oral administration of cyclosporine A for recipients of allogeneic marrow transplants: implications of clinical gut dysfunction. Br J Haematol 1984;56:223–31.

10. Merion RM, et al. Bile refeeding after liver transplantation and avoidance of intravenous cyclosporine. Surgery 1989;106:604.

11. Levy G, et al. Cyclosporine in liver transplant patients. Transplant Proc 1994;26: 3184–3187.

12. Gupta SK, et al. Pharmacokinetics of cyclosporine: influence of the rate-duration profile of an intravenous infusion in renal transplant patients. Br J Clin Pharmacol 1989;27:353.

13. Lindholm A, et al. Intraindividual variability in the relative systemic availability of cyclosporine after oral dosing. Eur J Clin Pharmacol 1988;34:461.

14. Ptachcinski RJ, et al. Cyclosporine kinetics in renal transplantation. Clin Pharmacol Ther 1985;38:296.

15. Yee GC, et al. Blood cyclosporine pharmacokinetics in patients undergoing marrow transplantation: influence of age, obesity, and hematocrit. Transplantation 1988;46:399.

16. Kahan BD, et al. The Neoral formulation: improved correlation between cyclosporine trough levels and exposure in stable renal transplant recipients. Transplant Proc 1994; 26:2940.

17. Levy G, Thervet E, Lake J, Uchida K. Patient management by Neoral® C2 monitoring: an international consensus statement. Transplantation 2002;73(Suppl):S12–S18.

18. Nashan B, Cole E, Levy G, Thervet E. Clinical validation studies of Neoral® C_2 monitoring: a review. Transplantation. 2002;73(Suppl):S3–S11.

19. Kershner RP, Fitzsimmons WE. Relationship of FK506 whole blood concentrations and efficacy and toxicity after liver and kidney transplantation. Transplantation 1996;62: 920–926.

20. Venkataramanan R, et al. Clinical pharmacokinetics of tacrolimus. Clin Pharmacokinet 1995;29:404–430.

21. Tuteja S, Alloway RR, Johnson JA. The effect of gut metabolism on tacrolimus bioavailability in renal transplant recipients. Transplantation 2001;71:1303–1307.

22. Mancinelli LM, et al. The pharmacokinetics and metabolic disposition of tacrolimus: a comparison across ethnic groups. Clin Pharmacol Ther 2001;69:24–31.

23. Kimikawa M, Kamoya K, Toma H, Teraoka S. Effective oral administration of tacrolimus in renal transplant recipients. Clin Transplant 2001;15:324–329.

24. Plosker GL, Foster RH. Tacrolimus: A further update of its pharmacology and therapeutic use in the management of organ transplantation. Drugs 2000;59:323–389.

25. Wallemacq PE, Verbeeck RK. Comparative clinical pharmacokinetics of tacrolimus in paediatric and adult patients. Clin Pharmacokinet 2001;40:283–295.

26. McDiarmid SV, Colonna JO, Shaked A, Vargas J, Ament ME, Busuttil RW. Differences in oral FK506 dose requirements between adult and pediatric liver transplant patients. Transplantation 1993;55:1328–1332.

27. Shaw LM, Kaplan B, Brayman KL. Advances in therapeutic drug monitoring for immunosuppressants: a review of sirolimus. Clin Ther 2000;22(Suppl B):B1–B13.

28. Kahan BD, et al. Therapeutic drug monitoring of sirolimus: correlations with efficacy and toxicity. Clin Transplant 2000;14:97–109.

29. Zimmerman J, Kahan BD. Pharmacokinetics of sirolimus in stable renal transplant patients after multiple oral dose administration. J Clin Pharmacol 1997;37:405–415.

30. Kaplan B, Meier-Kriesche HU, Napoli KL, Kahan BD. The effects of relative timing of sirolimus and cyclosporine microemulsion formation coadministration on the pharmacokinetics of each agent. Clin Pharmacol Ther 1998;63:48–53.

6

LIDOCAINE

Kevin Y. Ohara and Michael E. Winter

Lidocaine is a local anesthetic agent with antiarrhythmic properties; it is used for the acute treatment of severe ventricular arrhythmias.[1,2] In recent years the value of lidocaine versus other agents in acute cardiac arrest has been questioned. However, lidocaine is still one of the most common agents used for the acute treatment of ventricular arrhythmias. Lidocaine has poor oral bioavailability, is almost exclusively metabolized by the liver, and has a relatively short duration of action. For these reasons, lidocaine is almost always administered initially as a bolus dose of 1 to 1.5 mg/kg followed by a continuous infusion of approximately 1 to 4 mg/min. Because of the two-compartment modeling and rapid distribution of lidocaine, there are multiple schemes that have been used to rapidly achieve and then maintain the therapeutic effects. These usually include a combination of several small bolus doses of 0.5 to 1.0 mg/kg or an initial infusion rate of approximately 8 mg/min for 10 to 20 minutes followed by a reduction in the infusion rate to the usual maintenance rate of 1 to 4 mg/min.[3-5] Lidocaine has a narrow therapeutic index, and toxic effects are generally dose or concentration related. Furthermore, conditions such as congestive heart failure, liver dysfunction, severe trauma, critical illness, and concurrent medications may alter the pharmacokinetics of lidocaine and, therefore, the expected therapeutic responses to usual doses. The application of pharmacokinetic principles to the individualization of lidocaine dosing can be invaluable. Nevertheless, lidocaine's short half-life and use in acute treatment require a short assay turnaround time for optimal therapeutic drug monitoring.

THERAPEUTIC AND TOXIC PLASMA LEVELS

Lidocaine plasma concentrations of 1 to 5 mg/L are usually associated with therapeutic control of ventricular arrhythmias.[6-9] Minor central nervous system (CNS) side effects (e.g., dizziness, mental confusion, and blurred vision) can be observed in patients with plasma concentrations as low as 3 to 5 mg/L. Although seizures have occurred at plasma lidocaine concentrations as low as 6 mg/L, they are usually associated with concentrations exceeding 9 mg/L.[6-8,10,11] Lidocaine does not usually cause hemodynamic changes, but hypotension associated with myocardial depression has been observed in a patient whose plasma lidocaine concentration

KEY PARAMETERS: Lidocaine

Therapeutic Plasma Concentrations		1–5 mg/L	
F		1.0 (IV)	
S		0.87	
	Normal	CHF	Cirrhosis
Vi	0.5 L/kg	0.3 L/kg	0.61 L/kg
V	1.3 L/kg	0.88 L/kg	2.3 L/kg
$\alpha\ t\frac{1}{2}$	8 min	8 min	8 min
$\beta\ t\frac{1}{2}$	100 min	100 min	300 min
Cl	10 mL/kg/min	6 mL/kg/min	6 mL/kg/min

was 5.3 mg/L.[12] In addition, there are reports of sinus arrest following rapid intravenous injection[13] and conduction disturbances in patients with hyperkalemia.[14]

VOLUME OF DISTRIBUTION (V)

A two-compartment model can describe the distribution of lidocaine following an intravenous bolus (see Part I: Figure 9). The initial volume of distribution (Vi) appears to be approximately 0.5 L/kg, and the final volume following distribution (V) is approximately 1.3 L/kg.[10,11] The volume of distribution seems to increase in proportion to weight. Therefore, total body weight should be used to calculate the volume of distribution of lidocaine in obese subjects.[15] This volume of distribution, however, is not the initial or central compartment. Thus, it is not clear whether individual bolus doses that comprise the total loading dose ought to be adjusted. In addition, the volume of distribution reported in the previous study for both obese and non-obese subjects was approximately 2.7 L/kg. This value is larger than those normally reported and may be the result of dated analysis techniques or the specific patient populations studied. Unlike digoxin, the myocardium responds to lidocaine as though it is located in the initial volume (Vi). Therefore, the dose of each bolus injection of lidocaine should be based on Vi and not V. Plasma concentrations resulting from each bolus injection will fall as the drug distributes into the larger final volume of distribution. Therefore, the total loading dose should be calculated using the final volume of distribution (V). As stated previously, it is a common practice to initiate lidocaine therapy with a bolus dose of

1 to 1.5 mg/kg followed by a continuous infusion. It is often necessary to administer additional bolus doses to avoid loss of efficacy associated with the redistribution of the initial bolus into the tissue or peripheral compartment. Subsequent bolus doses are usually one-half of the initial bolus dose or in the range of 0.5 to 1.0 mg/kg. Because there is a residual lidocaine plasma concentration, smaller bolus doses minimize the potential risk of excessive distribution-phase concentrations and lidocaine toxicity.[3-5]

In congestive heart failure (CHF), both volumes of distribution for lidocaine are decreased: Vi is 0.3 L/kg and V is 0.88 L/kg.[11] This has also been seen in severe trauma and critically ill patients, in whom Vi is approximately 0.25 L/kg and V is approximately 0.75 L/kg[16,17] (critically ill was defined as ventilated patients in the intensive care unit suffering from systemic inflammatory response syndrome of various etiologies).[16] Both the total loading dose and the individual bolus injections should be reduced in these patients. In contrast, both volumes of distribution are increased with chronic liver disease: Vi is 0.61 L/kg and V is 2.3 L/kg.[11] Thus, slightly larger loading doses may be required in these patients. The increases in both volumes of distribution may be more prevalent with cirrhosis versus chronic active hepatitis.[18] Renal failure does not appear to alter the distribution of lidocaine.[11] In practice, the individual bolus dose is generally not adjusted for critical illness, severe trauma, CHF, or chronic liver disease; rather, the number of such doses required to achieve sustained antiarrhythmic effects would be expected to be fewer for critically ill patients and patients with severe trauma or CHF and greater for patients with chronic liver disease. For example, the total loading dose used in post-myocardial infarction patients with CHF should be approximately 40% lower than that used for similar patients without congestive failure.[11]

CLEARANCE (Cl)

Lidocaine has a high hepatic extraction ratio. Its clearance of 10 mL/kg/min (700 mL/min/70 kg) approximates plasma flow to the liver.[11,19,20] Less than 5% is cleared by the renal route. Because of the high first-pass effect, bioavailability (F) following oral administration is quite variable and F is usually in the range of 0.4.[21] This uncertainty in the systemic bioavailability by the oral route requires parenteral administration of lidocaine to ensure its efficacy.

CHF and hepatic cirrhosis decrease the clearance of lidocaine to about 6 mL/kg/min; therefore, a 40% reduction in the maintenance infusion is appropriate for patients with these conditions.[11,22,23] Severe trauma and critically ill patients also demonstrate a decrease in lidocaine clearance to about 6.8 mL/kg/min.[16,17] Because the drug is not cleared renally, no dose adjustment is required for patients with diminished kidney function. In obese subjects, the clearance of lidocaine appears to correlate more closely with the ideal body weight rather than total body weight. For this reason, maintenance infusions of lidocaine should be based on a subject's non-obese weight.[15]

Lidocaine is metabolized primarily to monoethylglycinexylidide (MEGX) and glycinexylidide (GX). MEGX appears to have activity similar to lidocaine. It is cleared by metabolism and, therefore, does not accumulate in renal failure. In contrast, approximately 50% of GX is cleared by the renal route and it, therefore, accumulates in patients with diminished renal function.[24] GX is less active than lidocaine and does not contribute to its therapeutic effect. The only known side effects of GX (i.e., headache and impaired mental performance) are dose related and occur at plasma concentrations >1.0 mg/L.[24] More serious toxicities have not been observed in patients with GX levels as high as 9 mg/L.[25]

HALF-LIFE (t½)

The lidocaine distribution half-life (α t$^1/_2$) of 8 minutes does not appear to be altered by heart failure, hepatic disease, or renal failure.

The elimination half-life (β t$^1/_2$) of lidocaine is a function of its volume of distribution and clearance as illustrated by Equation 6.1:

$$t\frac{1}{2} = \frac{(0.693)(V)}{Cl} \qquad \text{[Eq. 6.1]}$$

The usual elimination half-life for lidocaine is about 100 minutes.[11] It is unchanged in critically ill patients and patients with CHF or severe trauma, because both the volume of distribution and the clearance are reduced to a similar extent in these individuals.

Patients with liver disease have a lidocaine β half-life of about 300 minutes due to an increased volume of distribution and decreased clearance.[11] An elimination half-life of 200 minutes has been observed in healthy subjects following infusions lasting longer than 24 hours.[26] Because lidocaine concentrations continue to accumulate,[27,28] there is concern that patients receiving prolonged infusions of lidocaine may be at risk for lidocaine toxicity.[29] Also, the use of prophylactic lidocaine in acute myocardial infarction is not recommended.[2,30–32] For these reasons, the practice of using lidocaine prophylactically and continuing infusions longer than 24 hours is considered by some authors to carry a substantial risk of lidocaine toxicity and may increase mortality rates.[2,29–31]

TIME TO SAMPLE

Unless assay turnaround time is unusually short, lidocaine plasma concentrations should not be monitored until 4 to 8 hours have elapsed since the beginning of therapy. At this time, assay results should approximate steady-state concentrations. Plasma lidocaine concentrations obtained during the distribution phase following administration of a bolus dose may be useful to establish the relationship between lidocaine plasma concentration and efficacy. However, these plasma concentrations should not be used to adjust acute therapy unless the assay turnaround time is within minutes because plasma lidocaine concentrations change so rapidly. In most institutions, several hours and up to a day may be required for assay results; therefore, steady state for any given infusion dose will have been achieved by the time results are available (normal $t^{1}/_{2}$: 2 to 3 hours). For this reason, lidocaine assay results cannot be used to adjust the initial infusion or maintenance doses in most situations. Patients with cirrhosis who have a prolonged lidocaine half-life are an exception to this generalization. In most instances, lidocaine plasma concentrations are primarily used retrospectively to confirm clinical impressions. Lidocaine levels can also be used to assist in the evaluation of patients in whom the minor central nervous system side effects of dizziness or mental confusion are difficult or impossible to assess (e.g., those who are unconscious or are receiving other CNS depressant drugs). This would be especially true when the lidocaine infusion is likely to be continued for more than 12 to 24 hours. In these individuals, lidocaine levels might be used to evaluate slow accumulation toward concentrations that could be associated with seizures. This use of lidocaine concentrations is most applicable to patients whose cardiac output and, therefore, lidocaine clearance is declining.

Question #1. *P.M., a 55-year-old, 70-kg man, was admitted to the coronary care unit with a diagnosis of heart failure, probable myocardial infarction (MI), and hemodynamically compromising premature ventricular contractions (PVCs). Calculate a bolus dose of lidocaine that should achieve an immediate response for P.M. At what rate should this dose be administered?*

A lidocaine bolus dose can be calculated by using Equation 6.2 as shown below. Since lidocaine distribution follows a two-compartment model with the myocardium responding as though it were in the initial compartment, V in Equation 6.2 should be replaced with Vi (see the discussion on Lidocaine Volume of Distribution). The Vi for a patient with CHF is 0.3 L/kg (see Lidocaine Key Parameters) or 21 L for this 70 kg man.[11] S and F are assumed to be 0.87 and 1.0, respectively, for lidocaine. If it is assumed that peak levels should not exceed 3 mg/L to avoid toxicity, the appropriate bolus dose would be 70 mg:

$$\text{Loading Dose} = \frac{(V)(C)}{(S)(F)} \qquad \text{[Eq. 6.2]}$$

$$\text{Bolus Dose} = \frac{(Vi)(C)}{(S)(F)} \qquad \text{[Eq. 6.3]}$$

$$= \frac{(21\ L)(3\ mg/L)}{(0.87)(1)}$$

$$= 72\ mg\ or \approx 70\ mg$$

This bolus dose of 70 mg is essentially the same as the usually recommended dose of 1 to 1.5 mg/kg.[33] It should be given by slow IV push (25 to 50 mg/min).

Question #2. *Calculate a maintenance infusion rate that will achieve a steady-state plasma lidocaine concentration of 2 mg/L for P.M.*

The maintenance dose can be calculated from Equation 6.4. If it is assumed that a steady-state concentration of 2 mg/L is desired and if τ is assumed to be 1 minute, Cl to be 420 mL/min or 0.42 L/min (6 mL/kg/min $\times$ 70 kg) (see Lidocaine Key Parameters: CHF), S (0.87), and F (1), the maintenance dose would be calculated as follows:

$$\text{Maintenance Dose} = \frac{(Cl)(Css\ ave)(\tau)}{(S)(F)} \qquad \text{[Eq. 6.4]}$$

$$= \frac{(0.42\ L/min)(2\ mg/L)(1\ min)}{(0.87)(1)}$$

$$= 0.97\ mg/min$$

Although this calculated infusion is at the lower end of the frequently recommended infusion rates of 1 to 4 mg/min,[33] it is consistent with the conservative target steady-state level of 2 mg/L and the decreased clearance expected for P.M. who has CHF.

The assumed clearance value of 6 mL/kg/min for heart failure is an average value. Zito and Reid[34] have developed a scaling procedure in which the recommended lidocaine infusion rate is based on the degree of heart failure (Table 6.1). When lidocaine maintenance infusions were adjusted according to cardiac function in the clinical setting, significantly more patients were maintained within the usual therapeutic range for lidocaine. Although this study was restricted to individuals who had no evidence of heart failure or mild (clinical Class II) failure, it does point out the value of assessing cardiac status when determining a lidocaine maintenance infusion.[35] Others have also suggested utilizing cardiac output measurements to improve the predictive performance of population-based pharmacokinetic parameters.[36]

TABLE 6.1 Lidocaine Clearance Based on Degree of Heart Failure

Clinical Class	Symptoms	Apparent Lidocaine Clearance (mL/kg/min)
I	No heart failure	14.5
II	S₃ gallop and basilar pulmonary rales	5
III	Pulmonary edema	2.1
IV	Cardiogenic shock	2.1

Question #3. *P.M.'s PVCs were controlled by the 70 mg bolus dose of lidocaine and an infusion of 1 mg/min was begun. Fifteen minutes later, PVCs accompanied by a drop in blood pressure were again noted. What might account for the reappearance of the PVCs? What is an appropriate course of action at this point?*

The distribution half-life of lidocaine is about 8 minutes and the elimination half-life is 1.5 to 2 hours. Because 3 to 4 elimination half-lives (approximately 6 hours) must elapse before plasma lidocaine concentrations are at steady state, the recurrence of the PVCs 15 minutes after the bolus dose probably represents a declining plasma concentration caused by distribution rather than an inadequate maintenance dose. By rearranging the loading dose Equation 6.2:

$$\text{Loading Dose} = \frac{(V)(C)}{(S)(F)}$$

to form Equation 6.5 below, the plasma concentration (C°) resulting from the 70 mg bolus dose can be predicted by using the final volume of distribution (V) of 62 L (0.88 L/kg × 70 kg).

$$C^\circ = \frac{(S)(F)(\text{Loading Dose})}{(V)} \qquad \text{[Eq. 6.5]}$$

$$= \frac{(0.87)(1)(70 \text{ mg})}{(62 \text{ L})}$$

$$= 0.98 \text{ mg/L}$$

Since the predicted lidocaine concentration after distribution is approximately 1 mg/L, the total loading dose was probably too low and an additional bolus will be needed. It would be more rational to administer a second bolus dose rather than change the infusion rate. In practice, the second or third bolus doses are reduced by one-half to avoid excessive accumulation. In addition, some clinicians will increase the maintenance infusion for 20 to 30 minutes to allow for more rapid accumulation and then reduce the infusion back to the original rate.[3,5] An alternative approach to managing these breakthrough PVCs involves calculating the total loading dose required to achieve a final lidocaine concentration of 2 mg/L in V. The additional amount that would be required to fill this volume (total loading dose minus bolus doses already administered) could be administered over approximately 20 minutes. This approach prevents the breakthrough arrhythmias that result from tissue distribution of the initial intravenous bolus dose, but also reduces the CNS side effects caused by transiently elevated lidocaine concentrations associated with repeated bolus doses.[4,5,37]

If the PVCs had occurred several hours after starting the infusion, the most rational approach would have been to give a small bolus dose sufficient to increase the plasma concentration in the initial volume of distribution to 2 or 3 mg/L and to increase the infusion rate (maintenance dose) as well.

Question #4. *B.P., a 65-year-old, 70-kg man, was admitted with a diagnosis of hepatic encephalopathy and cirrhosis. On the fourth hospital day, he developed ventricular arrhythmias, and lidocaine was ordered. Calculate a bolus dose and a maintenance infusion rate that will achieve a steady-state lidocaine level of 2 mg/L.*

The following lidocaine pharmacokinetic parameters would be expected for a 70-kg patient with chronic liver disease:

Vi = 43 L (0.61 L/kg × 70 kg)

V = 161 L (2.3 L/kg × 70 kg)

Cl = 420 mL/min or 0.42 L/min or 25.2 L/hr (6 mL/kg/min × 70 kg)

As in Question 1, the initial bolus can be calculated from Equation 6.3, which replaces the term V in Equation 6.2 with Vi. Assuming a maximum plasma concentration of 3 mg/L in Vi is desired, the initial bolus should be 150 mg as calculated below:

$$\text{Bolus Dose} = \frac{(Vi)(C)}{(S)(F)}$$

$$= \frac{(43\ L)(3\ mg/L)}{(0.87)(1)}$$

$$= 148\ mg\ or \approx 150\ mg$$

This dose should be given no more rapidly than 25 to 50 mg/min. After final distribution, this 150 mg dose should result in a plasma level of 0.8 mg/L as shown below (Equation 6.5):

$$C^0 = \frac{(S)(F)(\text{Loading Dose})}{(V)}$$

$$= \frac{(0.87)(1)(150 \text{ mg})}{(161 \text{ L})}$$

$$= 0.8 \text{ mg/L}$$

Since this predicted plasma concentration is rather low, an additional bolus dose probably will be required. To avoid excessive accumulation, about one-half the original dose should be given.

The maintenance infusion can be calculated from Equation 6.4 using the expected clearance of 0.42 L/min and the desired steady-state lidocaine concentration of 2 mg/L:

$$\text{Maintenance Dose} = \frac{(Cl)(Css \text{ ave})(\tau)}{(S)(F)}$$

$$= \frac{(0.42 \text{ L/min})(2 \text{ mg/L})(1 \text{ min})}{(0.87)(1)}$$

$$= 0.97 \text{ mg/min}$$

Thus, a maintenance infusion of approximately 1 mg/min should achieve a steady-state plasma concentration of 2 mg/L.

Question #5. *Twelve hours after starting the infusion, B.P. appears to be more confused than usual. It is unclear whether his present condition is secondary to hepatic encephalopathy or lidocaine. Is it possible that the lidocaine is still accumulating and is causing the impaired mental state?*

The expected half-life for lidocaine in B.P. can be calculated from his assumed lidocaine Cl and V using Equation 6.1:

$$t\frac{1}{2} = \frac{(0.693)(V)}{Cl}$$

$$= \frac{(0.693)(161 \text{ L})}{25.2 \text{ L/hr}}$$

$$= 4.4 \text{ hr}$$

This calculated value of 4.4 hours is reasonably close to the value of 4.9 hours which is reported in the literature for patients with hepatic failure.[11] Since the expected half-life for lidocaine in this patient is 4 to 5 hours, steady-state levels may not have been achieved after 12 hours and his lidocaine levels may still be rising (see Part I: Half-Life) A STAT lidocaine concentration should be ordered to evaluate the contribution of lidocaine to B.P.'s altered mental status. If B.P.'s PVCs are well controlled, the maintenance infusion can also be decreased slowly with careful cardiac monitoring.

Question #6. *D.I., a 62-year-old, 60-kg man, has just had a myocardial infarction (MI) and has mild or Class II heart failure. On admission to the cardiac care unit, D.I. developed ventricular tachycardia and was treated successfully with an IV bolus dose of lidocaine followed by an infusion of 1.5 mg/min. D.I. had lidocaine levels at 24 and 48 hours of 3.5 mg/L and 4.5 mg/L, respectively. What are possible explanations for the 1 mg/L rise in the lidocaine level?*

Several studies have documented a slow rise in lidocaine concentrations in a number of patients. Even in healthy subjects, the apparent half-life of lidocaine after prolonged infusions appears to be increased.[22,23,26,27,29]

One very unlikely explanation for the slowly rising lidocaine levels is the possibility that the lidocaine level at 24 hours of 3.5 mg/L did not represent a steady-state concentration. If this were true, the volume of distribution for D.I. would have to be unrealistically large to account for the lidocaine concentration of 4.5 mg/L at 48 hours. It would be more realistic to assume an assay error of approximately 0.5 mg/L for each of the measured concentrations. Whereas this assay error exceeds the assumed confidence limit of 10%, it is more probable than an unusually large volume of distribution.

A change in clearance between the 24- and 48-hour time period that resulted in a change in the steady-state concentration could also explain this observation. Although this is possible, it would be more probable if one could identify a factor in D.I. associated with decreased clearance, such as a declining cardiac output or the addition of a beta-blocker to the medication regimen.[27]

The third and most likely explanation is that the plasma protein binding of lidocaine has changed as a result of an acute MI. Acute MI is only one of many conditions or disease states that have been associated with altered plasma binding of basic drugs (see Part I: Desired Plasma Concentrations). This rise in plasma binding is due to an increase in the α_1-acid glycoprotein (AAG) and it probably accounts for the slowly increasing concentrations of lidocaine in D.I. It is interesting to note that while the total lidocaine concentration is increased, the unbound concentration of lidocaine is relatively unaltered.[35,38] The rise in plasma protein occurs over the first 7 to 14 days and then declines slowly. Plasma protein concentrations remain elevated for 3 weeks following MI.[38,39]

Question #7. *D.F. is a 68-year-old, 60-kg woman with clinical Class II heart failure (see Table 6.1). She was given lidocaine for ventricular arrhythmias that occurred on postoperative day 1 following her car-*

diac surgery. She received an initial 60 mg bolus dose of lidocaine at 10:00 a.m. followed by 120 mg administered over the next 15 minutes (8 mg/min.) At 10:45 a.m. she was to be given a 2 mg/min constant infusion. Calculate her lidocaine concentration at the start of her maintenance infusion and at steady state.

To calculate D.F.'s lidocaine concentrations, it is first necessary to estimate her volume of distribution and clearance, taking into consideration her heart failure.

$$V = (0.88 \text{ L/kg})(60 \text{ kg}) = 52.8 \text{ L}$$

$$Cl = (5 \text{ mL/kg/min})(60 \text{ kg}) = 300 \text{ mL/min}$$

$$= (300 \text{ mL/min})(1 \text{ L/1000 mL}) = 0.3 \text{ L/min}$$

Next, using Equations 6.6 and 6.7, D.F.'s K and $t\frac{1}{2}$ can be calculated:

$$K = \frac{Cl}{V} \qquad \text{[Eq. 6.6]}$$

$$= \frac{0.3 \text{ L/min}}{52.8 \text{ L}}$$

$$= 0.0057 \text{ min}^{-1}$$

$$t\frac{1}{2} = \frac{0.693}{K} \qquad \text{[Eq. 6.7]}$$

$$= \frac{0.693}{0.0057 \text{ min}^{-1}}$$

$$= 122 \text{ min or} \approx 2 \text{ hr}$$

Note that the volume of distribution used was V rather than Vi because the plasma concentration was obtained approximately 30 minutes after the end of the infusion when distribution should be complete. To calculate the expected concentration at 10:45 a.m., Equations 6.8 and 6.9 can be combined. When the appropriate doses, times, and pharmacokinetic parameters are inserted into the equation, a lidocaine plasma concentration of 2.3 mg/L is calculated.

$$C_1 = \frac{(S)(F)(\text{Loading Dose})}{V}(e^{-Kt_1}) \qquad \text{[Eq. 6.8]}$$

$$C_1 = \frac{(S)(F)(Dose/t_{in})}{Cl}(1 - e^{-Kt_{in}})(e^{-Kt_1}) \qquad \text{[Eq. 6.9]}$$

$$C_1 = \frac{(S)(F)(\text{Loading Dose})}{V}(e^{-Kt_1}) + \frac{(S)(F)(Dose/t_{in})}{Cl}(1 - e^{-Kt_{in}})(e^{-Kt_1})$$

$$C_t = \frac{(0.87)(1)(60\ mg)}{52.8\ L}(e^{-(0.0057\ min^{-1})(45\ min)}) +$$

$$\frac{(0.87)(1)(120\ mg/15\ min)}{0.3\ L/min}(1 - e^{-(0.0057\ min^{-1})(15\ min)})(e^{-(0.0057\ min^{-1})(30\ min)})$$

$$= (0.99\ mg/L)(0.77) + (23.2\ mg/L)(1 - 0.92)(0.84)$$

$$= (0.76\ mg/L) + (1.56\ mg/L)$$

$$= 2.3\ mg/L$$

In the above, t_1 in the loading dose part of the equation is the time from the start of the 60 mg bolus dose to the time when the 2 mg/min infusion was started (i.e., 45 minutes). In the infusion part of the equation, tin refers to the duration of the infusion (i.e., 15 minutes), and t_1 is the time from the end of that 15 minute infusion until the start of the 2 mg/min maintenance infusion (i.e., 30 minutes). Note that Equations 6.8 and 6.9 are likely to underestimate the actual lidocaine concentration immediately after the bolus dose and during the 15-minute infusion. This is due to the two-compartment modeling and the fact that distribution is not yet complete.

The expected steady-state plasma concentration produced by the 2 mg/min infusion can be calculated using Equation 6.10.

$$\text{Css ave} = \frac{(S)(F)(Dose/\tau)}{Cl} \qquad \text{[Eq. 6.10]}$$

$$= \frac{(0.87)(1)(2\ mg/min)}{0.3\ L/hr}$$

$$= 5.8\ mg/min$$

This calculated steady-state lidocaine concentration of 5.8 mg/L is somewhat high and suggests that a reduction in the maintenance infusion may be warranted. Reducing the lidocaine infusion by one-half would reduce the steady-state plasma concentration by one-half to 2.9 mg/L. If the lidocaine infusion is not decreased, the patient should be monitored carefully for signs of lidocaine toxicity.

REFERENCES

1. Griffith MJ, et al. Relative efficacy and safety of intravenous drugs for termination of sustained ventricular tachycardia. Lancet 1990;336:670–673.

2. Guidelines 2000 for cardiopulmonary resuscitation and emergency cardiovascular care. Circulation 2000;102(Suppl I):I112–I128.

3. Greenblatt DJ, et al. Pharmacokinetic approach to the clinical use of lidocaine intravenously. JAMA 1976;236:273–277.

4. Riddell JG, et al. A new method for constant plasma drug concentration: application to lidocaine. Ann Intern Med 1984;100:25–28.

5. Salzer LB, et al. A comparison of methods of lidocaine administration in patients. Clin Pharmacol Ther 1981;29:617–624.

6. Gianelly R, et al. Effect of lidocaine on ventricular arrhythmias in patients with coronary heart disease. N Engl J Med 1967;277:1215–19.

7. Jewett DE, et al. Lidocaine in the management of arrhythmias after acute myocardial infarction. Lancet 1968;1:266.

8. Selden R, Sasahara AA. Central nervous system toxicity induced by lidocaine. JAMA 1967;202:908–9.

9. Lie KI, et al. Lidocaine in the prevention of primary ventricular fibrillation. N Engl J Med 1974;291:1324–1326.

10. Benowitz N. Clinical application of pharmacokinetics of lidocaine. In: Melmon K, ed. Cardiovascular Drug Therapy. Philadelphia: FM Davis, 1974:77–101.

11. Thomson PD. Lidocaine pharmacokinetics in advanced heart failure, liver disease, and renal failure in humans. Ann Intern Med 1973;78:499–508.

12. Stannard M, et al. Hemodynamic effects of lignocaine in acute myocardial infarction. Br Med J 1968;2:468.

13. Cheng TO, Wadhwa K. Sinus standstill following intravenous lidocaine administration. JAMA 1973;223:790–2.

14. Mclean SA, et al. Lidocaine-induced conduction disturbance in patients with systemic hyperkalemia. Ann Emerg Med. 2000;36:615–618.

15. Abernethy DR, Greenblatt DJ. Lidocaine disposition in obesity. Am J Cardiol 1984;53:1183–1186.

16. Berkenstadt H, et al. The pharmacokinetics of morphine and lidocaine in critically ill patients. Intensive Care Med 1999;25:110–112.

17. Berkenstadt H, et al. The pharmacokinetics of morphine and lidocaine in nine severe trauma patients. J Clin Anesth 1999;11:630–634.

18. Testa R, et al. Lidocaine elimination and monoethylglycinexylidide formation in patients with chronic hepatitis or cirrhosis. Hepatogastroenterology 1998;45:154–159.

19. Wilkinson GR. A physiological approach to hepatic drug clearance. Clin Pharmacol Ther 1975;18:377–90.

20. Pang KS, Rowland M. Hepatic clearance of drugs: I. Theoretical considerations of a "well-stirred" model and a "parallel tube" model. Influence of hepatic blood flow, plasma and blood cell binding and hepatocellular enzymatic activity on hepatic drug clearance. J Pharmacokinet Biopharm 1977;5:625–53.

21. Huet PM, et al. Bioavailability of lidocaine in normal volunteers and cirrhotic patients. Clin Pharmacol Ther 1979;25:229–230.

22. Prescott LF, et al. Impaired lignocaine metabolism in patients with myocardial infarction and cardiac failure. Br Med J 1976;1:939–41.

23. Prescott LF, Nimmo J. Plasma lidocaine concentrations during and after prolonged infusion in patients with myocardial infarction. In: Scott DB, Julian DG, eds. Lidocaine in the Treatment of Ventricular Arrhythmias. Edinburgh: E & S Livingstone, 1971:168.

24. Collingsworth KA, et al. Pharmacokinetics and metabolism of lidocaine in patients with renal failure. Clin Pharmacol Ther 1975;18:59–64.

25. Strong JM, et al. Pharmacological activity, metabolism, and pharmacokinetics of glycinexylidide. Clin Pharmacol Ther 1975;17:184–194.

26. Le Lorier J, et al. Pharmacokinetics of lidocaine after prolonged intravenous infusions in uncomplicated myocardial infarction. Ann Intern Med 1977;87:700–6.

27. Ochs HR, et al. Reduction in lidocaine clearance during continuous infusion and by coadministration of propranolol. N Engl J Med 1980;303:373–377.

28. Morgan DJ, et al. Prediction of acute myocardial disposition of antiarrhythmic drugs. J Pharm Sci 1989;78:384–388.

29. Zeisler JA, et al. Lidocaine therapy: time for re-evaluation. Clin Pharmacy 1993;12:527–528.

30. Hine LK, et al. Meta-analytic evidence against prophylactic use of lidocaine in acute myocardial infarction. Arch Intern Med 1989;149:2694–2698.

31. Sadowski ZP, et al. Multicenter randomized trial and a systematic overview of lidocaine in acute myocardial infarction. Am Heart J 1999;1137:792–798.

32. Alexander JH, et al. Prophylactic lidocaine use in acute myocardial infarction: incidence and outcomes from two international trials. Am Heart J 1999;137:799–805.

33. Anderson JL, et al. Anti-arrhythmic drugs: clinical pharmacology and therapeutic uses. Drugs 1978;15:271–309.

34. Zito RA, Reid P. Lidocaine kinetics predicted by indocyanine green clearance. N Engl J Med 1978; 298:1160–3.

35. Lopez LM, et al. Optimal lidocaine dosing in patients with myocardial infarction. Ther Drug Monit 1982;4:271–6.

36. Kuipers JA, et al. Modeling population pharmacokinetics of lidocaine: should cardiac output be included as a patient factor? Anesthesiology 2001;94:566–573.

37. Stargel WW, et al. Clinical comparison of rapid infusion and multiple injection methods for lidocaine loading. Am Heart J 1981;102:872–6.

38. Edwards DJ, et al. Alpha-1-acid glycoprotein concentration and protein binding in trauma. Clin Pharmacol Ther 1982;31:62–7.

39. Fremstad D, et al. Increased plasma binding of quinidine after surgery. A preliminary report. Eur J Clin Pharmacol 1976;10:441–4.

7

LITHIUM

Patrick R. Finley and Michael E. Winter

Lithium is a monovalent cation that has been used for more than 50 years in the treatment and prevention of various psychiatric conditions. Most commonly, lithium salts have been prescribed to prevent future manic or depressive episodes (i.e., maintenance or prophylactic therapy). Ordinarily, lithium is administered as the carbonate salt formulation which contains 8.12 mEq of lithium per 300 mg tablet or capsule. Lithium carbonate is also available as extended-release capsules, in strengths of 300 mg (8.12 mEq) or 450 mg (12.18 mEq), and lithium citrate is manufactured as an oral solution containing 8 mEq/5 mL. Whereas maintenance doses of lithium carbonate may be influenced considerably by a wide range of medical and physiologic factors (see below), the usual daily dose ranges from 600 to 1500 mg. Because lithium possesses a relatively narrow therapeutic range and exhibits fairly predictable pharmacokinetic behavior, it serves as an excellent candidate for routine therapeutic drug monitoring.

KEY PARAMETERS: Lithium	
Therapeutic Range	0.6–0.8 mEq/L
	(morning trough)
F	1 (100%)
V	0.7 L/kg
Cl	$0.25 \times Cl_{Cr}$
$t\frac{1}{2}$	
α	6 hr
β	20 hr

THERAPEUTIC AND TOXIC PLASMA CONCENTRATIONS

Extensive clinical and research experience with lithium has resulted in the identification of a well-defined plasma concentration range.[1-3] For the prevention of future manic or depressive episodes, the recommended plasma concentration range is approximately 0.6 to 0.8 mEq/L.[4] Occasionally, concentrations of 1.0 to 1.2 mEq/L are achieved for the acute treatment of mania, but the role of lithium in acute situations has diminished in recent years and the tolerability of these relatively high concentrations is rather poor.[1-3,5]

The most common acute side effects of lithium treatment are nausea, abdominal bloating, diarrhea, polyuria, polydipsia, muscle weakness, and somnolence. The gastrointestinal side effects seem to occur most commonly on initiation of treatment or when large doses of regular-release preparations are administered. These effects will subside over time but may also be minimized by administration with food or opting for extended-release products. The incidence and severity of acute adverse effects increase significantly with higher plasma concentrations (i.e., > 1.2 mEq/L). Nausea, vomiting, and diarrhea can become intractable; coarse tremors can develop; and profound central nervous system (CNS) deficits can ultimately occur, particularly when levels exceed 1.5 mEq/L.[5,6] In addition to these acute adverse effects, there are also a variety of long-term side effects that are commonly associated with plasma concentrations: fine intentional tremor, weight gain, thyroid abnormalities, and cognitive dulling.

BIOAVAILABILITY (F)

Lithium is rapidly absorbed, with peak plasma concentrations observed within 1 hour for the solution, 1 to 3 hours for the regular-release, and 3 to 6 hours for the extended-release preparations. Gastrointestinal absorption of lithium solution or regular-release tablets and capsules appears to be virtually complete (95% to 100%).[7,8] The absorption of sustained-release lithium products is more variable and ranges from 60% to 90%.[2]

VOLUME OF DISTRIBUTION (V)

Lithium is not protein bound and distributes throughout the bloodstream as a free ion. After absorption has occurred in the upper gastrointestinal tract, lithium undergoes a complex and prolonged distribution phase in the body. The usual volume of distribution for lithium is approximately 0.7 L/kg.[8] Although this volume of distribution is approximately equal to that of body water, lithium concentrates in various intracompartmental spaces and equilibrates very slowly with the extracellular fluid volume.[5] Overall, lithium disposition appears to conform to a two-compartment model with an initial volume of distribution of 0.25 to 0.3 L/kg and a final volume of distribution at equilibrium of ≈0.7 L/kg. The elevated plasma lithium concentrations observed during the distribution phase do not appear to correlate with either efficacy or toxicity.[3,7,8]

CLEARANCE (Cl)

Lithium is not metabolized and is eliminated from the body almost exclusively by the renal route, with negligible amounts lost through feces and sweat. Nearly 100% of the absorbed drug is filtered through the glomerulus, and 75% to 80% is reabsorbed in the proximal tubule.[3,8] The renal tubular reabsorption of lithium is very closely linked with sodium reabsorption and is influenced by the same factors regulating sodium balance (e.g., dehydration, hypotension, sodium depletion, etc.). In patients with a normal sodium balance, lithium clearance is ≈25% of creatinine clearance.[3,8]

A wide variety of medications and disease states can influence lithium clearance, most commonly through an alteration in renal function or sodium balance.[9] Certain diuretics (e.g., thiazides) have been shown to increase lithium levels dramatically, presumably through an influence on sodium homeostasis. This interaction appears to be much less significant with the more powerful loop diuretics.[9] Many nonsteroidal anti-inflammatory agents (NSAIDs; e.g., indomethacin, piroxicam, ketorolac, and naproxen) can also increase lithium concentrations, promoting signs and symptoms of toxicity by a mechanism that is not well understood.[10,11] This interaction is of greatest concern in patients taking NSAIDs at routine intervals (i.e., around the clock), and it does not occur with sulindac or acetaminophen. The angiotensin-converting enzyme (ACE) inhibitors can also increase lithium levels by 30% to 50% and are best avoided in lithium-treated patients if possible.[12]

Several factors have also been shown to accelerate lithium clearance and decrease plasma concentrations, potentially leading to a relapse in psychiatric illness.[9] Sodium loading, pregnancy, and acute mania can all decrease lithium levels to a significant extent. Among medications, theophylline and caffeine have been shown to have the same effect.

HALF-LIFE (t½)

The initial distribution or alpha half-life of lithium is approximately 6 hours, and the final elimination or beta half-life is 18 to 24 hours.[8] Plasma half-lives of 48 hours or longer have been demonstrated in patients with significant renal compromise.

SINGLE-POINT PREDICTIONS

A 24-hour serum lithium level obtained following a single specified dose (e.g., 1200 mg) can be used to predict maintenance dose requirements, although the clinical utility of this approach is limited.[13] One critical factor is the timing of the single plasma concentration measurement. For a one-compartment model drug, the optimal time to sample is ≈1.44 half-lives.[14] For this two-compartment drug, however, the 24-hour time interval appears to be appropriate because a significant amount of lithium is eliminated during the initial distribution phase. Patients for whom the single-point determination method is least likely to be successful include those who significantly differ from the average population in body size or lithium clearance. Therefore, the single-point determination method should be used with great caution in patients who are significantly larger or smaller than average, or in patients with an unusually high or low lithium clearance (i.e., patients who are predicted to require unusually high or low maintenance doses).

TIME OF SAMPLING

Since lithium distribution follows a two-compartment model, it is imperative that samples for lithium plasma levels be obtained at consistent and reproducible times. The current standard of practice is to obtain samples just before the first morning dose of lithium and at least 12 hours after the last evening dose.[3,6,15] The terminal or β half-life of 18 hours suggests that steady-state lithium levels should be attained within 3 to 5 days. Although lithium levels appear to plateau within 3 to 5 days, full therapeutic effects are not generally observed for 14 to 21 days after therapy has been initiated. Nevertheless, dosing adjustments may be implemented based on early steady-state plasma levels.

Question #1. *A.L., a 35-year-old, 72-kg man, is being treated with lithium (and olanzapine) for acute mania. He is receiving 300 mg of lithium carbonate at 9:00 a.m. and 5:00 p.m. His serum creatinine concentration is 1 mg/dL. Calculate the expected lithium concentration just before the morning dose on day 4 of therapy.*

Assuming A.L. has reasonably normal renal function and does not have an extended lithium half-life, steady state should be achieved in 3 days. The first step in calculating A.L.'s lithium concentration would be to approximate his renal function by use of Equation 7.1:

$$Cl_{cr} \text{ for males (mL/min)} = \frac{(140 - Age)(Weight \text{ in kg})}{(72)(SCr_{ss})} \quad \text{[Eq. 7.1]}$$

$$Cl_{cr} \text{ for males (mL/min)} = \frac{(140 - 35)(72)}{(72)(1)}$$

$$= 105 \text{ mL/min}$$

$$Cl_{cr} \text{ (L/hr)} = 105 \text{ mL/min} \left[\frac{60 \text{ min/hr}}{1000 \text{ mL/L}} \right]$$

$$= 6.3 \text{ L/hr}$$

The corresponding lithium clearance should be calculated next, using Equation 7.2 as follows:

$$\text{Lithium Clearance} = [0.25][\text{Creatinine Clearance}] \qquad [\text{Eq. 7.2}]$$

$$= [0.25][6.3 \text{ L/hr}]$$

$$= 1.6 \text{ L/hr}$$

A.L.'s total lithium dose of 600 mg corresponds to ≈16.2 mEq of lithium, based on the following calculation:

$$\frac{\text{Lithium Dose}}{(\text{mEq})} = \left[\text{Lithium Carbonate Dose} \atop (\text{mg})\right]\left[\frac{8.12 \text{ mEq}}{300 \text{ mg}}\right] \qquad [\text{Eq. 7.3}]$$

$$= [600 \text{ mg}]\left[\frac{8.12 \text{ mEq}}{300 \text{ mg}}\right]$$

$$= 16.2 \text{ mEq}$$

The average steady-state lithium concentration can then be calculated by using Equation 7.4. Note that F is 1 and S is 1, because the salt factor for the dose of lithium carbonate has already been corrected or accounted for in Equation 7.3.

$$\text{Css ave} = \frac{(S)(F)(\text{Dose}/\tau)}{Cl} \qquad [\text{Eq. 7.4}]$$

$$= \frac{(1)(1)(16.2 \text{ mEq}/24 \text{ hr})}{1.6 \text{ L/hr}}$$

$$= 0.42 \text{ mEq/L}$$

Question #2. *A.L.'s trough concentration on the morning of day 4 was 0.5 mEq/L. Calculate a new dosing regimen designed to achieve a trough concentration of 0.8 mEq/L.*

Equation 7.5 can be used to estimate A.L.'s lithium clearance:

$$Cl = \frac{(S)(F)(\text{Dose}/\tau)}{\text{Css ave}} \qquad [\text{Eq. 7.5}]$$

$$= \frac{(1)(1)(16.2 \text{ mEq}/24 \text{ hr})}{0.5 \text{ mEq/L}}$$

$$= 1.35 \text{ L/hr}$$

A.L.'s specific lithium clearance then can be used with Equation 7.6 to calculate the daily maintenance dose in mEq:

$$\text{Maintenance Dose} = \frac{(Cl)(Css\ ave)(\tau)}{(S)(F)} \quad \text{[Eq. 7.6]}$$

$$= \frac{(1.35\ \text{L/hr})(0.8\ \text{mEq/L})(24\ \text{hr})}{(1)(1)}$$

$$= 25.9\ \text{mEq}$$

Equation 7.7 can then be used to convert the lithium dose expressed as mEq/24 hours to the equivalent dose expressed in milligrams of lithium carbonate.

$$\frac{\text{Lithium Carbonate Dose}}{(mg)} = \left[\frac{\text{Lithium Dose}}{(mEq)}\right]\left[\frac{300\ mg}{8.12\ mEq}\right] \quad \text{[Eq. 7.7]}$$

$$= [25.9\ \text{mEq}]\left[\frac{300\ mg}{8.12\ mEq}\right]$$

$$= 957\ \text{mg or} \approx 900\ \text{mg}$$

This daily dose of 900 mg of lithium carbonate could be most conveniently administered as either three (300 mg) or two (450 mg) lithium carbonate tablets or capsules. Despite the long half-life, lithium is usually initiated in multiple daily doses to decrease acute gastrointestinal side effects. Once patients have achieved a desirable plasma concentration and their bipolar illness is under control, it has become a common practice to consolidate the total daily dose into single, once-daily administration of the extended-release product. There is evidence to suggest that this approach is associated with a decrease in the incidence and severity of polyuria and polydipsia, and a single daily dose may improve medication adherence as well.[16,17] The effects of this change on the interpretation of subsequent morning trough levels appear to be negligible.

An additional plasma level of lithium should be drawn once steady state is achieved on this new regimen. As A.L. has good renal function and his apparent lithium clearance is close to the predicted value, it is safe to assume that his half-life will be 24 hours or less and that steady-state dynamics will occur within 3 to 5 days.

One additional variable that should be taken into consideration is that lithium clearance values may increase by as much as 50% during the acute manic phase and fall to normal values once the patient's condition has stabilized.[17] Although the mechanism is not well understood, the clinical ramifications of this process may be that lithium levels appear to rise after patients are discharged from inpatient facilities. As a result, it is advisable to repeat lithium levels within 1 month after the resolution of symptoms.

Question #3. *M.C., a 55-year-old woman, is receiving 300 mg of lithium carbonate at 9:00 a.m. and 5:00 p.m. At 11:30 a.m. her lithium plasma concentration was 2.7 mEq/L. List six common reasons why lithium levels may be elevated (in general) and discuss how M.C. should subsequently be managed.*

Potential reasons for lithium elevation:

1. Plasma level obtained during distribution phase (i.e., less than 12 hours from last dose)
2. Overcompliance (e.g., confusion or administration of "prn" doses)
3. Drug interactions (e.g., diuretics, NSAIDs, ACE inhibitors)
4. Renal compromise
5. Dehydration
6. Sodium depletion

The successful management of M.C.'s situation involves, first, the appropriate interpretation of her lithium level. Thus, the first steps should be to confirm that the sample was drawn at the right time and to ensure that steady-state dynamics have been achieved. The significant two-compartmental modeling and the prolonged lithium α half-life of 6 hours dictate that lithium levels be obtained only before the first morning dose and at least 12 hours after the previous evening dose. If the level was drawn at an appropriate time, the next step would be to assess the patient's clinical presentation. Ordinarily, patients with levels in excess of 2.0 mEq/L will present with significant signs and symptoms of lithium toxicity (e.g., diarrhea, coarse tremor, ataxia, etc). If M.C.'s presentation is noncontributory, it is likely that this elevated lithium concentration of 2.7 mEq/L was obtained during the distribution phase. Plasma concentrations measured in this phase do not correlate with the efficacy or toxicity of lithium.

Question #4. *Immediately after the elevated lithium level is reported, M.C.'s physician examines her and finds that she is quite sluggish and slightly confused but responsive. She complains of intermittent vomiting and diarrhea and has difficulty walking down the hall. A neurologic examination reveals coarse intentional tremors in both hands and increased deep tendon reflexes. How should M.C. be managed at this time?*

Lithium intoxication is quite serious and often constitutes a medical emergency. If the exposure is acute (i.e., intentional or accidental overdose), gastric lavage is the first step to remove unabsorbed lithium from the gastrointestinal tract. A renal and electrolyte panel should also be drawn immediately, in addition to a plasma lithium level; an electrocardiogram (ECG) should be obtained. It is important to remember that, in the case of acute overdose, the lithium levels may be drawn during what is effectively the distribution phase, and interpretation of these elevated levels is impossible. Rehydration with normal saline is also vital to improve renal function and restore sodium balance, facilitating lithium clearance or removal. Although hemodialysis used to be recommended empirically whenever plasma levels exceeded 2.0 or 2.5 mEq/L, this decision should be based more on patient presentation. In general, hemodialysis should be reserved for patients with profound CNS deficits and/or acute renal failure. If hemodialysis is initiated, one should also remember that lithium will undergo an additional distribution phase at the end of the procedure (due to the removal of lithium from the central compartment). Thus, it is advisable to wait at least 6 to 8 hours before checking post-hemodialysis plasma levels.

In the case of M.C., her symptoms of lithium intoxication are moderate in severity and hemodialysis is not indicated.[18] Lithium should be discontinued for now, with a repeat level (and renal panel) obtained in a few hours to ensure that the plasma concentration is not increasing further (due to previously unabsorbed tablets or capsules in the gastrointestinal tract). Plasma lithium levels should also be obtained 24 to 48 hours later to estimate the lithium half-life and clearance. In the meantime, she should be rehydrated and every effort should be made (from patient interview and medical records) to determine the cause of her toxicity.

Question #5. *Are there any alternative methods for determining lithium concentrations?*

Although the effective compartment for lithium's therapeutic actions is believed to reside in the CNS, plasma levels are conveniently sampled as a guide to efficacy and toxicity. In theory, an alternative approach would be to quantify erythrocyte lithium concentrations because they represent an intracellular lithium concentration and may more directly correspond to the efficacy and toxicity of lithium. A number of studies have examined the relationship between efficacy and the erythrocyte lithium concentrations or the erythrocyte-plasma lithium concentration ratio and, unfortunately, the results are still inconclusive. Similarly, efforts have been made to correlate saliva concentrations with systemic effects but considerable variability has been found in the ratio of saliva to plasma concentrations.[19] In the future, lithium's therapeutic effects may be monitored through brain imaging techniques of the naturally occurring isotopes Li^6 and Li^7. Preliminary investigations have found a better correlation of clinical improvement with brain concentrations (quantified by magnetic resonance spectroscopy) than with serum levels.[20] The economic and clinical utility of this approach has yet to be elucidated.

REFERENCES

1. Consensus Development Panel. Mood disorders: pharmacologic prevention of recurrences. Am J Psychiatry 1985;142:469–476.

2. Carson SW. Lithium. In: Evans WE, et al., eds. Applied Pharmacokinetics: Principles of Therapeutic Drug Monitoring. 3rd Ed. Vancouver, WA: Applied Therapeutics, 1992;34:10–12.

3. Amdisen A. Lithium. In: Evans WE, Schentag JJ, Jusko WJ, eds. Applied Pharmacokinetics: Principles of Therapeutic Drug Monitoring. 2nd Ed. Spokane: Applied Therapeutics, 1986:978–1002.

4. American Psychiatric Association: Practice Guideline for the Treatment of Patients with Bipolar Disorder (Revision). Am J Psychiatry 2002;159(Suppl 4):20–21.

5. Elizur A, et al. Intra: extracellular lithium ratios and clinical course in affective states. Clin Pharm Ther 1972;13:947–53.

6. Salem RB. A pharmacist's guide to monitoring lithium drug-drug interactions. Drug Intell Clin Pharm 1982;16:745–7.

7. Sugita ET, et al. Lithium carbonate absorption in humans. Clin Pharm 1973;13:264–70.

8. Groth U, et al. Estimation of pharmacokinetic parameters of lithium from saliva and urine. Clin Pharmacol Ther 1974;16:490–8.

9. Finley PR, Warner MD, Peabody CA. Clinical relevance of drug interactions with lithium. Clin Pharmacokinet 1995;29:172–191.

10. Frolich JC, et al. Indomethacin increases plasma lithium. Med J 1979;1:1115–1116.

11. Ragheb M, Powell AL. Lithium interaction with sulindac and naproxen. J Clin Psychopharmacol 1986;6:150–154.

12. Balwin CM, Safferman AZ. A case of lisinopril-induced lithium toxicity. DICP Ann Pharmacother 1990;24:946–947.

13. Cooper TB, et al. The 24-hour serum lithium level as a prognosticator of dosage requirements. Am J Psychiatry 1973;130:601–603.

14. Unadkat JD, Rowland M. Further considerations of the "single-point, single-dose" method to estimate individual maintenance dosage requirements. Ther Drug Monit 1982;4:201–8.

15. Bergner PE, et al. Lithium kinetics in man: effect of variation in dosage pattern. Br J Pharmacol 1973;49:328–39.

16. Miller AL, Bowden CL, Plewes J. Lithium and impairment of renal concentrating ability. J Affect Disord 1985;9:115–119.

17. Bowden CL. Key treatment studies of lithium in manic-depressive illness: efficacy and side effects. J Clin Psychiatry 1998;59(Suppl 6):13–19.

18. Sadosty AT, Groleau GA, Atcherson MM. The use of lithium levels in the emergency department. J Emerg Med 1999;17:887–891.

19. McKeage MJ, Maling TJB. Saliva lithium: a poor predictor of plasma and erythrocyte levels. N Z Med J 1989;102:559–560.

20. Kato T, Inubushi T, Takahashi S. Relationship of lithium concentrations in the brain measured by lithium-7 magnetic resonance spectroscopy to treatment response in mania. J Clin Psychopharmacol 1994;14:330–335.

8

METHOTREXATE (MTX)

Betsy L. Althaus and Michael E. Winter

Methotrexate is a folic acid anti-metabolite that competitively inhibits di-hydrofolate reductase, the enzyme responsible for converting folic acid to the reduced or active folate cofactors. Methotrexate is used to treat a number of neoplasms, including leukemia, osteogenic sarcoma, breast cancer, and non-Hodgkin's lymphoma. Methotrexate is administered by the parenteral route when doses exceed 30 mg/m^2 because oral absorption is limited.[1] Current dosing regimens range from as low as 2.5 mg to as high as 12 gm/m^2 or more. High-dose methotrexate is administered over a period as short as 3 to 6 hours to as long as 40 hours.[2,3]

Approximately 50% of methotrexate is bound to plasma proteins.[1,2] Methotrexate is primarily renally cleared. It is a weak acid with a pKa of 5.4. At low pH, the drug has limited solubility and may precipitate in the urine, causing renal damage. Therefore, a patient receiving high-dose methotrexate should receive hydration, and the urine pH should be maintained above 7. Methotrexate has some minor metabolites with weak activity, the most important of which is 7-hydroxy-methotrexate. The concentration of this metabolite may become significant with high doses of methotrexate. Although 7-hydroxy-methotrexate has only about 1/200th the clinical activity of methotrexate, it is one-third to one-fifth as soluble. As a result, it may precipitate in the renal tubules causing acute nephrotoxicity.[4] This solubility problem is an additional reason why patients receiving large doses of methotrexate should be adequately hydrated and have their urine alkalinized.[2,3]

THERAPEUTIC AND TOXIC PLASMA CONCENTRATIONS

The therapeutic and toxic effects of methotrexate are closely linked to its plasma concentrations. Since the goal of therapy is to inhibit dihydrofolate reductase (DHFR) and ultimately to deplete the reduced folate cofactors, the relative ability to inhibit DHFR and the time course required to deplete the cofactors is critical to the relationship between the drug's efficacy and its toxicity.

Units

Methotrexate is generally administered in mg or gm doses and the plasma concentrations are reported in units of mg/L, μg/mL, and molar or micromolar units. When methotrexate concentrations are reported in molar units, they usually range from values of 10^{-8} to 10^{-2} molar. In addition, they are commonly reported in micromolar (or 10^{-6} molar) units. To interpret methotrexate concentrations accurately, it is important to establish which units are being reported and how those units correspond to the generally accepted therapeutic or toxic values. Methotrexate has a molecular weight of 454 gm/mole; therefore, a value of 0.454 mg/L is equal to 1×10^{-6} molar or 1 micromolar. To convert methotrexate concentrations in units of mg/L to molar concentrations, the following equation can be used:

$$\text{Methotrexate Concentration in } 10^{-6} \text{ Molar} = \frac{\text{Methotrexate Concentration in mg/L}}{0.454} \quad \text{[Eq. 8.1]}$$

KEY PARAMETERS: Methotrexate

Therapeutic Plasma Concentration	Variable
Toxic Concentration	
Plasma	$> 1 \times 10^{-7}$ molar for > 48 hours $> 1 \times 10^{-6}$ molar at > 48 hours requires increased leucovorin rescue doses
CNS	Continuous CNS methotrexate concentrations $> 10^{-8}$ molar

F
  Dose < 30 mg/m^2
  Dose > 30 mg/m^2
	
	100%
	Variable

Vi (initial)	0.2 L/kg
V AUC	0.7 L/kg
Cl	$[1.6][Cl_{Cr}]$

t½
  α[a]
  β[b]
	
	3 hr
	10 hr

[a] t½ of 3 hours generally employed with methotrexate plasma concentrations greater than 5×10^{-7} molar.
[b] t½ of 10 hours generally employed with methotrexate plasma concentrations of less than 5×10^{-7} molar.

In the above equation, the factor 0.454 is the number of mg/L equal to 10^{-6} molar or 1 micromolar. Methotrexate concentrations reported in molar units should first be converted to 10^{-6} molar and then multiplied times the factor 0.454 to calculate the equivalent methotrexate concentration in units of mg/L:

$$\frac{\text{Methotrexate Concentration}}{\text{in mg/L}} = \left(\frac{\text{Methotrexate Concentration}}{\text{in } 10^{-6} \text{ Molar}}\right)(0.454) \quad \text{[Eq. 8.2]}$$

Methotrexate concentrations in the units of molar, micromolar, or mg/L are interchangeable, as long as the correct unit adjustment and interpretation of the reported concentration are made. For example, a methotrexate concentration of 1 micromolar would be equivalent to the following:

$$0.01 \times 10^{-4} \text{ molar}$$

$$0.1 \times 10^{-5} \text{ molar}$$

$$1 \times 10^{-6} \text{ molar}$$

$$1 \ \mu M \text{ (micromolar)}$$

$$10 \times 10^{-7} \text{ molar}$$

$$0.454 \text{ mg/L}$$

Although all the concentrations listed above represent the same value, the units differ. For example, the concentration, 0.01×10^{-4} molar, is expressed in units that are 100 times more concentrated than 10^{-6}. Therefore, when interpreting methotrexate plasma concentrations, it is important to determine whether a value of 1.0 represents micromolar units (10^{-6} molar) or some other unit value.

Therapeutic Plasma Concentrations

Most therapeutic regimens are designed to achieve concentrations above 1×10^{-7} molar (0.1 micromolar) for < 48 hours. Concentrations of methotrexate that have been associated with successful treatment of various neoplasms range from 10^{-6} up to 10^{-3} or 10^{-2} molar. Although the relationship of the methotrexate concentration to tumor kill is somewhat empiric, Evans et al. have documented that methotrexate concentrations in the range of 16×10^{-6} molar are successful in the treatment of leukemic patients.[5] These high methotrexate levels are not usually associated with serious methotrexate toxicity as long as adequate hydration and renal function are maintained, and the methotrexate concentration falls below 1×10^{-7} molar (0.1 micromolar) within 48 hours following the initiation of therapy or the discontinuation of leucovorin rescue.

Toxic Plasma Concentration

Plasma concentrations exceeding 1×10^{-7} molar for 48 hours or more are associated with methotrexate toxicity.[6] The most common toxic effects of methotrexate include myelosuppression, oral and gastrointestinal mucositis, and acute hepatic dysfunction.[1,2,6]

LEUCOVORIN RESCUE. To ensure that methotrexate toxicities do not occur in moderate and high-dose treatment regimens, leucovorin is administered every 4 to 6 hours in doses that range from 10 to 100 mg/m²[2,3,6] The usual course of rescue therapy is from 12 to 72 hours, or until the plasma concentration of methotrexate falls below the critical value of 1×10^{-7} molar. In some rescue protocols, concentrations of 5×10^{-8} (0.05 micromolar) are considered to be the value indicating the rescue is complete.[3]

Methotrexate concentrations in excess of 1×10^{-6} molar (1 micromolar) at 48 hours are associated with an increased incidence of methotrexate toxicity, even in the face of leucovorin rescue doses of 10 mg/m². When the methotrexate concentration exceeds 1×10^{-6} molar at 48 hours, increasing the leucovorin rescue dose to 50 to 100 mg/m² or more reduces methotrexate toxicity.[6] Presumably, this increased dose enables leucovorin factor to compete successfully with methotrexate for intracellular transport and to thereby rescue host tissues.

Although rescue regimens vary considerably, most employ a leucovorin dosing regimen of ≈10 mg/m² administered every 6 hours for 72 hours. If the methotrexate concentration falls below 1×10^{-7} molar (0.1 micromolar) or 5×10^{-8} (0.05 micromolar) before the completion of the 72-hour rescue period, then the rescue factor can be discontinued. If the methotrexate concentrations are still greater than 1×10^{-7} but less than 1×10^{-6} at 48 hours, then rescue with leucovorin is continued at doses of ≈10 mg/m² every 6 hours until the methotrexate concentration falls below the rescue value of 1×10^{-7} molar (0.1 micromolar) or 5×10^{-8} (0.05 micromolar).

Goals of Monitoring

One of the primary goals of methotrexate plasma monitoring is to ensure that all patients receive adequate doses of rescue factor to prevent serious toxicity. Because most high-dose rescue regimens are designed to "save" the average patient, the vast majority of methotrexate plasma levels that are obtained for monitoring will be routine and are unlikely to require intervention. Nevertheless, plasma concentration monitoring can be used to detect unusual methotrexate disposition characteristics that could result in serious toxicity.

Methotrexate Assays

There are a number of methotrexate assays that use differing methodologies; however, none of these appear to be clearly superior to the others. All assays used should have the ability to measure plasma concentrations below the rescue value of 5×10^{-8} (0.05 micromolar) and above 1×10^{-6} molar. When methotrexate plasma levels are still elevated at 48 hours, the dose of rescue factor must be increased.[7,8]

BIOAVAILABILITY (F)

Methotrexate oral absorption is complete and rapid, with peak concentrations occurring 1 to 2 hours following doses of < 30 mg/m^2. At higher doses, the extent of methotrexate absorption declines, and bioavailability is incomplete.[1] For this reason, moderate- and high-dose methotrexate regimens must be administered by the parenteral route. Low-dose methotrexate (< 30 mg/m^2) may be administered parenterally or orally.

VOLUME OF DISTRIBUTION (V)

The relationship between methotrexate plasma concentrations and volume of distribution is complex. The drug displays at least a bi-exponential elimination curve, indicating that there is an initial plasma volume of distribution of about 0.2 L/kg and a second larger volume of distribution of 0.5 to 1.0 L/kg following complete distribution.[9,10] The evaluation of the apparent volume of distribution for methotrexate is further complicated by the fact that it appears to increase at higher plasma concentrations.[9] This phenomenon may reflect an active transport system that becomes saturated at high plasma concentrations and reverts to passive intracellular diffusion of methotrexate. The multi-compartmental modeling, as well as the variable relationship between the plasma concentration and apparent volume of distribution of methotrexate, make calculation of methotrexate loading doses somewhat speculative. Nevertheless, when loading doses are required, a volume of distribution of 0.2 to 0.5 L/kg is usually employed.

The presence of third-space fluids such as ascites, edema, or pleural effusions can also influence the volume of distribution of methotrexate.[11] Although pleural effusions do not substantially increase the volume of distribution, the high concentrations of methotrexate that accumulate in these spaces can be important because equilibration with plasma is delayed. In patients with pleural effusions, the initial elimination half-life appears to be normal; however, the second elimination phase is prolonged.[12] Prolongation of this terminal elimination phase is significant because the time required for patients to achieve a methotrexate plasma concentration of less than 1×10^{-7} can be extended. In this situation, additional doses of rescue factor may have to be administered beyond the usual rescue period [see Fig. 8.1 and Methotrexate Half-Life (t½)].

CLEARANCE (Cl)

The vast majority of methotrexate is eliminated by the renal route.[12,13] Methotrexate clearance ranges from 1 to as much as 2 times the creatinine

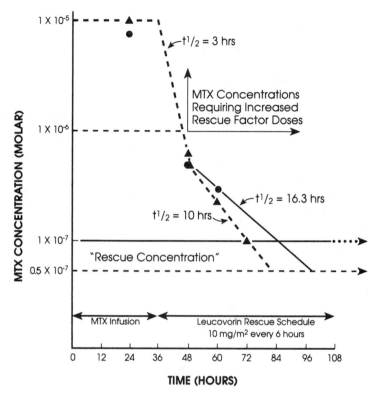

FIGURE 8.1. Methotrexate. This figure represents a semilog plot of the expected (▲) and measured (●) methotrexate (MTX) plasma concentrations during and following a 36-hour infusion. Levels were obtained at 24, 48, and 60 hours after the start of the infusion. Note that leucovorin rescue should be continued as long as the methotrexate concentration is greater than the rescue value, represented here as either 1×10^{-7} molar (0.1 micromolar) or 0.05×10^{-6} molar (0.05 micromolar), and that the rescue dose should be increased for methotrexate levels greater than 1×10^{-6} molar at 48 hours and beyond.

clearance.[2,4,12,13] (The author uses a factor of 1.6 to estimate methotrexate clearance in the clinical setting.) Methotrexate clearance by an active transport mechanism that may be saturable results in a renal clearance value that varies (relative to creatinine clearance) with methotrexate plasma concentrations.[4]

The renal clearance of methotrexate also is influenced by a number of compounds (e.g., probenecid and salicylates influence weak acid secretion). In addition, sulfisoxazole and other weak acids have been reported to diminish the renal transport of methotrexate.[4,14] Because methotrexate renal clearance may be inhibited, all drugs should be added cautiously to the regimen of a patient receiving methotrexate therapy. Although early reports attributed salicylate-induced methotrexate toxicity to plasma protein displacement of methotrexate, the most likely mechanism is an alteration in renal clearance. An alteration in plasma binding is an unlikely explanation because methotrexate is only 50% bound to plasma proteins.[4,14]

Changes in renal function are important when designing and monitoring methotrexate therapy. Therefore, all patients receiving moderate and high-dose methotrexate therapy should have their plasma level of methotrexate and their renal function monitored. Although the therapeutic dose of methotrexate may range over several grams, serious toxicity and death have been attributed to doses as low as 10 mg of methotrexate when administered to a patient with inadequate renal function.[15,16]

Concomitant administration of the prostaglandin inhibitors indomethacin and ketoprofen with methotrexate has been associated with an acute decrease in renal function and a greatly prolonged exposure to high methotrexate concentrations.[17,18] This interaction presumably results from the combined renal effects of the nonsteroidal anti-inflammatory agent with methotrexate. Although this interaction has not been described for all nonsteroidal anti-inflammatory agents, these agents should be avoided in patients receiving methotrexate therapy.

A relatively small percentage of methotrexate is metabolized; nevertheless, significant amounts of methotrexate metabolites can be found in the urine when large doses are administered. This is especially true during the late phase of methotrexate elimination when the majority of the parent compound has been eliminated. The most extensively studied metabolite is the 7-hydroxy-methotrexate compound, which is considered to be potentially nephrotoxic because of its low water solubility.[4]

HALF-LIFE (t½)

The relationship between methotrexate's volume of distribution and clearance is complex. Because of the potential for capacity-limited intracellular transport and capacity-limited renal clearance, the apparent half-lives for methotrexate are determined by both a changing volume of distribution and a changing clearance. Consequently, the elimination of methotrexate is not accurately described by linear pharmacokinetic modeling. Given these problems, a relatively simple two-compartment model with an initial α half-life of 2 to 3 hours and a β or terminal half-life of approximately 10 hours appears to represent the elimination phase reasonably well.[10,12,13] The terminal or β half-life of approximately 10 hours often does not become apparent until plasma concentrations decline into the range of 5×10^{-7} molar (0.5×10^{-6} or 0.5 micromolar). Since the terminal phase is also independent of the dose administered, it probably reflects a change in the distribution and elimination of methotrexate.

Whereas the apparent terminal half-life of methotrexate is somewhat variable, it does not appear to increase with increasing doses. Unlike most other two-compartmental drugs, significant methotrexate is eliminated during the α phase. In fact, a very large percentage of the total methotrexate dose may be eliminated during the α phase. Nevertheless, the terminal phase is also important, because retention of even a very small amount of the administered dose can be potentially toxic to the patient.[10,11]

Pleural effusions or other third space fluid collections can significantly prolong the terminal half-life of methotrexate, and leucovorin rescue regimens may need to be extended over a longer period in these situations. Some patients may unexpectedly develop acute changes in renal function or prolonged elimination characteristics that are unpredictable and independent of renal function. For this reason, continued monitoring of methotrexate is essential, even if early plasma level monitoring indicates that an adjustment of the methotrexate dose or leucovorin regimen is unnecessary.

TIME TO SAMPLE

Methotrexate plasma concentrations can be used to evaluate the potential efficacy of a given dosing regimen and to determine if the quantity and/or duration of leucovorin rescue is adequate. There are two situations when monitoring methotrexate levels for efficacy is useful. The first is in patients who are to receive prolonged methotrexate infusions, since in these cases the infusion rate can be adjusted. The second is in patients who are going to receive repeated methotrexate doses, in which case future doses can be adjusted to achieve the desired target concentration.

When using methotrexate levels to evaluate the leucovorin rescue dosage regimen, samples are obtained 24 to 48 hours following the initiation of therapy to determine whether additional leucovorin will be required, either in quantity or duration of administration. For example, plasma levels greater than 1×10^{-6} molar at 48 hours are usually associated with increased methotrexate toxicity unless leucovorin rescue doses are increased from 10 mg/m² every 6 hours to 50 to 100 mg/m² every 4 to 6 hours. For patients with plasma levels below 1×10^{-6} but above 1×10^{-7} molar, a leucovorin rescue dose of 10 mg/m² every 6 hours is generally adequate to prevent toxicity if continued until the plasma concentration drops below 1 to 0.5×10^{-7} molar.

Plasma samples obtained before the critical 48-hour time period may indicate whether the elimination of methotrexate is normal; however, because of the potential toxicity associated with even small amounts of retained methotrexate, all patients should have documented methotrexate concentrations below 1×10^{-7} molar or 0.5×10^{-7} molar before leucovorin rescue is discontinued. Calculating the critical rescue value may be acceptable in some cases, but extrapolating the data to more than one or two methotrexate half-lives is hazardous because the half-life of methotrexate tends to increase during the final decay periods. In most protocols, methotrexate levels are monitored sometime during the IV infusion, at 48 hours, and then every 24 hours until levels drop below the concentration at which the patient is considered to be "rescued," usually to less than 1×10^{-7} molar. As an added precaution, many institutions use 0.5×10^{-7} molar as the target rescue concentration.

Question #1. *P.J., a 61-year-old, 69-kg man (SCr = 1.1 mg/dL), is to re-ceive a course of methotrexate therapy for acute lymphoblastic leukemia. His regimen will consist of a 400-mg methotrexate loading dose to be administered over 15 minutes, followed by an IV infusion of 50 mg/hr for the next 36 hours. He will then receive a 100 mg (≈50 mg/m²) dose of leucovorin every 6 hours intravenously for the first 4 doses followed by 8 doses orally of 20 mg (≈10 mg/m²) at 6-hour inter-vals or until the methotrexate concentration is < 0.5 × 10⁻⁷ molar. The leucovorin regimen will begin immediately after the 36-hour methotrex-ate infusion has been discontinued and is scheduled to continue for the next 72 hours, with the last dose given 102 hours after initiation of the methotrexate therapy. Methotrexate levels are scheduled to be obtained 24 hours after the beginning of the 50-mg/hr infusion, at 48 hours (12 hours after the end of the 36-hour infusion), and at 60 hours (24 hours after the end of the methotrexate infusion). Calculate the anticipated methotrexate concentrations at the scheduled sampling times.*

Before the anticipated methotrexate concentrations can be calcu-lated, it is first necessary to determine P.J.'s creatinine clearance, using Equation 8.3:

$$\frac{Cl_{cr} \text{ for males}}{\text{(mL/min)}} = \frac{(140 - \text{Age})(\text{Weight})}{(72)(SCr_{ss})} \qquad \text{[Eq. 8.3]}$$

$$= \frac{(140 - 61)(69)}{(72)(1.1)}$$

$$= 68.8 \text{ mL/min}$$

The creatinine clearance of 68.8 mL/min can be converted to 4.13 L/hr:

$$\frac{Cl_{cr}}{\text{(L/hr)}} = \left[\frac{Cl_{cr}}{\text{(mL/min)}}\right]\left[\frac{60 \text{ min/hr}}{1000 \text{ mL/L}}\right]$$

$$= [68.8 \text{ mL/min}]\left[\frac{60 \text{ min/hr}}{1000 \text{ mL/L}}\right]$$

$$= 4.13 \text{ L/hr}$$

This creatinine clearance of 4.13 L/hr can then be placed into Equation 8.4 to calculate a methotrexate clearance (Cl_{MTX}) of 6.6 L/hr.

$$Cl_{MTX} = (1.6)(Cl_{cr}) \qquad \text{[Eq. 8.4]}$$

$$= [1.6][4.13 \text{ L/hr}]$$

$$= 6.6 \text{ L/hr}$$

The 24-hour concentration represents an average steady-state level. The steady-state level of methotrexate in mg/L can then be calculated by using the equation for steady-state concentration (Equation 8.5):

$$\text{Css ave} = \frac{(S)(F)(\text{Dose}/\tau)}{Cl} \qquad \text{[Eq. 8.5]}$$

$$= \frac{(1)(1)(50 \text{ mg}/1 \text{ hr})}{6.6 \text{ L/hr}}$$

$$= 7.6 \text{ mg/L}$$

The values of S and F were assumed to be 1, and this methotrexate concentration in mg/L can be converted to a concentration in the units of micromoles or 10^{-6} molar by use of Equation 8.1:

$$\frac{\text{Methotrexate Concentration}}{\text{in } 10^{-6} \text{ Molar}} = \frac{\text{Methotrexate Concentration}}{\dfrac{\text{in mg/L}}{0.454}}$$

$$= \frac{7.6 \text{ mg/L}}{0.454}$$

$$= 16.7 \times 10^{-6} \text{ molar or } 1.67 \times 10^{-5} \text{ molar}$$

The resultant methotrexate concentration of approximately 16.7×10^{-6} or 1.67×10^{-5} molar assumes that steady state has been achieved 24 hours after the infusion rate of 50 mg/hr has been initiated. Steady state is assumed to have been achieved because the methotrexate plasma concentrations are relatively high. At concentrations greater than 10^{-7} molar, a half-life of 2 to 3 hours appears to determine the elimination and accumulation of most of the methotrexate in the body. As noted earlier, this model is not consistent with the traditional view of a two-compartment model in which the terminal half-life plays an important role in the accumulation toward steady state. Although there is the possibility of some continued accumulation, this generally appears to be minor, and use of the shorter, 2- to 3-hour methotrexate half-life in evaluating initial methotrexate loss or accumulation is satisfactory in most cases.

Assuming, then, that the plasma concentration at the end of the 36-hour infusion is 16.7×10^{-6} molar, a plasma concentration of 1.04×10^{-6} molar (10.4×10^{-7} molar) at 48 hours (or 12 hours after the infusion has been discontinued) can be calculated using Equation 8.6.

$$C_2 = C_1(e^{-Kt}) \qquad \text{[Eq. 8.6]}$$

C_1 is the methotrexate plasma concentration at the end of the infusion, and t is the 12-hour time interval spanning from the end of the 36-hour infusion to the time of sampling at 48 hours. K is the elimination rate constant calculated from a rearrangement of the equation for $t\frac{1}{2}$ (Equation 8.7) and using the shorter elimination half-life of 3 hours.

$$t\frac{1}{2} = \frac{0.693}{K} \qquad \text{[Eq. 8.7]}$$

$$K = \frac{0.693}{t\frac{1}{2}} \qquad \text{[Eq. 8.8]}$$

$$K = \frac{0.693}{t\frac{1}{2}}$$

$$= \frac{0.693}{3 \text{ hr}}$$

$$= 0.231 \text{ hr}^{-1}$$

$$C_2 = C_1(e^{-Kt})$$

$$C_2 = (16.7 \times 10^{-6} \text{ molar})(e^{-(0.231 \text{ hr}^{-1})(12 \text{ hr})})$$

$$= (16.7 \times 10^{-6} \text{ molar})(0.0625)$$

$$= 1.04 \times 10^{-6} \text{ molar or } 10.04 \times 10^{-7} \text{ molar}$$

Because this methotrexate concentration is 1×10^{-6} molar 48 hours after starting the methotrexate therapy, the leucovorin rescue dose does not have to be increased. The planned leucovorin rescue schedule should be continued until the concentration falls to 0.5×10^{-7}.

Calculation of the methotrexate concentration 60 hours after the infusion has been initiated (24 hours after the infusion has been concluded) is more problematic. The half-life for methotrexate tends to increase as the methotrexate concentration approaches 0.2 to 0.7×10^{-6} (2 to 7×10^{-7}) molar. Therefore, use of a traditional two-compartment model for this drug is inappropriate because the more prolonged terminal half-life correlates more closely with a specific concentration range than with a specific time interval following discontinuation of the infusion. This unusual phenomenon may be related to a change in the active transport system that is influenced by plasma concentration.

One technique that is used to predict methotrexate concentrations several hours after the infusion has been discontinued is to decay the methotrexate concentration to a range of 0.2 to 0.7×10^{-6} molar using a half-life of 3 hours. The longer or β half-life of 10 hours is then used to predict subsequent decay. If a plasma concentration of 0.5×10^{-6} is arbitrarily selected as the cut-off concentration for using a half-life of 3 hours, the time required for the initial decay can be calculated using Equation 8.9:

$$t = \frac{\ln\left(\dfrac{C_1}{C_2}\right)}{K} \qquad \text{[Eq. 8.9]}$$

C_1 represents the initial plasma concentration of 16.7×10^{-6} molar, C_2 the arbitrary cut-off plasma concentration of 0.5×10^{-6} molar, and K the elimination rate constant corresponding to the initial half-life of 3 hours (0.231 hr^{-1}). Using Equation 8.9, the time (t) required for the methotrexate concentration to fall to 0.5×10^{-6} molar would be 15.2 hours after the end of the infusion or 51.2 hours after the methotrexate regimen is begun:

$$t = \frac{\ln\left(\dfrac{16.7 \times 10^{-6}\ \text{molar}}{0.5 \times 10^{-6}\ \text{molar}}\right)}{0.231\ \text{hr}^{-1}}$$

$$= \frac{3.5}{0.231\ \text{hr}^{-1}}$$

$$= 15.2\ \text{hr}$$

To calculate the plasma concentration at 60 hours, the plasma level at 51.2 hours (36-hour infusion + 15.2-hour decay) would have to be decayed for an additional 8.8 hours. In this case, however, the elimination rate constant that corresponds to the terminal elimination half-life of 10 hours would be used (Equation 8.8):

$$K = \frac{0.693}{t_{1/2}}$$

$$= \frac{0.693}{10\ \text{hr}}$$

$$= 0.0693\ \text{hr}^{-1}$$

Using these values and the equation for first-order elimination of a drug from the body (Equation 8.6), a methotrexate concentration of 2.7×10^{-7} molar at 60 hours can be calculated.

$$C_2 = (C_1)(e^{-Kt})$$

$$= (0.5 \times 10^{-6}\ \text{molar})(e^{-(0.0693\ \text{hr}^{-1})(8.8\ \text{hr})})$$

$$= 0.27 \times 10^{-6}\ \text{molar or } 2.7 \times 10^{-7}\ \text{molar}$$

These calculations suggest that an additional 24 hours will be required to decay the concentration to 0.5×10^{-7} molar:

$$t = \frac{\ln\left(\dfrac{0.27 \times 10^{-6} \text{ molar}}{0.05 \times 10^{-6} \text{ molar}}\right)}{0.0693 \text{ hr}^{-1}}$$

$$= \frac{1.68}{0.0693 \text{ hr}^{-1}}$$

$$= 24 \text{ hr}$$

Since this concentration will decay to a concentration below 0.5×10^{-7} (0.05 micromolar) (the rescue value) in a little more than 2 half-lives, it would appear from our calculations that P.J. will have been rescued by leucovorin successfully.

Therefore, the rescue concentration will be achieved before leucovorin is scheduled to be discontinued. Nevertheless, these predicted concentrations are only approximations and cannot replace measured methotrexate concentrations. A graphic representation of the expected methotrexate concentrations [▲] is plotted in Figure 8.1. Unless there is a dramatic increase in the methotrexate half-life, the concentration will be well below 1×10^{-7} molar long before the leucovorin is scheduled to be discontinued.

Question #2. *P.J.'s methotrexate levels were reported as 13.5×10^{-6} molar at 24 hours, 0.83×10^{-6} molar (8.3×10^{-7} molar) at 48 hours, and 0.44×10^{-6} molar (4.4×10^{-7} molar) at 60 hours. How would one interpret each of these methotrexate values? What would be an appropriate course of action regarding P.J.'s rescue therapy?*

The initial plasma concentration of 13.5×10^{-6} is lower than the predicted concentration calculated in Question 1 (16.7×10^{-6} molar). The lower-than-predicted concentration suggests that P.J.'s methotrexate clearance is greater than expected; however, the difference between the predicted and actual concentrations is well within the expected variation.

The plasma level of 8.3×10^{-7} molar at 48 hours (12 hours after the end of the infusion) suggests that P.J. is progressing as expected during the initial elimination phase. The difference between the expected (10.4×10^{-7} molar) and observed concentrations is minimal, considering the fact that the initial plasma level was slightly lower than predicted (see Fig. 8.1). Because the observed plasma level is below 1×10^{-6} molar at 48 hours, it is unnecessary to increase the leucovorin dose.

The measured methotrexate concentration of 4.4×10^{-7} molar (0.44 micromolar) at 60 hours is greater than the predicted concentration of 2.7×10^{-7} molar (0.27 micromolar). Although the differences are not remarkable, it is of some concern that P.J.'s half-life is longer than anticipated. P.J.'s elimination rate constant of 0.053 hr^{-1} can be calculated using these two methotrexate concentrations, the time interval between the concentration and rearranging Equation 8.9 to form Equation 8.10.

$$K = \frac{\ln\left(\dfrac{C_1}{C_2}\right)}{t} \qquad \text{[Eq. 8.10]}$$

$$= \frac{\ln\left(\dfrac{8.3 \times 10^{-7}\ \text{molar}}{4.4 \times 10^{-7}\ \text{molar}}\right)}{12\ \text{hr}}$$

$$= \frac{0.63}{12\ \text{hr}}$$

$$= 0.053\ \text{hr}^{-1}$$

P.J.'s corresponding methotrexate t$\frac{1}{2}$ of 13.1 hours can be calculated using the K value of 0.053 hr^{-1} and Equation 8.7.

$$t\tfrac{1}{2} = \frac{0.693}{K}$$

$$= \frac{0.693}{0.053\ \text{hr}^{-1}}$$

$$= 13.1\ \text{hr}$$

Although the increased methotrexate half-life appears to be substantial, the accuracy of the half-life calculation is uncertain because the plasma levels used are separated by a time interval that is less than one half-life. The increase in this terminal half-life of methotrexate could be attributed to any of the following: an assay error, accumulation of methotrexate in a pleural effusion or other third-space fluid, a drug-induced reduction in the renal clearance of methotrexate (e.g., salicylates), or a normal variance in methotrexate elimination.

Regardless of the cause, it is important to determine whether P.J. will achieve a plasma concentration of less than 0.5×10^{-7} molar by the time the leucovorin rescue is scheduled to be discontinued. Using the patient-specific or revised elimination rate constant of 0.053 hr^{-1} and Equation 8.9, it appears as though P.J.'s methotrexate concentration will fall to 0.5×10^{-7} molar after an additional 41 hours (101 hours after starting the methotrexate therapy). This is just at the time scheduled for the last dose of leucovorin (102 hours after starting the methotrexate infusion).

$$t = \frac{\ln\left(\frac{C_1}{C_2}\right)}{K}$$

$$= \frac{\ln\left(\frac{4.4 \times 10^{-7} \text{ molar}}{0.5 \times 10^{-7} \text{ molar}}\right)}{0.053 \text{ hr}^{-1}}$$

$$= \frac{2.17}{0.053 \text{ hr}^{-1}}$$

$$= 41 \text{ hr}$$

This calculation should not be used as the sole criterion for evaluating the success of rescue therapy because the elimination rate constant calculation is uncertain and the methotrexate terminal half-life may become more prolonged as the plasma concentration declines. In this particular case, additional methotrexate plasma levels should be obtained to ensure that the actual plasma concentration is below the critical value of 0.5×10^{-7} before leucovorin rescue is discontinued. If this critical value has not been achieved by 102 hours, then additional doses of leucovorin will have to be administered until P.J. has achieved a plasma level below 0.5×10^{-7} molar (see Fig. 8.1). Note that the observed methotrexate levels suggest P.J. has a more prolonged terminal half-life.

Question #3. *C.T. is a 50-year-old, 60-kg man with a serum creatinine of 1.0 mg/dL. He has osteogenic sarcoma and is to receive 24 gm IV methotrexate infused over 4 hours, followed at 24 hours by leucovorin 20 mg orally every 6 hours until the methotrexate levels are less than 0.05 micromolar. Calculate the methotrexate concentration at the end of the 4-hour infusion, 12 hours after the end of the infusion, and 48 hours after the start of the infusion (44 hours after ending the infusion).*

To calculate the expected concentrations, one first needs to estimate C.T.'s methotrexate clearance by calculating his creatinine clearance (Equation 8.3).

$$\frac{\text{Cl}_{cr} \text{ for males}}{\text{(mL/min)}} = \frac{(140 - \text{Age})(\text{Weight})}{(72)(\text{SCr}_{ss})}$$

$$= \frac{(140 - 50)(60 \text{ kg})}{(72)(1.0 \text{ mg/dL})}$$

$$= 75 \text{ mL/min}$$

$$\frac{\text{Cl}_{cr}}{\text{(L/hr)}} = \left[\frac{\text{Cl}_{cr}}{\text{(mL/min)}}\right]\left[\frac{60 \text{ min/hr}}{1000 \text{ mL/L}}\right]$$

$$= [75 \text{ mL/min}]\left[\frac{60 \text{ min/hr}}{1000 \text{ mL/L}}\right]$$

$$= 4.5 \text{ L/hr}$$

and then his corresponding methotrexate clearance of 7.2 L/hr (Equation 8.4).

$$Cl_{MTX} = (1.6)(Cl_{cr})$$

$$= (1.6)(4.5 \text{ L/hr})$$

$$= 7.2 \text{ L/hr}$$

To calculate the methotrexate concentration obtained at the end of the infusion and 12 hours after the infusion, the shorter elimination half-life of 3 hours should be used to calculate the elimination rate constant (Equation 8.8).

$$K = \frac{0.693}{t\frac{1}{2}}$$

$$= \frac{0.693}{3 \text{ hr}}$$

$$= 0.231 \text{ hr}^{-1}$$

To predict the methotrexate concentration (C_2) at the end of the infusion and 12 hours later, Equation 8.11 can be used, where t_{in} represents the time over which the dose was infused and t_2 represents the time from the end of the infusion to the drug concentration.

$$C_2 = \frac{(S)(F)(Dose/t_{in})}{Cl}(1 - e^{-Kt_{in}})(e^{-Kt_2}) \qquad \text{[Eq. 8.11]}$$

$$= \frac{(1)(1)(24{,}000 \text{ mg/4 hr})}{7.2 \text{ L/hr}}(1 - e^{-(0.231)(4 \text{ hr})})(e^{-(0.231)(t_2)})$$

$$= (833.3 \text{ mg/L})(1 - 0.4)(e^{-(0.231)(t_2)})$$

$$= 500 \text{ mg/L} (e^{-(0.231)(t_2)})$$

Where $t_2 = 0$ hours for the level drawn at the end of the infusion:

$$= 500 \text{ mg/L} (e^{-(0.231)(0)})$$

$$= 500 \text{ mg/L}$$

and $t_2 = 12$ hours, for the level drawn 12 hours after the end of the infusion:

$$= 500 \text{ mg/L} (e^{-(0.231)(12)})$$

$$= 500 \text{ mg/L} (0.063)$$

$$= 31.5 \text{ mg/L}$$

Using Equation 8.1, one can convert the methotrexate concentrations from mg/L to micromolar (10^{-6} molar) at the end of the 4-hour infusion:

$$\text{Methotrexate Concentration in } 10^{-6} \text{ Molar} = \frac{\text{Methotrexate Concentration in mg/L}}{0.454}$$

$$= \frac{500 \text{ mg/L}}{0.454}$$

$$= 1101 \times 10^{-6} \text{ molar}$$

And 12 hours later:

$$= \frac{31.5 \text{ mg/L}}{0.454}$$

$$= 69.4 \times 10^{-6} \text{ molar}$$

To calculate the plasma concentration at 48 hours (44 hours after ending the infusion), it will be necessary to use Equation 8.9 to decay the plasma concentration to the point at which the half-life changes from 3 hours to approximately 10 hours.

$$t = \frac{\ln\left(\dfrac{C_1}{C_2}\right)}{K}$$

$$= \frac{\ln\left(\dfrac{69.4 \times 10^{-6} \text{ molar}}{0.5 \times 10^{-6} \text{ molar}}\right)}{0.231 \text{ hr}^{-1}}$$

$$= \frac{\ln(138.8)}{0.231 \text{ hr}^{-1}}$$

$$= \frac{4.93}{0.231 \text{ hr}^{-1}}$$

$$= 21.3 \text{ hr}$$

Therefore, 21.3 hours after the 12-hour sample, or at $\approx$37 hours from the start of the infusion (4 hour infusion + 12 hours + 21 hours), the methotrexate concentration would be approximately 0.5×10^{-6} molar. To calculate the concentration at 48 hours, the plasma concentration of 0.5×10^{-6} molar should be decayed for another 11 hours. At this concentration range, however, one anticipates the half-life of methotrexate to be approximately 10 hours, corresponding to an elimination rate constant of 0.0693 hr^{-1} (Equation 8.8).

$$K = \frac{0.693}{t\frac{1}{2}}$$

$$= \frac{0.693}{10 \text{ hr}}$$

$$= 0.0693 \text{ hr}^{-1}$$

Now, using Equation 8.6 and the new elimination rate constant, the methotrexate concentration 14 hours later (48 hours after starting the infusion) can be calculated.

$$C_2 = (C_1)(e^{-Kt})$$

$$= (0.5 \times 10^{-6} \text{ molar})(e^{-(0.0693)(11 \text{ hr})})$$

$$= (0.5 \times 10^{-6} \text{ molar})(0.47)$$

$$= 0.24 \times 10^{-6} \text{ molar or 0.24 micromolar}$$

The expected methotrexate concentration of approximately 0.24 micromolar is well below the concentration range at which an increase in the leucovorin rescue dose is required, but still above the concentration range at which it could be discontinued. Assuming the rescue concentration is approximately 0.05 micromolar, it can be seen that approximately a little more than 2 half-lives will be required to reach the concentration of methotrexate at which leucovorin can be discontinued.

Because methotrexate pharmacokinetic parameters are subject to considerable variability, these estimated plasma concentrations would have to be confirmed with actual plasma level measurements. In most clinical institutions, an early plasma concentration is obtained near the end of the methotrexate infusion to ensure that high and potentially therapeutic methotrexate levels are achieved. Additional levels are drawn approximately every 24 hours to track the methotrexate decline and to guide the leucovorin dosing requirements.

Question #4. *R.J., an 18-year-old, 50-kg woman with leukemia, is to be treated every 7 days with intrathecal methotrexate to prevent central nervous system (CNS) spread of her bone marrow disease. What would be an appropriate dose for R.J., considering her age and body size?*

There is considerable evidence that regardless of body size, patients older than 3 years of age should receive a standard 12 mg dose of intrathecal methotrexate. This dose disregards body size, because the cerebrospinal fluid volume approaches 80% to 90% of its maximum value within the first 3 years of life. Furthermore, the size of the CNS compartment does not correlate well with either total body weight or body surface area.[19,20]

Question #5. *When patients are receiving intrathecal methotrexate, what factors should be considered in evaluating the risk of methotrexate toxicity?*

Intrathecally administered doses of methotrexate are first cleared from the CNS into the systemic circulation and then eliminated from the systemic circulation by the usual renal route. Since the standard intrathecal dose of methotrexate is only 12 mg, the risk of systemic methotrexate toxicity is relatively low unless the patient develops renal dysfunction. Therefore, the patient's renal function should be evaluated. It is also important to assure that the patient has not received drugs that are known to inhibit the renal clearance of methotrexate. In patients with severe renal dysfunction, serious systemic toxicity and even death can result from intrathecally administered methotrexate because of the patient's inability to eliminate the drug from the body.[15,16]

CNS toxicities can be mild to severe and include mild weakness, minor transient paralysis, and, in rare instances, severe leukoencephalopathy.[21,22] Serious CNS toxicities are associated with CNS methotrexate levels that are continuously maintained at a concentration above 10^{-8} molar.[21] For this reason, CNS methotrexate levels should be monitored to ensure that the CNS level has declined to an acceptable value before the weekly dose is administered. Patients who are most likely to retain methotrexate and have high CNS concentrations after intrathecal or intraventricular injections are those with active CNS disease (e.g., meningeal leukemia) or other defects in cerebrospinal flow.[19,21,22] An additional point to be made, although not a pharmacokinetic one, is that intraventricular or intrathecal doses of methotrexate are frequently given concomitantly with intravenous vincristine to increase tumor cell kill. Vincristine cannot be administered intraventricularly, as this route of vincristine administration is reported to be 100% fatal. It is therefore critical to recognize that although these two drugs are frequently given at the same time during a course of therapy, vincristine is never administered directly into the CNS.[23]

REFERENCES

1. Wan SH, et al. Effect of route of administration and effusions on methotrexate pharmacokinetics. Cancer Res 1974;34:3487.
2. Bleyer WA. The clinical pharmacology of methotrexate. Cancer 1978;41:36.
3. Bleyer WA. Methotrexate: clinical pharmacology, current status and therapeutic guidelines. Cancer Treat Rev 1977;4:87.
4. Shen DD, Azarnoff DL. Clinical pharmacokinetics of methotrexate. Clin Pharmacokinet 1978;3:1.
5. Evans WE, et al. Clinical pharmacodynamics of high-dose methotrexate in acute lymphocytic leukemia. N Engl J Med 1986;314:471.
6. Stoller RG, et al. Use of plasma pharmacokinetics to predict and prevent methotrexate toxicity. N Engl J Med 1977;297:630.

7. Buice RG. Evaluation of enzyme immunoassay, radioassay and radioimmunoassay of serum methotrexate, as compared with liquid chromatography. Clin Chem1980;26:1902.

8. Crom WR, Evans WE. Methotrexate. In: Evans WE et al., eds. Applied Pharmacokinetics: Principles of Therapeutic Drug Monitoring. 3rd Ed. Vancouver: Applied Therapeutics,1992:1–42.

9. Leme PR, et al. Kinetic model for the disposition and metabolism of moderate and high-dose methotrexate (NSC-740) in man. Cancer Chemother Rep 1975;59:811.

10. Pratt CB, et al. High-dose methotrexate used alone and in combination for measurable primary or metastatic osteosarcoma. Cancer Treat Rep 1980;64:11.

11. Evans WE, Pratt CB. Effect of pleural effusion on high-dose methotrexate kinetics. Clin Pharmacol Ther 1978;23:68.

12. Isacoff WH, et al. Pharmacokinetics of high-dose methotrexate with citrovorum factor rescue. Cancer Treat Rep 1977;61:1665.

13. Stoller RG, et al. Pharmacokinetics of high-dose methotrexate (NSC-740). Cancer Chemother Rep 1975;6(Pt. III):19.

14. Liegler DG, et al. The effect of organic acids on renal clearance of methotrexate in man. Clin Pharmacol Ther 1969;10:849.

15. Cadman EC, et al. Systemic methotrexate toxicity. Arch Intern Med 1976;136:1321.

16. Ahmad S, et al. Methotrexate-induced renal failure and ineffectiveness of peritoneal dialysis. Arch Intern Med 1978;138:1146.

17. Ellison NM, Servi RJ. Acute renal failure and death following sequential intermediate-dose methotrexate and 5-FU: a possible adverse effect due to concomitant indomethacin administration. Cancer Treat Rep 1985;69:342.

18. Thyss A, et al. Clinical and pharmacokinetic evidence of a life-threatening interaction between methotrexate and ketoprofen. Lancet 1986;1:256.

19. Bleyer WA. Clinical pharmacology of intrathecal methotrexate. II. An improved dosage regimen derived from age-related pharmacokinetics. Cancer Treat Rep 1977;61:1419.

20. Bonati M, et al. Clinical pharmacokinetics of cerebrospinal fluid. Clin Pharmacokinet 1982;7:312.

21. Bleyer WA, et al. Neurotoxicity and elevated cerebrospinal fluid methotrexate concentration in meningeal leukemia. N Engl J Med 1973;289:770.

22. Duffner PK, et al. CT abnormalities and altered methotrexate clearance in children with CNS leukemia. Neurology 1984;34:229.

23. Solimando DA, Wilson JT. Prevention of accidental intrathecal administration of vincristine sulfate. Hosp Pharm 1982;17:540.

9

PHENOBARBITAL

John E. Murphy and Michael E. Winter

Phenobarbital is a long-acting barbiturate used in the treatment of seizure disorders, insomnia, and anxiety. It is most commonly administered orally, but it may be administered intramuscularly and intravenously as well.

The usual adult maintenance dose of 2 mg/kg/day produces a steady-state concentration of approximately 20 mg/L. Limited evidence suggests that dosing should be based on total body weight.[1] Phenobarbital has a half-life of approximately 5 days; therefore, therapeutic concentrations are not achieved for 2 to 3 weeks following the initiation of a maintenance regimen. When therapeutic concentrations of 20 mg/L are required immediately, a loading dose of 15 mg/kg can be administered, usually in 3 divided doses of 5 mg/kg given every 2 to 3 hours.

KEY PARAMETERS: Phenobarbital	
Therapeutic Concentrations	15–40 mg/L
Bioavailability (F)	1.0 (> 0.9)
S (for Na salt)	0.9

V
  Neonates
  Children and Adults
	
	0.9 L/kg (0.7–1.0)
	0.7 L/kg (0.6–0.7)

Cl[a]
  Children
 	
  Adults and neonates
	
	0.008 L/kg/hr
	(0.2 L/kg/day)
	0.004 L/kg/hr
	(0.1 L/kg/day)

t½
  Children
  Adults
	
	2.5 days
	5 days

Fraction Unbound (fu)	0.5

[a]Primarily metabolized by the liver, 20% cleared renally. Clearance in children older than 1 year of age is approximately twice the adult value.

THERAPEUTIC AND TOXIC CONCENTRATIONS

In adults, phenobarbital concentrations of 10 to 30 mg/L are required for seizure control.[2] The overall therapeutic range is now considered to be 15 to 40 mg/L.[3] The upper end of the therapeutic range is limited by the appearance of side effects such as central nervous system (CNS) depression and ataxia.[4] Patients may exhibit no symptoms of chronic toxicity even when phenobarbital concentrations exceed 40 mg/L.[5] Phenobarbital concentrations in excess of 100 to 150 mg/L are considered potentially lethal, although patients with higher concentrations have survived.[5-7] Many patients develop excessive sedation when phenobarbital concentrations are rapidly pushed into the therapeutic range. For this reason, when it is clinically feasible many prescribers prefer to start patients on about 25% of the target maintenance dose for the first week of therapy and then increase the maintenance dose by another 25% for each of the subsequent 3 weeks, finally achieving the full maintenance dose regimen on the fourth week of therapy. The technique of slowly increasing the maintenance dose allows many patients to adjust to their phenobarbital concentrations; however, it does prolong the time required to achieve concentrations in the usually accepted therapeutic range.[8] With adequate monitoring, slow administration (if given intravenously), and concern for the sedative effects of phenobarbital, full loading doses have been used to quickly bring a patient to the therapeutic range.

BIOAVAILABILITY (F)

Although it has not been well studied, available data indicate that at least 80% and probably > 90% of phenobarbital administered orally is absorbed. Complete bioavailability ($F = 1.0$) is supported by the observation that similar concentrations are observed when the same dose of phenobarbital is given orally and parenterally. Intramuscular dosing has been shown to be 100% bioavailable,[9] and administration of the injectable product as a rectal solution results in 90% bioavailability.[10]

Phenobarbital is frequently administered as the sodium salt, which is approximately 91% phenobarbital acid ($S \cong 0.91$); however, a correction for the salt form is seldom made, because the degree of error is small and the therapeutic range is relatively broad. When phenobarbital is administered parenterally, it is usually administered at a rate of no more than 50 mg/min to avoid toxicities associated with the propylene glycol diluent.[11] Proportionally slower infusion rates based on the size of the patient should be used in children.

VOLUME OF DISTRIBUTION (V)

The volume of distribution for phenobarbital in children and adults is approximately 0.7 L/kg.[12,13] In newborns it is slightly higher at approximately 0.9 L/kg (0.7 to 1 L/kg).[14,15]

CLEARANCE (Cl)

Phenobarbital is primarily metabolized by the liver; less than 20% is eliminated by the renal route.[16] The average total clearance for phenobarbital in adults and newborns is $\approx$4 mL/kg/hr (0.004 L/kg/hr) or 0.1 L/kg/day. This clearance value of approximately 0.1 L/kg/day results in the following clinical observation: for every 1 mg/kg/day of phenobarbital sodium administered, a steady-state phenobarbital concentration of about 10 mg/L is achieved.

$$\text{Css ave} = \frac{(S)(F)(\text{Dose}/\tau)}{Cl} \qquad \text{[Eq. 9.1]}$$

$$= \frac{(0.9)(1)(1 \text{ mg/kg/day})}{0.1 \text{ L/kg/day}}$$

$$= 9 \text{ mg/L } or \approx 10 \text{ mg/L}$$

This clinical guideline suggests that in adult and newborn patients, maintenance doses of 2 mg/kg/day should result in steady-state concentrations of $\approx$20 mg/L. The clearance in children 1 to 18 years of age is approximately twice the average adult clearance.[17-19] Therefore, these patients generally require maintenance doses of phenobarbital that are about twice those of the average adult, or a maintenance dose of 4 to 5 mg/kg/day will be needed to achieve steady-state concentrations of 20 mg/L.

HALF-LIFE (t½)

The half-life of phenobarbital is $\approx$5 days in most adult patients, but may be as short as 2 to 3 days in some individuals, especially children.

TIME TO SAMPLE

Phenobarbital has a half-life of approximately 5 days; as a result, samples obtained within the first 1 to 2 weeks of therapy yield relatively little information about the eventual steady-state concentrations. For this reason, routine phenobarbital concentrations should be monitored 2 to 3 weeks after the initiation or a change in the phenobarbital regimen. Samples obtained before this time should be used either to determine whether an additional loading dose is needed (e.g., when concentrations are much lower than desired), or whether the maintenance dose should be withheld (e.g., phenobarbital concentrations are much greater than desired).

Once steady state has been achieved, the time of sampling within a dosing interval of phenobarbital is not critical; concentrations can be obtained at almost any time relative to the phenobarbital dose. As a matter of consistency, however, trough concentrations are generally recommended. If phenobarbital is being administered by the intravenous (IV) route, care should be taken to sample at least 1 hour after the end of the infusion to avoid the distribution phase.

Question #1. *P.M., a 2-week-old, 3.2-kg neonate, has developed idiopathic tonic–clonic seizure activity. An IV loading dose of phenobarbital sodium of 20 mg/kg was given followed by maintenance doses of 1.5 mg/kg every 12 hours. Estimate the post-load phenobarbital concentration and the average steady-state concentration from the maintenance dose.*

Since this is a loading dose problem and there is no existing initial drug concentration, Equation 9.2 should be used to estimate C^o:

$$C^o = \frac{(S)(F)(\text{Loading Dose})}{V} \qquad \text{[Eq. 9.2]}$$

F can be assumed to be 1.0 since this is an IV dose and S = 0.9 for phenobarbital sodium. V is estimated to be 0.9 L/kg (see Key Parameters: Phenobarbital) or 2.9 L. After the loading dose of 64 mg (20 mg/kg · 3.2 kg), the predicted post-load concentration (ideally taken about 1 hour after the loading dose to avoid any distribution phase) is:

$$C^o = \frac{(0.9)(1)(64 \text{ mg})}{2.88 \text{ L}}$$

$$C^o = 19.9, \approx 20 \text{ mg/L}$$

The loading dose and volume of distribution could each be used without multiplying by the patient's weight to get the dose in mg (64 mg) and the volume in L (2.9 L) since weight will cancel out of the numerator and denominator.

$$C^o = \frac{(0.9)(1)(20 \text{ mg/kg})}{0.9 \text{ L/kg}}$$

$$C^o = 20 \text{ mg/L}$$

Although representative of the situation, it is not necessary to use Equation 9.4 to account for the difference between the concentration drawn at 1 hour and that assumed to have occurred at C^o since very little elimination will occur in such a short time when the drug has a very long half-life. The estimated half-life is:

$$t\frac{1}{2} = \frac{(0.693)(V)}{Cl} \qquad \text{[Eq. 9.3]}$$

$$t\frac{1}{2} = \frac{(0.693)(0.9 \text{ L/kg})}{0.004 \text{ L/kg/hr}} = 156 \text{ hours or 6.5 days}$$

$$C_1 = \frac{(S)(F)(\text{Loading Dose})}{V}(e^{-Kt_1}) \qquad \text{[Eq. 9.4]}$$

The fraction of drug or concentration remaining (e^{-kt}) after t time (1 hour in this case) would be 0.996, indicating negligible elimination. The difference in prediction would be 20 mg/L versus 20 mg/L $\times$ 0.996 = 19.92 mg/L. As with many aspects of equation use in pharmacokinetics, when one event occurs quickly relative to another, the equations may be simplified with little error.[20]

Because clearance is the major determinant of the eventual steady-state concentrations achieved by the maintenance dose, this parameter must be estimated for P.M. Whereas, there is intersubject variability, the average clearance of phenobarbital in newborns is 4 mL/kg/hr or 0.004 L/kg/hr. Thus, the expected clearance for P.M., who is 3.2 kg, is 0.013 L/hr:

$$\text{Clearance Newborn Phenobarbital} = (0.004 \text{ L/kg/hr})(\text{Weight in kg}) \qquad \text{[Eq. 9.5]}$$

$$= (0.004 \text{ L/kg/hr})(3.2 \text{ kg})$$

$$= 0.013 \text{ L/hr}$$

The predicted average steady-state concentration of the maintenance dose of 1.5 mg/kg (4.8 mg) every 12 hours is determined from Equation 9.1:

$$\text{Css ave} = \frac{(S)(F)(\text{Dose}/\tau)}{Cl}$$

$$= \frac{(0.9)(1)(4.8 \text{ mg}/12 \text{ hr})}{(0.013 \text{ L/h})}$$

$$= 28 \text{ mg/L}$$

With the long half-life estimated in this patient, the dose could easily be given once daily. However, the elixir is not readily taken by infants because of the taste and volume (5 ml delivers either 15 or 20 mg depending on the manufacturer). Mixing the smaller volume that can be used with twice daily dosing in formula or breast milk seems to increase palatability.

Question #2. *P.M. has a post-load concentration of 22 mg/L, one hour after the dose. Because the baby is still having seizures, the team monitoring P.M.'s progress decides to increase his concentration to 30 mg/L. Calculate an additional loading dose to take his concentration to 30 mg/L (assume that little elimination has occurred in the time from sample collection to the decision to increase P.M.'s phenobarbital concentration) and adjust his maintenance dose to provide a predicted Css ave of 30 mg/L.*

It is important to remember that the patient's volume of distribution can now be determined, and this should be used rather than the population average volume to determine the new dose. A second critical point to remember is that the baby should not be given a dose to take him from 0 mg/L to 30 mg/L, but rather from the concentration of 22 mg/L to 30 mg/L, or an incremental change in concentration of 8 mg/L.

Calculate the baby's volume of distribution using Equation 9.6 below:

$$V = \frac{(S)(F)(\text{Loading Dose})}{C} \qquad [\text{Eq. 9.6}]$$

$$= \frac{(0.9)(1)(64 \text{ mg})}{22 \text{ mg/L}}$$

$$= 2.62 \text{ L}$$

$$= 2.62 \text{ L} \div 3.2 \text{ kg} = 0.8 \text{ L/kg}$$

The additional incremental loading dose is then determined using Equation 9.7:

$$\text{Incremental Loading Dose} = \frac{(V)(C_{desired} - C_{initial})}{(S)(F)} \qquad [\text{Eq. 9.7}]$$

$$= \frac{(2.62 \text{ L})(30 \text{ mg/L} - 22 \text{ mg/L})}{(0.9)(1)}$$

$$= 23 \text{ mg}$$

Since doses and concentrations are proportional for first-order drugs like phenobarbital, the dose could simply have been solved by ratio. The loading dose of 64 mg produced a post-load concentration of 22 mg/L. To increase the concentration by 8 mg/L, the ratio is:

$$(64 \text{ mg})\left(\frac{8 \text{ mg/L}}{22 \text{ mg/L}}\right) = 23 \text{ mg}$$

The new maintenance dose can also be solved this way:

$$(4.8 \text{ mg q12h})\left(\frac{30 \text{ mg/L}}{28 \text{ mg/L}}\right) = 5.1 \text{ mg every 12 hrs}$$

Or, the revised desired Css ave of 30 mg/L can be put into Equation 9.8.

$$\text{Maintenance Dose} = \frac{(Cl)(Css \text{ ave})(\tau)}{(S)(F)} \qquad \text{[Eq. 9.8]}$$

$$= \frac{(0.004 \text{ L/kg/hr})(3.2 \text{ kg})(30 \text{ mg/L})(12 \text{ hours})}{(0.9)(1)}$$

$$= 5.1 \text{ mg every 12 hours}$$

Question #3. *P.M. has his concentration measured half-way through the dosage interval (Css ave) after 6 weeks of dosing at 5.1 mg of phenobarbital elixir every 12 hours; it is reported as 23 mg/L. The baby now weighs 4 kg. Determine the baby's phenobarbital clearance assuming that the concentration is at steady state. S = 1, assume F = 1.*

By rearranging Equations 9.1 we can solve for clearance:

$$Cl = \frac{(S)(F)(Dose/\tau)}{(Css \text{ ave})} \qquad \text{[Eq. 9.9]}$$

$$= \frac{(1)(1)(5.1 \text{ mg/12 hr})}{(23 \text{ mg/L})}$$

$$= 0.0185 \text{ L/hr} \div 4 \text{ kg}$$

$$= 0.0046 \text{ L/kg/hr}$$

Due to the baby's weight gain and continuation of the 5.1 mg dose, the concentration dropped despite no difference in clearance per body weight from predicted. If necessary, because of continuing seizure activity, a small loading dose could be given followed by an increase in maintenance dose to bring the concentration back to near 30 mg/L (or to any other desired concentration).

Question #4. *W.R., a 39-year-old, 70-kg man, developed generalized seizures several months after an automobile accident in which he* *sustained head injuries. Phenobarbital is to be initiated. Calculate an oral loading dose of phenobarbital to produce a concentration of 20 mg/L.*

Because this is a loading dose problem and there is no existing initial drug concentration, Equation 9.10 should be used:

$$\text{Loading Dose} = \frac{(V)(C)}{(S)(F)} \qquad [\text{Eq. 9.10}]$$

If F and S are assumed to be 1 and the volume of distribution is assumed to be 0.7 L/kg (see Key Parameters: Phenobarbital) or 49 L, the calculated loading dose will be 980 mg or approximately 1 gm as shown below.

$$\text{Loading Dose} = \frac{(49\ \text{L})(20\ \text{mg/L})}{(1)(1)}$$

$$= 980\ \text{mg or} \approx 1\ \text{gm}$$

This 1 gm dose is very close to the usual loading dose of 15 mg/kg. It may be administered orally, intramuscularly, or intravenously.

Generally, the loading dose is divided into three or more portions and administered over several hours. The necessity for dividing the loading dose when administered orally or intramuscularly is not clear. It is probably done to act as a precaution against toxicity should a two-compartmental distribution exist or to avoid cardiovascular toxicity from the propylene glycol diluent in the injectable dosage form (see Chapter 10: Phenytoin).

Question #5. *Calculate an oral maintenance dose for W.R. that will maintain a phenobarbital concentration of 20 mg/L. How should the dose be administered?*

Because clearance is the major determinant of the maintenance dose, this parameter must be estimated for W.R. Although there is some intersubject variability, the average clearance of phenobarbital in adults is 4 mL/kg/hr or 0.1 L/kg/day. Thus, the expected clearance for W.R., who is 70 kg, is 7 L/day.

If S and F are assumed to be 1, the maintenance dose of phenobarbital can be calculated using Equation 9.8:

$$\text{Maintenance Dose} = \frac{(Cl)(Css\ ave)(\tau)}{(S)(F)}$$

$$= \frac{(7\ \text{L/day})(20\ \text{mg/L})(1\ \text{day})}{(1)(1)}$$

$$= 140\ \text{mg}$$

In practice, the daily dose is often divided into two or more portions; however, with a half-life of 5 days (Equation 9.3), once daily dosing should suffice.[12] If the entire dose is given at bedtime, some of the side effects associated with sedation may be reduced.

$$t\frac{1}{2} = \frac{(0.693)(V)}{Cl}$$

$$= \frac{(0.693)(49\ L)}{7\ L/day}$$

$$= 4.85\ days\ or\ \approx 5\ days$$

Interestingly, the calculated dose corresponds to an empiric clinical guideline that has been used for many years: the phenobarbital steady-state concentration produced by a maintenance dose will be approximately equal to 10 times the daily dose in mg/kg:

$$W.R.'s\ Maintenance\ Dose\ (mg/kg) = \frac{140\ mg}{70\ kg}$$

$$= 2\ mg/kg$$

According to the clinical guideline, the concentration in mg/L produced by this dose will be 20 mg/L (2 × 10).

Question #6. *If W.R. does not receive a loading dose, how long will it take to achieve a minimum therapeutic concentration of 15 mg/L following the initiation of the maintenance dose? How long will it take to achieve a steady-state concentration of 20 mg/L?*

To answer a question involving time, knowledge of the half-life is required. The half-life for phenobarbital in W.R. is approximately 5 days, as calculated in Question #5. If it is assumed that 3 to 5 half-lives are a sufficient approximation of steady state (87.5% to 96.9% of steady state), approximately 15 to 25 days will be required to approach the final plateau concentration of 20 mg/L. Because the minimum therapeutic concentration of 15 mg/L is three-quarters (75%) of the predicted steady-state concentration of 20 mg/L, two half-lives or 10 days will be required for the phenobarbital concentration to accumulate to 15 mg/L.

$$K = \frac{0.693}{t\frac{1}{2}}$$ [Eq. 9.11]

$$= \frac{0.693}{5\ days}$$

$$= 0.139\ days^{-1}$$

$$C_1 = \frac{(S)(F)(Dose/\tau)}{Cl}\left(1 - e^{-Kt_1}\right) \qquad \text{[Eq. 9.12]}$$

Where $\dfrac{(S)(F)(Dose/\tau)}{Cl}$ is the Css ave (in this case 20 mg/L), and t_1 is the duration of the maintenance dose therapy, in this case 10 days.

$$= (20\ mg/L)(1 - e^{-(0.139d^{-1})(10\ days)})$$
$$= (20\ mg/L)(0.75)$$
$$= 15\ mg/L$$

The time can also be calculated by manipulating Equation 9.12.

After the passage of sufficient time to reach steady state (i.e., 3 to 5 $t_{1/2}$'s where e^{-kt} approaches 0, leaving $1 - e^{-kt}$ to approximately $1 - 0$, or 1), Equation 9.12:

$$C_1 = \frac{(S)(F)(Dose/\tau)}{Cl}(1 - e^{-Kt_1})$$

becomes Equation 9.1:

$$Css\ ave = \frac{(S)(F)(Dose/\tau)}{Cl}$$

Therefore, Equation 9.12 can be rewritten as:

$$C_1 = Css\ ave(1 - e^{-Kt_1}) \qquad \text{[Eq. 9.13]}$$

And then, it follows that:

$$\frac{C_1}{Css\ ave} = 1 - e^{-Kt_1} \qquad \text{[Eq. 9.14]}$$

By taking the natural log (ln) of both sides of Equation 9.14 and re-arranging the terms, the time to achieve a certain C_1 can be estimated:

$$t = \frac{-\ln\left(1 - \dfrac{C_1}{Css\ ave}\right)}{K}$$ [Eq. 9.15]

$$= \frac{-\ln\left(1 - \dfrac{15}{20}\right)}{0.139\ d^{-1}}$$

$$= 10\ days$$

Question #7. *If W.R. had felbamate added to his overall therapy, how would this affect the original maintenance dose prediction?*

The use of felbamate is not common because it is only recommended in patients with seizures unresponsive to conventional first-line therapy. However, when used it is often with other agents, and the drug–drug interactions with other anticonvulsants are potentially significant. Felbamate has been reported to increase the $AUC_{0\ to\ 24\ hours}$ and Css max of phenobarbital by 22% and 24%, respectively.[21] This would indicate a reduction in clearance of approximately 20% (or ~0.8 of normal). The dose suggested could be empirically decreased by 20% to account for the interaction, and the patient could be told that if felbamate is discontinued, a phenobarbital dose increase might be necessary. Since the interaction is of moderate impact and the predicted concentration at the lower end of the therapeutic range, it would also be reasonable to simply monitor the steady-state concentrations and make dosing adjustments if necessary.

Question #8. *K.P., a 62-year-old, 57-kg woman, was admitted for poor seizure control. Before admission she had been receiving an unknown dose of phenobarbital. On admission, the phenobarbital concentration was 5 mg/L, and she was started on 60 mg of phenobarbital every 8 hours (180 mg/day). Five days later, the phenobarbital trough concentration was 17 mg/L. Calculate her final steady-state concentration on the present regimen.*

There are several ways to approach this problem. Since Css ave is defined by clearance, one could use the average clearance for phenobarbital (0.1 L/kg/day $\times$ 57 kg = 5.7 L/day) and insert this value into Equation 9.1:

$$Css\ ave = \frac{(S)(F)(Dose/\tau)}{Cl}$$

$$= \frac{(1)(1)(180\ mg/day)}{5.7\ L/day}$$

$$= 31.6\ mg/L$$

Another method could be used to estimate the steady-state value. The concentration of 17 mg/L reported on the fifth day is assumed to represent the sum of the fraction of the initial concentration (5 mg/L) remaining at this time plus the accumulated concentration resulting from five daily doses of 180 mg. If K.P.'s half-life for phenobarbital is 5 days, the fraction of the initial concentration remaining after 1 half-life will be 0.5 and contribution to the reported concentration at 5 days will be 2.5 mg/L (5 mg/L × 0.5). The remaining portion of the reported concentration (14.5 mg/L) represents 50% of the steady-state concentration that will be produced by the 180 mg/day dose (after one half-life, 50% of steady-state has been achieved). Therefore, the predicted Css ave would be 29 mg/L (2 × 14.5 mg/L).

One also could use the empiric clinical guideline discussed in Question #5 regarding the prediction of Css ave from the mg/kg dose of phenobarbital. In this case the mg/kg dose would be 180 mg/57 kg or 3.16 mg/kg. The predicted Css ave would be 31.6 mg/L (3.16 × 10).

All these estimates are based on the assumption that K.P.'s pharmacokinetic parameters for phenobarbital are similar to those reported in the literature. Since the estimates for Css ave are at the upper end of the therapeutic range, it would be reasonable to obtain another concentration 15 to 20 days after the initiation of the maintenance dose. Also, because the repeat concentration will be obtained after more than 2 half-lives have passed, K.P.'s clearance for phenobarbital can be estimated more reliably (see Part I: Interpretation of Plasma Drug Concentrations).

If the concentration on the fifth day was predicted from the average pharmacokinetic parameters, the value would be quite close to what was measured (see below). Thus, it appears her parameters are similar to the averages. The approach below can be used when the measured concentration does not conveniently fall exactly on a multiple of the half-life as in the example above.

Equation 9.16 is used to calculate the concentration (C_1) remaining from initial 5 mg/L:

$$C_1 = C^o(e^{-Kt_1}) \qquad\qquad \text{[Eq. 9.16]}$$

$$C_{1 \text{ at 5 days}} = 5 \text{ mg/L}(e^{-(K)(5 \text{ days})})$$

$$= 5 \text{ mg/L}\left(e^{-\left(\frac{0.693}{5 \text{ days}}\right)(5 \text{ days})}\right)$$

$$= 2.5 \text{ mg/L}$$

Although there are a number of models, Equation 9.17, which describes the concentration C_2 following the Nth dose, can be used to determine the contribution of the five doses of 180 mg given each day (see Part I: Selecting the Appropriate Equation: Series of Individual Doses).

$$C_2 = \left[\frac{\left(\frac{(S)(F)(Dose)}{V} \right)}{(1 - e^{-K\tau})} \right] (1 - e^{-K(N)\tau})(e^{-Kt_2}) \qquad \text{[Eq. 9.17]}$$

$$C_2 = \left[\frac{\left(\frac{(1)(1)(180 \text{ mg})}{(0.7 \text{ L/kg})(57 \text{ kg})} \right)}{(1 - e^{-(0.139 \text{ days}^{-1})(1 \text{ day})})} \right] (1 - e^{-(0.139 \text{ days}^{-1})(5)(1 \text{ day})})(e^{-(0.139 \text{ days}^{-1})(1 \text{ day})})$$

$C_2 = 15.2$ mg/L

$C_1 + C_2 = 2.5$ mg/L $+ 15.2$ mg/L

$\qquad = 17.7$ mg/L (vs. measured concentration of 17 mg/L)

Question #9. *N.P., a 35-year-old, 80-kg man, is being treated for a seizure disorder secondary to a motor vehicle accident. He has been receiving 200 mg/day of phenobarbital (100 mg BID) for the past 15 days. The phenobarbital serum concentration just before the morning dose on day 16 (i.e., at the trough of the 30th and just before to the 31st dose) was reported to be 29 mg/L. Calculate the phenobarbital concentration you would have predicted on that day if N.P. has average pharmacokinetic parameters for phenobarbital.*

The average pharmacokinetic parameters for N.P. are as follows: Cl = 8 L/day (0.1 L/kg/day × 80 kg); V = 56 L (0.7 L/kg × 80 kg).

Using the values above for Cl and V, Equation 9.18 can be used to calculate an elimination rate constant (K) of 0.143 days^{-1}:

$$K = \frac{Cl}{V} \qquad \text{[Eq. 9.18]}$$

$$= \frac{8 \text{ L/day}}{56 \text{ L}}$$

$$= 0.143 \text{ day}^{-1}$$

and using the K value from above in Equation 9.19 below, a half-life of 4.85 days is calculated:

$$t\frac{1}{2} = \frac{0.693}{K} \qquad \text{[Eq. 9.19]}$$

$$t\frac{1}{2} = \frac{0.693}{0.143 \text{ day}^{-1}}$$

$$= 4.85 \text{ days}$$

Since N.P. has been receiving his phenobarbital maintenance dose for 15 days or approximately 3 half-lives, the phenobarbital concentration is assumed to be a steady-state concentration. Equation 9.20 can be used to predict the trough concentration at steady state. Using the previously calculated parameters, the steady-state trough concentration should be approximately 24 mg/L based on the calculation below.

$$\text{Css min} = \left[\dfrac{\dfrac{(S)(F)(Dose)}{V}}{(1 - e^{-K\tau})} \right] (e^{-K\tau}) \qquad \text{[Eq. 9.20]}$$

$$= \left[\dfrac{\dfrac{(1)(1)(100 \text{ mg})}{56 \text{ L}}}{(1 - e^{-(0.143 \text{ days}^{-1})(0.5 \text{ days})})} \right] (e^{-(0.143 \text{ days}^{-1})(0.5 \text{ days})})$$

$$= \left[\dfrac{1.78 \text{ mg/L}}{0.069} \right] [0.93]$$

$$= [25.9 \text{ mg/L}][0.93]$$

$$= 24 \text{ mg/L}$$

Question #10. *Considering the measured phenobarbital concentration of 29 mg/L in N.P., what method is most appropriately used to adjust his pharmacokinetic parameters? Do these patient-specific parameters suggest that a maintenance dose adjustment is necessary if the goal is to maintain the phenobarbital concentration at 25 mg/L?*

The measured trough concentration of phenobarbital is greater than the predicted concentration; therefore, N.P.'s phenobarbital clearance is likely to be lower than expected. If this is true, then his phenobarbital half-life is likely to be longer than 5 days (see Equation 9.3 below), and a nonsteady-state approach will have to be used to revise his clearance value.

$$\uparrow t\tfrac{1}{2} = \frac{(0.693)(V)}{\downarrow Cl}$$

Although there are a number of models, Equation 9.17, which describes the concentration (C_2, t_2 hours following the Nth dose, fits this situation nicely (see Part I: Selecting the Appropriate Equation: Series of Individual Doses).

$$C_2 = \left(\dfrac{\dfrac{(S)(F)(Dose)}{V}}{(1 - e^{-K\tau})} \right) (1 - e^{-K(N)\tau})(e^{-Kt_2})$$

Tau (τ) is the dosing interval of 0.5 days, N is the number of doses administered (30), and t_2 is the time elapsed since the last dose (0.5 days). To calculate the concentration at the time of sampling (C_2), the elimination rate constant will have to be adjusted first by reducing the expected clearance value in Equation 9.18.

$$K = \frac{Cl}{V}$$

Unfortunately, there is not a direct solution to this problem, and a trial and error method must be used to find the clearance value that will predict the observed phenobarbital concentration of 29 mg/L. For example, if a phenobarbital clearance of 6 L/day is used in Equation 9.18 and volume is assumed to be equal to the average value, an elimination rate constant of 0.107 days^{-1} is calculated.

$$K = \frac{Cl}{V}$$

$$= \frac{6\ \text{L/day}}{56\ \text{L}}$$

$$= 0.107\ \text{days}^{-1}$$

and

$$t\frac{1}{2} = \frac{0.693}{K}$$

$$= \frac{0.693}{0.107\ \text{days}^{-1}}$$

$$= 6.5\ \text{days}$$

The elimination rate constant, (0.107 days^{-1}) when placed in Equation 9.17, results in an expected phenobarbital concentration of approximately 26 mg/L.

$$C_2 = \left(\frac{\frac{(S)(F)(Dose)}{V}}{(1 - e^{-K\tau})} \right)(1 - e^{-K(N)\tau})(e^{-Kt_2})$$

$$= \left(\frac{\frac{(1)(10(100\ \text{mg})}{56\ \text{L}}}{(1 - e^{-(0.107d^{-1})(0.5\ \text{days})})} \right)(1 - e^{-(0.107\ d^{-1})(30)(0.5\ \text{days})})(e^{-(0.107\ d^{-1})(0.5\ \text{days})})$$

$$= \frac{1.78\ \text{mg/L}}{0.052}(1 - 0.2)(0.948)$$

$$= 25.9\ \text{mg/L or} \approx 26\ \text{mg/L}$$

Further decreasing the phenobarbital clearance to 5 L/day in Equation 9.18 results in an elimination rate constant of 0.0893 days^{-1}, and when this elimination rate constant is used in Equation 9.17, a phenobarbital concentration of 28.7 mg/L is calculated.

$$K = \frac{Cl}{V}$$

$$= \frac{5 \text{ L/day}}{56 \text{ L}}$$

$$= 0.0893 \text{ days}^{-1} \text{ and}$$

$$t_{\frac{1}{2}} = \frac{0.693}{K} = \frac{0.693}{0.0893 \text{ days}^{-1}}$$

$$= 7.8 \text{ days}$$

$$C_2 = \left(\frac{\frac{(S)(F)(\text{Dose})}{V}}{(1 - e^{-K\tau})} \right) (1 - e^{-K(N)\tau})(e^{-Kt_2})$$

$$= \left(\frac{\frac{(1)(1)(100 \text{ mg})}{0.0893 \text{ L}}}{(1 - e^{-(0.0893 \text{ d}^{-1})(0.5 \text{ days})})} \right) (1 - e^{-(0.0893 \text{ d}^{-1})(30)(0.5 \text{ days})})(e^{-(0.0893 \text{ d}^{-1})(0.5 \text{ days})})$$

$$= \frac{1.78 \text{ mg/L}}{0.0437} (0.738)(0.956)$$

$$= 28.7 \text{ mg/L or} \approx 29 \text{ mg/L}$$

The convergence of the predicted and observed concentration suggests that N.P.'s phenobarbital clearance is approximately 5 L/day. Assuming that this clearance is reasonably accurate, the predicted steady-state phenobarbital concentration (Equation 9.1) would then be approximately 40 mg/L on the current dosing regimen of 200 mg/day as calculated below.

$$\text{Css ave} = \frac{(S)(F)(\text{Dose}/\tau)}{Cl}$$

$$= \frac{(1)(1)(200 \text{ mg/day})}{5 \text{ L/day}}$$

$$= 40 \text{ mg/L}$$

If a steady-state concentration of approximately 25 mg/L is desired, a reduction in the maintenance dose to approximately 125 mg/day would be necessary as shown below (Equation 9.8).

$$\text{Maintenance Dose} = \frac{(Cl)(Css\ ave)(\tau)}{(S)(F)}$$

$$= \frac{(5\ L/day)(25\ mg/L)(1\ day)}{(1)(1)}$$

$$= 125\ mg$$

This could also be solved by the ratio of concentration change to dose (since 40 mg/L is predicted to occur with a 200 mg/day dose, a 25 mg/L concentration requires a proportionally smaller dose):

$$\left(\frac{25\ mg/L}{40\ mg/L}\right)(200\ mg) = 125\ mg$$

Since N.P.'s revised phenobarbital clearance is based on a measured drug concentration obtained very close to two estimated half-lives (i.e., 2 × 7.8 days ≈ 15 days) after therapy was initiated, the revision and expected steady-state concentration must be considered somewhat uncertain.

Although it may be appropriate to reduce the phenobarbital dose, additional concentration monitoring would be prudent in 24 to 40 days to ensure that the steady-state concentration is actually about 25 mg/L on a daily dose of 125 mg.

Question #11. *Calculate a revised concentration for N.P. using a nonsteady-state continuous infusion model.*

Because of the relatively long half-life and short dosing interval, the continuous infusion model (Eq. 9.1) is usually satisfactory when predicting steady-state phenobarbital. In this case Equation 9.12 will have to be used because the phenobarbital concentration was obtained before steady state had been achieved (see Fig. 9.1 and Part I: Figure 31).

$$C_1 = \frac{(S)(F)(Dose/\tau)}{Cl}(1 - e^{-Kt_1})$$

An important check in using Equation 9.12 is to multiply the duration of the infusion (t_1) by the infusion rate (dose divided by τ). This product should equal the total amount of drug that has been administered to the patient. For example, in N.P. the infusion rate of 100 mg divided by 0.5 days times the duration of the infusion of 15 days results in a total administered dose of 3000 mg.

$$\text{Total amount of drug administered} = (Dose/\tau)(t_1) \qquad \text{[Eq. 9.21]}$$

$$= (100\ mg/0.5\ days)(15\ days)$$

$$= 3000\ mg$$

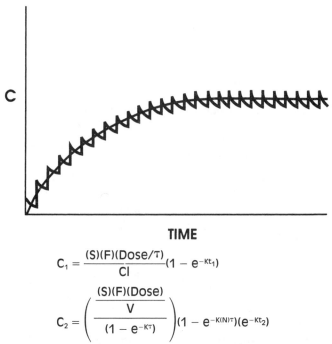

$$C_1 = \frac{(S)(F)(Dose/\tau)}{Cl}(1 - e^{-Kt_1})$$

$$C_2 = \left(\frac{\dfrac{(S)(F)(Dose)}{V}}{(1 - e^{-K\tau})} \right)(1 - e^{-K(N)\tau})(e^{-Kt_2})$$

FIGURE 9.1. Concentration-time curve for the accumulation and eventual attainment of steady state for a drug administered with a dosing interval that is much shorter than the elimination half-life. The solid smooth line represents the accumulation pattern during a continuous input model as expressed in Equation 9.12, and the sawtoothed pattern indicates the accumulation pattern for a drug administered intermittently, as in Equation 9.17. Note that the concentrations predicted by the intermittent input model are very similar to the accumulation pattern of the continuous input model.

This amount (3000 mg) is equal to the total amount of phenobarbital actually administered (i.e., 100 mg × 30 doses). Early in a regimen, the total amount of drug administered and the duration of the theoretical infusion are somewhat disparate. For example, immediately after the administration of the second phenobarbital dose, a total of 200 mg has been administered, while the total time elapsed is only one-half day. However, use of Equation 9.21 suggests that only 100 mg has been administered. Whereas this problem is most apparent early in therapy, it is seldom an issue after multiple doses have been administered. This is because a variation in one dosing interval represents a relatively small percentage error with respect to the total amount of drug administered.

Using Equation 9.12, the previously calculated clearance of 5 L/day, and the corresponding elimination rate constant of 0.0893 day^{-1}, a phenobarbital concentration of 29.6 mg/L is calculated.

$$C_1 = \frac{(1)(1)(100 \text{ mg/0.5 days})}{5 \text{ L/day}} (1 - e^{-(0.0893 \text{ days}^{-1})(15 \text{ days})})$$

$$= (40 \text{ mg/L})(0.74)$$

$$= 29.6 \text{ mg/L}$$

The similarities between the predicted phenobarbital concentration using the continuous infusion and the intermittent bolus model suggest that either model could be used, with the continuous infusion model requiring fewer computations.

Question #12. *J.R., an epileptic male who has been managed chronically with phenobarbital 120 mg/day, has recently developed hypoalbuminemia secondary to nephrotic syndrome. Will his phenobarbital concentration be affected by decreases in his albumin concentration or renal function?*

Only 40% to 50% of phenobarbital is bound to plasma proteins; therefore, fu (the fraction of phenobarbital that is unbound) is 0.5 to 0.6.[22,23] The concentration of a drug that is bound to protein to the extent of 50% or less is not likely to be significantly affected by changes in plasma protein concentrations or protein binding affinity.

The renal clearance for phenobarbital is probably less than 20% of the total clearance in patients with normal renal function and an uncontrolled urine pH (i.e., the urine pH is not intentionally adjusted).[16] Therefore, it is unlikely that patients with renal failure will require significant adjustments in their phenobarbital dosage regimens.

To summarize, J.R.'s phenobarbital concentrations are not likely to be significantly affected by his hypoalbuminemia or poor renal function.

Question #13. *R.T. is a 28-year-old, 70-kg man with chronic renal failure and a seizure disorder. He has been maintained with 60 mg of phenobarbital BID and has steady-state concentrations of 20 mg/L. Over the past 3 months, his renal function has progressively worsened and he is to be started on 3 hours of high-flux hemodialysis 3 times weekly. Will he require an adjustment of his maintenance regimen? (See Part I: Dialysis of Drugs.) If he were eventually switched to continuous peritoneal dialysis, would that create a need for adjustment of his maintenance regimen?*

To determine whether a significant amount of drug is lost during each dialysis period, the three steps outlined in Part I: Dialysis of Drugs should be examined. First, the apparent volume of distribution for unbound drug should be estimated using Equation 9.22. Using a volume of distribution of 0.7 L/kg or 49 L for this 70 kg patient and a free fraction or fu of 0.5 for phenobarbital, the apparent unbound volume of distribution for phenobarbital in R.T. is approximately 98 L. Since this is less than the upper limit of 250 L for a dialyzable drug, dialysis possibly could remove a significant amount of phenobarbital.

$$\text{Unbound Volume of Distribution} = \frac{V}{fu} \qquad \text{[Eq. 9.22]}$$

$$= \frac{49 \text{ L}}{0.5}$$

$$= 98 \text{ L}$$

R.T.'s clearance of phenobarbital must be estimated next. The usual clearance of 0.1 L/kg/day, or 7 L/day for the 70 kg patient, represents a total body clearance of approximately 5 mL/min. This value is low enough (i.e., < 500 to 700 mL/min) that dialysis could significantly increase the total clearance.

$$\text{Clearance (ml/min)} = (7 \text{ L/day})\left(\frac{1000 \text{ ml/L}}{1440 \text{ min/day}}\right)$$

$$= 4.9 \text{ mL/min or} \approx 5 \text{ mL/min}$$

Finally, estimate the drug's half-life using Equation 9.3. The apparent half-life for phenobarbital of approximately 5 days is much longer than the lower limit of 1 to 2 hours set in Criterion 3 (i.e., hemodialysis is unlikely to significantly alter the dosing regimen if the drug half-life is very short).

$$t\tfrac{1}{2} = \frac{(0.693)(V)}{Cl}$$

$$= \frac{(0.693)(49 \text{ L})}{7 \text{ L/day}}$$

$$= 4.9 \text{ days}$$

Since the unbound volume of distribution and phenobarbital clearance of R.T. are relatively small, and the half-life is much greater than the lower limit of 1 to 2 hours, a significant amount of phenobarbital could be cleared during a dialysis period. For this reason, the actual clearance of phenobarbital during standard hemodialysis will have to be determined from the literature. The clearance of phenobarbital by hemodialysis has not been studied extensively; however, two older cases on the use of "standard" hemodialysis in the treatment of phenobarbital overdoses indicated that the clearance of phenobarbital by standard hemodialysis was approximately 3 L/hr.[7,24] A recent case report of an overdose indicated that newer high-flux, high-efficiency polysulfone hemodialysis membranes are much more efficient. For this patient, the first step would be to calculate his phenobarbital clearance (Cl) using Equation 9.9:

$$CI = \frac{(S)(F)(Dose/\tau)}{Css\ ave}$$

$$= \frac{(1)(1)(60\ mg/0.5\ day)}{20\ mg/L}$$

$$= 6\ L/day\ or\ 0.25\ L/hr$$

Using Equation 9.23, an estimate of 10 L/hr[25] as the clearance by high-flux dialysis (Cl_{dial}) and the patient's calculated clearance (Cl_{pat}) of 0.25 L/hr, a dialysis replacement dose can be calculated. Equation 9.23 was selected to calculate the replacement dose because of the long half-life and relatively short dosing interval for phenobarbital (see Part I: Dialysis of Drugs and Figure 33).

$$\text{Post Dialysis Replacement Dose} = (V)(Css\ ave)\left(1 - e^{-\left(\frac{Cl_{pat} + Cl_{dial}}{V}\right)(T_{dial})}\right) \qquad \text{[Eq. 9.23]}$$

$$= (49\ L)(20\ mg/L)\left(1 - e^{-\left(\frac{0.25\ L/hr + 10\ L/hr}{49\ L}\right)(3\ hr)}\right)$$

$$= (980\ mg)(1 - e^{-(0.209\ hr^{-1})(3\ hr)})$$

$$= (980\ mg)(1 - 0.53)$$

$$= 460\ mg$$

This replacement dose of approximately 450 mg represents the amount of drug eliminated from the body during the dialysis period by both metabolic and dialysis clearance. In this case, the vast majority of the drug eliminated during the 3-hour dialysis period represents drug eliminated by the dialysis route. For this reason, the total daily phenobarbital dose on days of dialysis would be 120 mg (maintenance dose) plus the postdialysis dose of ≈450 mg. If less efficient dialyzers are used, the post-dialysis dose would be less. For example, if the clearance of 3 L/hr from the older case reports is used in the above calculations with a 3-hour dialysis period, the replacement dose would be approximately 175 mg. This illustrates one of the problems of using literature on dialysis clearance to predict doses. That is, dialyzers and dialysis procedures have become more efficient over time. It is therefore important to seek data on the actual dialysis membrane and procedures being used or to measure before and after concentrations to determine actual loss in a given patient. In addition, it is possible that the actual drug loss during high-flux dialysis will be less for R.T. than was estimated. One possible flaw in the estimation is that the amount eliminated in Equation 9.23 assumes that the Cl_{dial} is eliminating phenobarbital from the entire volume of distribution, when, in fact, it is the plasma that is being cleared. If plasma is cleared faster than it can re-equilibrate from the deeper tissues, the amount of drug loss will be less than predicted and there will be a significant rebound in the plasma concentration following dialysis. The more efficient the dialysis membrane, the more likely it is that Equation 9.23 will overestimate the amount of drug loss.

Standard replacement doses of phenobarbital after dialysis are frequently in the range of 200 to 300 mg. While this replacement dose appears to be large when compared with the maintenance dose, it is not unusual. If there is concern about the size of the postdialysis replacement dose, one could administer a smaller dose of 100 to 200 mg after dialysis and continue to monitor the patient during subsequent dialysis periods to ensure that the phenobarbital concentration does not continue to decline due to additional elimination by the dialysis route.

If R.T. receives continuous peritoneal dialysis (CAPD), then further dose adjustments will be needed. In hemodialysis, where dialysis is intermittent, the majority of the phenobarbital clearance during dialysis is primarily Cl_{dial} and hence the need for a replacement dose post-dialysis. With CAPD, the dialysis clearance values are lower but continuous. As a result, both the clearance by CAPD and the patient's metabolism are important contributors to the elimination of phenobarbital. With continuous peritoneal dialysis, it appears that 35% to 50% of the daily dose is removed in the dialysate. Thus, the predicted daily dose would usually be increased by about 40% to compensate for the additional loss due to peritoneal dialysis.[26] The clearance due to dialysis in CAPD is greatly affected by dextrose concentration, dwell time, and number of cycles. For example, in the case cited, loss of phenobarbital was only ~7 mg during a 12-hour daytime period with one cycle versus ~45 mg during six cycles at night.[26] Thus, steady-state concentrations should be used to guide therapy, and if the peritoneal exchange process is altered significantly (i.e., volume or exchange dwell time), additional dose adjustments may be necessary.

Question #14. *H.P., a 7-year-old, 30-kg boy, is to be given phenobarbital for his seizure disorder. Calculate the maintenance dose of phenobarbital that will produce a steady-state concentration of ≈25 mg/L.*

To calculate H.P.'s phenobarbital maintenance dose, one would first assume his clearance to be ≈6 L/day (0.2 L/kg/day × 30 kg). This clearance value, although larger than the usual adult value, is consistent for children. Using Equation 9.8 with a target concentration of 25 mg/L, and a salt form (S) fraction of 1, a daily maintenance dose of 150 mg can be calculated.

$$\text{Maintenance Dose} = \frac{(Cl)(Css\ ave)(\tau)}{(S)(F)}$$

$$= \frac{(6 \text{ L/day})(25 \text{ mg/L})(1 \text{ day})}{(1)(1)}$$

$$= 150 \text{ mg}$$

Depending on the clinical situation, one could administer a loading dose to rapidly achieve therapeutic concentrations or start the patient on his maintenance dose without a loading dose. In the latter situation, the urgency of the clinical situation will determine whether the initial maintenance dose should be 150 mg/day or one quarter of the target maintenance dose ($\approx$38 mg/day) for the first week, increased by $\approx$38 mg/day weekly until the final maintenance dose of 150 mg/day is being administered. As noted previously, excessive sedation can be a consequence of starting the patient with the full maintenance dose. H.P. should be monitored for both therapeutic and potential side effects during this period of dose titration.

Question #15. *H.P. is able to take phenobarbital tablets and is given the commercially available dose of 65 mg twice daily for a total daily dose of 130 mg. What impact would the use of this dose have on the predicted Css ave?*

With use of Equation 9.1, the Css ave can be predicted from the actual dose used:

$$\text{Css ave} = \frac{(S)(F)(\text{Dose}/\tau)}{Cl}$$

$$= \frac{(1)(1)(130 \text{ mg/day})}{6 \text{ L/day}}$$

$$= 21.7 \text{ mg/L}$$

Or, because in Equation 9.1, Css ave and dose are proportional so long as S, F, and τ are held constant, the new Css ave could have been calculated as a ratio of the doses times the predicted concentration:

$$\text{Css ave} = (25 \text{ mg/L})\left(\frac{130 \text{ mg}}{150 \text{ mg}}\right) = 21.7 \text{ mg/L}$$

Question #16. *S.M., a 45-year-old, 60-kg woman, was recently prescribed 120 mg/day of phenobarbital. Ten days ago her concentration was 15 mg/L; today her phenobarbital concentration is 24 mg/L. Based on the data provided, what would you calculate her steady-state phenobarbital concentration to be?*

To calculate S.M.'s phenobarbital concentration, one will first have to determine her clearance. Unfortunately, because phenobarbital has a long half-life, it is unlikely that the present concentration of 24 mg/L represents steady state. Therefore, some type of iterative search or indirect procedure must be used to extract clearance. One method is to combine Equations 9.16 and 9.12 where C^o is the initial phenobarbital concentration of 15 mg/L and, in Equation 9.12, the infusion rate is essentially represented by the daily dose of 120 mg/day. In both Equations 9.16 and 9.12, the time interval "t" between C^o and the current concentration of 24 mg/L would be 10 days.

$$C_1 = C^o(e^{-Kt}) + \frac{(S)(F)(Dose/\tau)}{Cl}(1 - e^{-Kt_1})$$

$$24 \text{ mg/L} = (15 \text{ mg/L})(e^{-(K)(10 \text{ days})}) + \left[\frac{(1)(1)(120 \text{ mg/day})}{Cl}\right](1 - e^{-(K)(10 \text{ days})})$$

Unfortunately, the resolution to this problem first requires assuming S.M.'s volume of distribution (0.7 L/kg × 60 kg or = 42 L) and then iteratively solving for the clearance (Cl) and K (Cl/V = Cl/42 L) until the result is a calculated concentration equal to the observed C_1 of 24 mg/L. As discussed previously, this is a sometimes laborious procedure, and an alternative approach that could be of use is the mass balance equation, Equation 9.24:

$$Cl = \frac{\left(\dfrac{SFD}{\tau}\right) - \left(\dfrac{(C_2 - C_1)V}{t}\right)}{C \text{ ave}} \qquad [\text{Eq. 9.24}]$$

In the above equation, if one substitutes S.M.'s maintenance dose of phenobarbital, the corresponding C_1 of 15 mg/L and C_2 of 24 mg/L, and assumes that the C ave is ≈19.5 mg/L, or halfway between the initial and present phenobarbital concentrations [(15 mg/L + 24 mg/L)/2], a clearance of ≈4.2 L/day is calculated.

$$Cl = \frac{\left(\dfrac{(1)(1)(120 \text{ mg})}{1 \text{ day}}\right) - \left(\dfrac{(24 \text{ mg/L} - 15 \text{ mg/L})(42 \text{ L})}{10 \text{ days}}\right)}{19.5 \text{ mg/L}}$$

$$= \frac{120 \text{ mg/day} - \dfrac{378 \text{ mg}}{10 \text{ days}}}{19.5 \text{ mg/L}}$$

$$= \frac{82.2 \text{ mg/day}}{19.5 \text{ mg/L}}$$

$$= 4.2 \text{ L/day}$$

This clearance value of 4.2 L/day corresponds to a half-life of approximately 7 days (Equation 9.3, using 42 L as the assumed V).

$$t_{1/2} = \frac{(0.693)(V)}{Cl}$$

$$= \frac{(0.693)(42 \text{ L})}{4.2 \text{ L/day}}$$

$$= 6.9 \text{ days}$$

Using Equation 9.11 and the $t_{1/2}$ from above, the elimination rate constant (K) can be calculated:

$$K = \frac{0.693}{t_{1/2}}$$

$$= \frac{0.693}{6.9 \text{ days}}$$

$$= 0.1 \text{ days}^{-1}$$

As discussed in Part I, there are several conditions that should be met if the prediction calculated by use of the mass balance equation is to be reasonably accurate. First, the time between the first and second concentrations should be at least 1 but no longer than 2 drug half-lives. Second, if concentrations are rising, C_2 should be less than twice C_1. Third, the rate of drug administration should be reasonably regular and smooth. By examining the drug half-life, the change in concentrations, and the dosing regimen, it is clear that we have met all three of these conditions; therefore, one would anticipate that the clearance value predicted should be reasonably accurate.

If there was concern about the validity of the revised clearance derived from the mass balance equation, the clearance value of 4.2 L/day along with the corresponding elimination rate constant of 0.1 days^{-1} could be used in Equations 9.16 and 9.12 to confirm that both the iterative search and mass balance equations generate essentially the same answer.

$$C_1 = C^0(e^{-Kt}) + \frac{(S)(F)(Dose/\tau)}{Cl}(1 - e^{-Kt_1})$$

$$= (15 \text{ mg/L})(e^{-(0.1 \text{ days}^{-1})(10 \text{ days})}) + \left[\frac{(1)(1)(120 \text{ mg/day})}{4.2 \text{ L/day}} \right](1 - e^{-(0.1 \text{ days}^{-1})(10 \text{ days})})$$

$$= [15\text{mg/L} (0.368)] + [(28.57 \text{ mg/L})(1 - 0.368)]$$

$$= 5.52 \text{ mg/L} + 18 \text{ mg/L}$$

$$= 23.52 \text{ mg/L}$$

As can be seen from this calculation, the predicted concentration using the exponential equations results in a value very close to the observed concentration of 24 mg/L. This comparison is useful when there is concern that the assumptions implicit in the mass balance equation have oversimplified a more complex problem. Our comparison indicates that both approaches are equivalent.

To calculate the expected steady-state concentration of approximately 29 mg/L, Equation 9.1 would be used in conjunction with our revised phenobarbital clearance of 4.2 L/day.

$$\text{Css ave} = \frac{(S)(F)(\text{Dose}/\tau)}{Cl}$$

$$= \frac{(1)(1)(120 \text{ mg/day})}{4.2 \text{ L/day}}$$

$$= 28.57 \text{ or } \approx 29 \text{ mg/L}$$

REFERENCES

1. Wilkes L, Danziger LH, Rodvold KA, et al. Phenobarbital pharmacokinetics in obesity. A case report. Clin Pharmacokinet 1992;22:481–484.

2. Buchthal F, et al. Relation of EEG and seizures to phenobarbital in serum. Arch Neurol 1968;19:567.

3. Jannuzzi G, Cian P, Fattore C, et al. A multicenter randomized controlled trial on the clinical impact of therapeutic drug monitoring in patients with newly diagnosed epilepsy. Epilepsia 2000;41:222–230.

4. Plass GL, Hine CH. Hydantoin and barbiturate blood levels observed in epileptics. Arch Int Pharmacodyn Ther 1960;128:375.

5. Sushine I. Chemical evidence of tolerance to phenobarbital. J Lab Clin Med 1957;50:127.

6. Baselt RC, et al. Therapeutic and toxic concentrations of more than 100 toxicologically significant drugs in blood, plasma, or serum: a tabulation. Clin Chem 1975;21:44.

7. Kennedy AC, et al. Successful treatment of three cases of very severe barbiturate poisoning. Lancet 1969;1:995.

8. Levy RE, et al. Carbamazepine, valproic acid, phenobarbital and ethosuximide. In: Evans WE, et al. eds. Applied Pharmacokinetics: Principles of Therapeutic Drug Monitoring. 3rd Ed. Vancouver: Applied Therapeutics Inc, 1992.

9. Wilensky AJ, et al. Kinetics of phenobarbital in normal subjects and epileptic patients. Eur J Clin Pharmacol 1982;23:87–92.

10. Graves NM, et al. Relative bioavailability of rectally administered phenobarbital sodium parenteral solution. Drug Intell Clin Pharm 1989;23:565–568.

11. Gal P. Phenobarbital and primidone. In: Taylor WJ, Diers-Caviness MH, eds. A Text Book for the Clinical Application of Therapeutic Drug Monitoring. Irving: Abbott Laboratories Diagnostics Division, 1986:237–252.

12. Havidberg E, Dam M. Clinical pharmacokinetics of anticonvulsants. Clin Pharmacokinet 1976;1:151.

13. Alvin J, et al. The effect of liver disease in man on the disposition of phenobarbital. J Pharmacol Exp Ther 1975;192:224.

14. Battino D, Estienne M, Avanzini G. Clinical pharmacokinetics of antiepileptic drugs in paediatric patients. Part I: Phenobarbital, primidone, valproic acid, ethosuximide and mesuximide. Clin Pharmacokinet 1995;29:257–286.

15. Touw DJ, et al. Clinical pharmacokinetics of phenobarbital in neonates. Eur J Pharmaceut Sci 2000;12:111–116.

16. Linton AL, et al. Methods of forced diuresis and its application in barbiturate poisoning. Lancet 1967;2:377.

17. Heimann G, Gladtke E. Pharmacokinetics of phenobarbital in childhood. Eur J Clin Pharmacol 1977;12:305.

18. Painter MJ, et al. Phenobarbital and diphenylhydantoin levels in neonates with seizures. J Pediatr 1978;92:315.

19. Botha JH, Gray AL, Miller R. Determination of phenobarbitone population clearance values for South African children. Eur J Clin Pharmacol 1995;48:381–383.

20. Murphy JE, Winter ME. Clinical pharmacokinetic pearls: using bolus vs infusion equations. Pharmacotherapy 1996;16:698–700.

21. Reidenberg P, et al. Effects of felbamate on the pharmacokinetics of phenobarbital. Clin Pharmacol Ther 1995;58:279–287.

22. Waddell WJ, Butler TC. The distribution of phenobarbital. J. Clin Invest 1957;36:1217.

23. Houghton GW, et al. Brain concentrations of phenytoin, phenobarbitone, and primidone in epileptic patients. Eur J Clin Pharmacol 1975;9:73.

24. Henderson LW, Merrill JP. Treatment of barbiturate intoxication. Ann Intern Med 1966;64:876.

25. Palmer BF. Effectiveness of hemodialysis in the extracorporeal therapy of phenobarbital overdose. Am J Kidney Dis 2000;36:640–643.

26. Porto I, John EG, Heilliczer J. Removal of phenobarbital during continuous cycling peritoneal dialysis in a child. Pharmacotherapy 1997;17:832–835.

10

PHENYTOIN

Michael E. Winter

Phenytoin is primarily used as an anticonvulsant and has been used in the treatment of certain types of cardiac arrhythmias.[1] It is usually administered orally in single or divided doses of 200 to 400 mg/day. When a rapid therapeutic effect is required, a loading dose of 15 mg/kg can be administered by oral or intravenous (IV) routes. Although phenytoin for injection can be administered intramuscularly, this route should be avoided because of slow and erratic absorption. Fosphenytoin is a more soluble ester of phenytoin and can be administered by the IV or intramuscular (IM) route. Absorption of fosphenytoin by the IM route is more rapid than the oral route but slower than the IV route of administration.[2]

KEY PARAMETERS: Phenytoin	
Therapeutic Plasma Concentration	10–20 mg/L
F[a]	1
S[b]	0.92, 1
V	0.65 L/kg

Cl
    Vm[c]
    Km[d]
	
	7 mg/kg/day
	4 mg/L

$t_{1/2}$[e]	Concentration-dependent
fu (Fraction Unbound in Plasma)	0.1

[a]Oral bioavailability is generally assumed to be 1 (100% absorbed). However, bioavailability is difficult to estimate, and different drug products are not considered to be interchangeable or therapeutically equivalent.
[b]Capsules and the injectable preparations (phenytoin and fosphenytoin), S = 0.92; for the suspension and chewable tablet, S = 1.
[c]Adult value, Vm values are > 7 mg/kg/day and age dependent for children.
[d]Adult value, Km values are variable for children.
[e]See $t_{1/2}$ section for time to steady state.

Individualizing the dose of phenytoin is beset by two major problems. First, binding of phenytoin to plasma proteins is decreased in patients with renal failure or hypoalbuminemia. Second, the metabolic capacity of phenytoin is limited; therefore, changes in the maintenance dose result in disproportionate changes in steady-state plasma concentrations. The capacity-limited metabolism of phenytoin also eliminates the clinical usefulness of half-life ($t\frac{1}{2}$) as a pharmacokinetic parameter and makes estimates of the time required to achieve steady state difficult.

THERAPEUTIC AND TOXIC PLASMA CONCENTRATIONS

Phenytoin plasma concentrations of 10 to 20 mg/L are generally accepted as therapeutic.[3-8] Plasma concentrations in the range of 5 to 10 mg/L can be therapeutic for some patients, but concentrations < 5 mg/L are not likely to be effective.[9]

A number of phenytoin side effects, such as gingival hyperplasia, folate deficiency, and peripheral neuropathy, do not appear to be easily related to plasma phenytoin concentrations. In contrast, central nervous system (CNS) side effects do correlate with plasma concentration. Far-lateral nystagmus usually occurs in patients with plasma phenytoin concentrations > 20 mg/L. The concentration range associated with this effect, however, is broad, with some patients showing symptoms at concentrations of 15 mg/L and others having no nystagmus at concentrations > 30 mg/L. While far-lateral nystagmus is often used to monitor phenytoin therapy, it is seldom considered a true drug side effect or toxicity and is not a reason to reduce the phenytoin dose. Other CNS symptoms such as ataxia and diminished mental capacity are frequently observed in patients with concentrations exceeding 30 mg/L and 40 mg/L, respectively.[4] In addition, precautions should be taken when phenytoin for injection is administered by the IV route because the propylene glycol diluent has cardiac depressant properties.[3] Fosphenytoin is more soluble than phenytoin for injection and does not contain propylene glycol as a diluent. However, fosphenytoin does have similar effects on the myocardium and cardiovascular system (bradycardia and hypotension) but to a lesser extent. Clinicians should be aware that the maximum recommended rate of IV administration is 50 mg/min for phenytoin for injection and 150 mg/min for fosphenytoin.

Alterations in Plasma Protein Binding

The usual phenytoin therapeutic range of 10 to 20 mg/L represents the total drug concentration, which consists of unbound (or free) drug concentration plus phenytoin, which is bound to plasma albumin. The usual fu or free fraction of phenytoin is 0.1. Therefore, approximately 90% of phenytoin in the plasma is bound to serum albumin; about 10% is unbound and free to equilibrate with the tissues where the pharmacologic effects and metabolism occur. It is important to keep in mind that while most of the phenytoin in plasma is bound to plasma albumin, most of the phenytoin is not in plasma. Therefore, any phenytoin displaced off the plasma albumin, while a large percentage of the drug in plasma, is a small percentage of phenytoin in the tissue. The displaced phenytoin will re-equilibrate with the tissue, resulting in very little change in the unbound or free plasma phenytoin concentration and very little change in the pharmacologic effect. Following re-equilibration of the displaced phenytoin, the unbound plasma phenytoin concentration will be relatively unchanged, but the total plasma phenytoin concentration will be decreased because the bound concentration has decreased. As a result the total level will appear to be low relative to its potential for pharmacologic effect (therapeutic and/or toxic).

There are two approaches one can use to interpret phenytoin levels when protein binding is significantly altered. The first is to adjust all the parameters (i.e., therapeutic range, volume of distribution, and Km) to those that would be observed in the presence of altered plasma binding. The second is to convert the measured or observed plasma concentration with low binding into that which would be observed under normal binding conditions (C Normal Binding). In this instance, the parameters (i.e., therapeutic range, volume of distribution, and Km) associated with normal plasma protein binding would also be used in any calculations. While either of these approaches is acceptable, it is the author's belief that the second method is least likely to result in calculation errors. Therefore, this latter approach will be used throughout this chapter when alterations in plasma binding are encountered.

The three factors that are known to significantly alter the plasma protein binding of phenytoin are hypoalbuminemia, renal failure, and displacement by other drugs.

HYPOALBUMINEMIA. In patients with low serum albumin, Equation 10.1 can be used to determine the plasma concentration that would have been observed with a normal plasma protein concentration.

$$\text{C Normal Binding} = \frac{C'}{(1 - fu)\left[\dfrac{P'}{P_{NL}}\right] + fu} \qquad \text{[Eq. 10.1]}$$

C' is the observed plasma concentration reported by the laboratory; fu is the normal free fraction of drug (phenytoin fu = 0.1);[10–12] P' is the patient's serum albumin in units of gm/dL; P_{NL} is the normal serum albumin (4.4 gm/dL); and C Normal Binding is the plasma drug concentration that would have been observed if the patient's serum albumin concentration had been normal. Placing the corresponding values for fu and a normal serum albumin results in Equation 10.2 below.

$$\frac{\text{Phenytoin Concentration}}{\text{Normal Plasma Binding}} = \frac{\text{Patient's Phenytoin Concentration with Altered Plasma Binding}}{\left[0.9 \times \dfrac{\text{Patient's Serum Albumin}}{4.4 \text{ gm/dL}}\right] + 0.1} \qquad \text{[Eq. 10.2]}$$

This equation is most useful when a patient has a low serum albumin concentration but does not have significantly diminished renal function and is not taking other drugs known to displace phenytoin.

RENAL FAILURE. In patients with end-stage renal disease, the free fraction of phenytoin increases from 0.1 to 0.2 to 0.35.[10,13-16] Some of this change in plasma binding is due to the decrease in serum albumin concentration associated with end-stage renal disease, and some of the binding changes are due to a change in the binding affinity of phenytoin to serum albumin. When the creatinine clearance is > 25 mL/min, the change in the binding affinity is minimal, no adjustment for renal function need be made, and Equation 10.2 should be used. However, if the creatinine clearance is < 10 mL/min and the patient is undergoing hemodialysis treatments, binding changes can be significant.[17]

In the latter circumstance, Equation 10.2 can be altered to accommodate changes in both the serum albumin concentration and the affinity of phenytoin for serum albumin. Hence, Equation 10.3:

$$\frac{\text{Phenytoin Concentration}}{\text{Normal Plasma Binding}} = \frac{\text{Dialysis Patient's Phenytoin Concentration with Altered Plasma Binding}}{\left[(0.9)(0.48) \times \dfrac{\text{Patient's Serum Albumin}}{4.4 \text{ gm/dL}}\right] + 0.1} \qquad \text{[Eq. 10.3]}$$

The above equations should only be used in patients with end-stage renal disease receiving hemodialysis treatments because the factor that represents the decreased affinity for phenytoin binding to serum albumin (0.48) was derived from this type of patient. Note that, in Equation 10.3, fu is again assumed to be 0.1 [i.e., $0.9 = (1 - fu)$] because the Phenytoin Concentration Normal Plasma Binding (C Normal Binding) calculated by Equation 10.3 corrects for both serum albumin and renal dysfunction. In addition, it should be recognized that Equations 10.2 and 10.3 are only approximate estimates of normal plasma binding phenytoin concentrations and there can be considerable variance among individual patients. The general concept, however, that phenytoin binding needs to be considered when evaluating phenytoin concentration, is important to remember when using phenytoin concentrations to adjust a patient's dosing regimen. In patients with diminished renal function who are not undergoing intermittent hemodialysis, binding affinity is unpredictably altered when the creatinine clearance is between 10 and 25 mL/min. The plasma concentration of drugs cannot be interpreted accurately for this group of patients using Equation 10.3.[17]

When discussing alterations in plasma binding with a non-pharmacist clinician it is often useful to consider what would be the target phenytoin in a patient with decreased plasma binding. That is, what is the lower and upper concentration in your patient with altered binding that would be equivalent to the usual range of 10 to 20 mg/L when binding is normal. These values can be calculated by rearranging the Equations 10.2 and 10.3.

For patients with hypoalbuminemia and a creatinine clearance > 25 mL/min, the equivalent lower and upper end of the concentration range would be:

$$\text{Patient's Therapeutic Range With Low Albumin that would be Equal to 10 mg/L} = \quad [\text{Eq. 10.4}]$$

$$10 \text{ mg/L} \times \left[\left(0.9 \times \frac{\text{Patient's Serum Albumin}}{4.4 \text{ gm/dL}} \right) + 0.1 \right]$$

$$\text{Patient's Therapeutic Range With Low Albumin that would be Equal to 20 mg/L} = \quad [\text{Eq. 10.5}]$$

$$20 \text{ mg/L} \times \left[\left(0.9 \times \frac{\text{Patient's Serum Albumin}}{4.4 \text{ gm/dL}} \right) + 0.1 \right]$$

For patients with hypoalbuminemia who are receiving dialysis, the equivalent lower and upper end of the concentration range would be:

$$\text{Patient's Therapeutic Range With Low Albumin and on Dialysis that would be Equal to 10 mg/L} = \quad [\text{Eq. 10.6}]$$

$$10 \text{ mg/L} \times \left[\left(0.9 \times 0.48 \times \frac{\text{Patient's Serum Albumin}}{4.4 \text{ gm/dL}} \right) + 0.1 \right]$$

$$\text{Patient's Therapeutic Range With Low Albumin and on Dialysis that would be Equal to 20 mg/L} = \quad [\text{Eq. 10.7}]$$

$$20 \text{ mg/L} \times \left[\left(0.9 \times 0.48 \times \frac{\text{Patient's Serum Albumin}}{4.4 \text{ gm/dL}} \right) + 0.1 \right]$$

DRUG DISPLACEMENT. Drugs also can displace phenytoin from plasma protein binding sites. As explained in Part I: Desired Plasma Concentration, it is usually difficult to estimate the extent of drug displacement from protein-binding sites because the concentration of the displacing agent is seldom known. One exception to this rule is the situation in which serum concentrations of both valproic acid and phenytoin are being monitored. When the serum valproic acid concentration is < 20 mg/L, the displacement of phenytoin appears to be minimal and adjustment of the phenytoin concentration is probably not warranted. When the valproic acid concentration increases, the extent of phenytoin displacement from plasma-protein binding sites increases. At valproic acid concentrations of approximately 70 mg/L, phenytoin serum concentrations decrease by 40% (see Valproic Acid).[18,19]

In a study by Kerrick, Wolff, and Graves,[20] an equation was developed to help correct or adjust for the displacement of phenytoin by valproic acid. Equation 10.8 below is a modification of their original equation:

$$\frac{\text{Phenytoin Concentration}}{\text{Normal Plasma Binding}} = \frac{[0.095 + (0.001)(\text{Valproic Acid Concentration})](\text{Phenytoin Concentration})}{0.1} \quad \text{[Eq. 10.8]}$$

Where the Phenytoin Concentration Normal Plasma Binding is the concentration that would have been reported if there had been no displacement by valproic acid (i.e., fu = 0.1). The valproic acid and phenytoin concentrations are the concentrations that are reported by the laboratory. Note, however, that Equation 10.8 has the requirement that the two drug concentrations be measured (obtained) at the same time. In addition, there should not be any other factors present that would alter plasma binding (e.g., hypoalbuminemia, renal failure, other displacing drugs).

BIOAVAILABILITY (F)

Phenytoin is completely absorbed (F = 1.0) from most currently available products[21]; however, the various dosage forms and different manufacturers' products are not considered to be interchangeable.[6,22–25] In addition there are different salt forms of phenytoin. The capsule and injectable preparations consist of the sodium salt (S = 0.92) of phenytoin, whereas the chewable tablet and suspension contain the acid form (S = 1.0) of phenytoin. Although the fosphenytoin injectable product has a salt factor different than 0.92, the content of the fosphenytoin vial is labeled as mg of P.E. or "Phenytoin Equivalent"; therefore, a salt factor (S) of 0.92 should be used in calculations with this product. The rate of phenytoin absorption following oral administration is slow because of the limited aqueous solubility of phenytoin. This is true regardless of whether the prompt or extended absorption oral products are used.[22] Serum concentrations of phenytoin extended absorption products usually peak 3 to 12 hours after oral administration when given as the usual daily maintenance doses.[22]

Phenytoin is absorbed slowly and the bioavailability could be less than 100% in patients with rapid gastrointestinal transit times.[26] Phenytoin concentrations are significantly decreased in patients receiving liquid dietary supplements (nasogastric feedings) and neonates.[27–29] Presumably, rapid gastrointestinal motility decreases the apparent bioavailability of phenytoin, although the specific mechanism has not been identified. In some patients receiving nasogastric feedings, phenytoin doses of up to 1200 mg/day were required to achieve therapeutic concentrations. Discontinuation of the enteral feedings resulted in a significant increase in the phenytoin plasma concentrations. It is recommended that patients receiving nasogastric feedings be closely monitored as concentrations within the usual therapeutic range are difficult to achieve and maintain. Similar potential problems may occur when phenytoin is administered concomitantly with antacids.[27,30]

The bioavailability of phenytoin is difficult to evaluate because of the drug's capacity-limited metabolism.[31] The slow absorption of phenytoin also tends to diminish the change in concentration following an oral dose. In most patients receiving oral phenytoin, the change in concentration (ΔC) will be about half that observed when giving the drug by the IV route. The slow rate of absorption also results in delayed peak concentrations that occur between 3 and 12 hours after administration of normal maintenance doses. When loading doses of 1 gm are administered orally as the extended absorption product, serum concentrations usually peak in about 24 hours; if the dose is increased to 1600 mg, the peak may be delayed as much as 30 hours.[32,33] The time required to achieve the peak concentration can be decreased if a phenytoin "prompt absorption" product is administered.[25] However, the time to peak is still delayed, and the IV route is preferred when rapid achievement of therapeutic concentrations is required.

While the absorption of phenytoin is almost certainly a complex process, one approach the author has used is to assume an absorption rate of approximately 50 mg/hr for the extended absorption product Dilantin Kapseals. This absorption rate is consistent with the observations stated above and is sometimes useful when estimating a time when the peak concentration will occur following oral administration. In addition, although it is common practice to divide large doses into 5 mg/kg increments administered every 2 hours, there are no studies documenting that this procedure is optimal in terms of the dose size or interval between doses.

VOLUME OF DISTRIBUTION (V)

The volume of distribution of phenytoin in patients with normal renal function and with normal serum albumin concentrations is approximately 0.65

L/kg.[10,34,35] Although the volume of distribution for phenytoin is increased in patients with diminished plasma binding, the loading dose should not be changed because changes in the volume of distribution resulting from changes in plasma binding are accompanied by equal and opposite changes in the desired phenytoin concentration. Also, the amount of phenytoin in the plasma represents only a small fraction of the total amount of phenytoin in the body. The approach taken in this chapter is to correct any measured concentrations altered by binding to the concentration that would be observed under normal plasma binding conditions. Under these conditions a volume of distribution of 0.65 L/kg, which represents normal plasma binding (fu = 0.1), should be used in all computations.

In obese patients the volume of distribution for phenytoin is a complex relationship between plasma protein binding, lipid solubility, and tissue perfusion. Equation 10.9 below is based on a study by Abernathy and Greenblatt.[36]

For obese patients:

$$V_{Phenytoin\ in\ L} = 0.65\ L/kg[IBW + 1.3(TBW - IBW)] \qquad \text{[Eq. 10.9]}$$

Where TBW is the patient's total body weight in kg and IBW is the patient's ideal body weight in kg.

$$\frac{\text{Ideal Body Weight}}{\text{for males in kg}} = 50 + (2.3)(\text{Height in Inches} > 60) \qquad \text{[Eq. 10.10]}$$

$$\frac{\text{Ideal Body Weight}}{\text{for females in kg}} = 45 + (2.3)(\text{Height in Inches} > 60) \qquad \text{[Eq. 10.11]}$$

CAPACITY-LIMITED METABOLISM

For most drugs, the rate of metabolism (and/or excretion) is proportional to the plasma concentration. Clearance is defined as the volume of plasma that is completely cleared of drug per unit of time [see Part I: Clearance (Cl)]. For first-order drugs, clearance can be viewed as a fixed proportionality constant that makes the steady-state plasma concentration equal to the rate of drug administration (R_A) as illustrated by Equation 10.12:

$$R_A = (Cl)(Css\ ave) \qquad \text{[Eq. 10.12]}$$

R_A is $(S)(F)(Dose/\tau)$. This view of first-order pharmacokinetics, however, does not apply to phenytoin because the clearance of phenytoin decreases as Css ave increases.

The clearance of phenytoin from plasma occurs primarily by metabolism, and the rate of phenytoin metabolism approaches its maximum at therapeutic concentrations. Thus, the metabolism of phenytoin is described as being capacity-limited.[4,35,37–40] Capacity-limited metabolism results in clearance values that decrease with increasing plasma concentrations. Therefore, when the maintenance dose is increased, the plasma concentration rises disproportionately[37,41–46] (Fig. 10.1). This disproportionate rise in the steady-state plasma level makes dosage adjustment difficult.

The model that appears to fit the metabolic pattern for phenytoin elimination is the one originally proposed by Michaelis and Menten. The velocity (v) or rate at which an enzyme system can metabolize a substrate (S) can be described by the following equation:

$$v = \frac{(Vm)(S)}{Km + S}$$

[Eq. 10.13]

Vm is the maximum metabolic capacity or maximum rate of metabolism, and Km is the substrate concentration at which v will be one-half of Vm. When the average steady-state phenytoin concentration (Css ave) is substituted for the substrate concentration (S) and the daily dose or administration rate of phenytoin [R_A or (S)(F)(Dose/τ)] for v,[42,44–46] Equation 10.13 can be rewritten as:

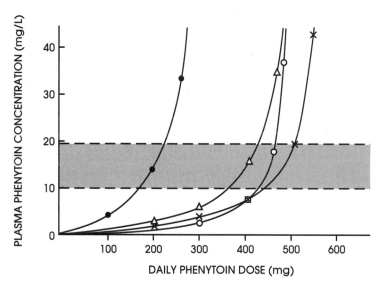

FIGURE 10.1. Changes in steady-state phenytoin plasma concentrations with maintenance dose. Note that for each patient the plasma phenytoin concentration at steady state increases disproportionately with an increase in the rate of administration, especially as the dose approaches Vm. The patients in Figure 10.1 represent the following Vm, Km values: (●) 300 mg/day, 7 mg/L; (Δ) 500 mg/day, 4 mg/L, (○) 500 mg/day and 2 mg/L, and (×) 600 mg/day, 4 mg/L. Also note that for those patients with a low Km value, the range of doses that will result in a Css ave between 10 and 20 mg/L is very narrow.

$$(S)(F)(Dose/\tau) = \frac{(Vm)(Css\ ave)}{Km + Css\ ave} \qquad [Eq.\ 10.14]$$

In Equation 10.14 the "clearance" that makes $(S)(F)(Dose/\tau)$ equal to Css ave is a value that will change as the Css ave changes. As a result, there will be a disproportionate change in the Css ave resulting from a change in the administration rate:

$$(S)(F)(Dose/\tau) = \frac{(Vm)}{Km + Css\ ave}(Css\ ave)$$

Equation 10.14 can also be rearranged as follows:

$$Css\ ave = \frac{(Km)[(S)(F)(Dose/\tau)]}{Vm - [(S)(F)(Dose/\tau)]} \qquad [Eq.\ 10.15]$$

In accordance with the original definition of Vm and Km for Equations 10.13 through 10.15, Vm is the maximum rate of metabolism (metabolic capacity) and Km is the plasma concentration at which the rate of metabolism is one-half the maximum. The units for Vm and Km are usually mg/day and mg/L, respectively.

Equation 10.15 illustrates the sensitive and disproportionate relationship between the rate of phenytoin administration and Css ave when the rate of administration approaches Vm, the maximum metabolic capacity. If the maintenance dose were equal to Vm, then Vm-$(S)(F)(Dose/\tau)$ would be 0 and Css ave would be infinity:

$$Css\ ave = \frac{(Km)[(S)(F)(Dose/\tau)]}{Vm - [(S)(F)(Dose/\tau)]}$$

$$= \frac{(Km)[(S)(F)(Dose/\tau)]}{0}$$

$$= [\ \infty\ ]$$

If $(S)(F)(Dose/\tau)$ is greater than Vm, Css ave will be a negative number indicating that steady state can never be achieved. Equation 10.15 is therefore invalid as a predictor of Css ave when $(S)(F)(Dose/\tau)$ is equal to or exceeds Vm.

As can be seen from Equation 10.15, the relationship between steady-state phenytoin concentrations and the maintenance dose can be extremely sensitive. Understanding and being able to use pharmacokinetic parameters for phenytoin helps clinicians make initial dose adjustments and use clinical guidelines more effectively. For example, the following dose increments have been suggested using phenytoin concentrations as a guide: increasing the daily dose by 100 mg/day when Css ave concentrations are < 7 mg/L; by 50 mg/day when Css ave concentrations are 7 to < 12 mg/L; and a maximum increase of 30 mg/day when Css ave concentrations are > 12 mg/L.[47] While these guidelines are consistent with the usual pharmacokinetic parameters, any increase in dose should be considered carefully in the context of patient compliance and any potential alterations in plasma binding. One should also keep in mind that adding 100 mg/day to patients with a Css ave of 6 mg/L taking 200 mg/day will probably result in a more dramatic rise in the new steady-state phenytoin concentration than for patients with a Css ave of 6 mg/L taking 400 mg/day.

Km values are usually between 1 and 20 mg/L.[41,43–45,48] Vm (the maximum metabolic capacity) appears to be between 5 and 15 mg/kg/day in most patients.[41,44,45] The relationship between Km and Vm is not clear, but if one of these parameters is low, the other is frequently also low.[41,42,45] The average values for Km and Vm are difficult to establish. It is the author's opinion that approximately 4 mg/L for Km and 7 mg/kg/day for Vm are reasonable initial estimates for the average adult patient.

For pediatric patients, the Vm is usually larger than 7 mg/kg/day. Vm values are approximately 10 to 13 mg/kg/day for children 6 months through 6 years of age, and 8 to 10 mg/kg/day for children 7 through 16 years of age.[49–51] Km values for children vary considerably in the literature; some authors have suggested values of 2 to 3 mg/L,[50,52] and others have suggested that a Km value of 6 to 8 mg/L is more appropriate.[49,51] An average Km value of 7 mg/L, although uncertain, is not an unreasonable estimate for children between the ages of 6 months and 16 years of age.

CONCENTRATION-DEPENDENT CLEARANCE

The relationship between phenytoin clearance and phenytoin plasma concentration (Css ave) can be seen by studying Equation 10.14 and comparing it to the equivalent first-order equation. In the first-order equation below, clearance (Cl) is a constant value and can be thought of as the proportionality constant that makes the Css ave equal to $(S)(F)(Dose/\tau)$.

$$(S)(F)(Dose/\tau) = (Cl)(Css\ ave) \qquad \text{[Eq. 10.16]}$$

If we replace (Cl) in the equation for a first-order drug with the term $(Vm)/(Km + Css\ ave)$, we again have Equation 10.14:

$$(S)(F)(Dose/\tau) = \frac{(Vm)(Css\ ave)}{Km + Css\ ave}$$

where the clearance of phenytoin is:

$$Cl_{Phenytoin} = \frac{Vm}{Km + C} \qquad \text{[Eq. 10.17]}$$

Note that in Equation 10.17 the Css ave has been replaced by C to represent any phenytoin concentration. If C is very small compared to Km, clearance will be a relatively constant value (Vm/Km) and the metabolism will appear to follow first-order pharmacokinetics. Most drugs that are metabolized appear to fall into this category (i.e., the concentrations used therapeutically are well below the value of Km). However, if the drug concentration approaches or exceeds Km, clearance will decrease and the metabolism will no longer appear to follow a first-order process. As clearance decreases with increasing phenytoin concentration, the velocity or metabolic rate will increase, but not in proportion to the increase in plasma concentration (see Fig. 10.1). Since Km values for phenytoin are generally below the usual therapeutic range, nearly all patients will display capacity-limited metabolism for phenytoin.

Alterations in plasma binding will also alter the apparent Km value. This is because Km values are reported as total phenytoin concentration, and it is only the unbound concentration that can cross cell membranes and be available for metabolism. Again as previously discussed, changes in plasma binding have a profound effect on the total phenytoin concentration but not the unbound phenytoin concentration. The general approach taken in this chapter is to adjust the measured concentration to that which would be observed under normal plasma binding conditions and to use pharmacokinetic parameters (V, Km, and C or Css ave) which are based on normal plasma binding.

CONCENTRATION-DEPENDENT HALF-LIFE

The usual reported half-life (t½) for phenytoin is ≈22 hours[38]; however, the t½ is not a constant value because the clearance of phenytoin changes with the plasma concentration. If Equation 10.17 (the clearance equation for phenytoin):

$$Cl_{Phenytoin} = \frac{Vm}{Km + C}$$

is substituted into the usual equation for half-life:

$$t\frac{1}{2} = \frac{(0.693)(V)}{Cl} \qquad \text{[Eq. 10.18]}$$

the half-life of phenytoin can be derived:

$$t \; \tfrac{1}{2}_{\text{Phenytoin}} = \frac{(0.693)(V)}{Vm}(Km + C) \qquad \text{[Eq. 10.19]}$$

Based on Equation 10.19 it can be predicted that the half-life of phenytoin will increase as the plasma concentration increases, an observation that has been confirmed.[39] The value and applicability of this observation are very limited, however.

Limited Utility of Half-Life

The clinical usefulness of the phenytoin half-life is limited because the time required to achieve steady state can be much longer than the usual 3 to 4 times the apparent half-life. Likewise, the time required for a plasma concentration to decay following discontinuation of the maintenance dose will be less than predicted by the apparent half-life. The problems associated with capacity-limited metabolism can best be explained by first examining the relationship between the rate of drug administration and elimination for a first-order drug. For a first-order drug, when the rate of administration (R_A) exceeds the rate of drug elimination from the body (R_E), the amount of drug in the body will increase and the drug accumulates. If the rate of elimination exceeds the rate of drug administration, the amount of drug in the body will decrease.

$$R_A - R_E = \frac{\Delta \text{ Amount of Drug in Body}}{t} \qquad \text{[Eq. 10.20]}$$

The rate of drug elimination for a first-order drug is the product of clearance (Cl) and plasma concentration (C). When the pharmacokinetic parameter, clearance, and plasma concentration are substituted into Equation 10.20, the change in the amount of drug in the body per unit of time (Δ Amount in body/t) is small when the product of Cl times C approaches the rate of drug administration. This proportional relationship between C and rate of elimination is the key to the usefulness of $t\tfrac{1}{2}$. Inspecting Equation 10.21:

$$R_A - (Cl)(C) = \frac{\Delta \text{ Amount of Drug in Body}}{t} \qquad \text{[Eq. 10.21]}$$

it can be see that when C is 50% of Css ave, Δ Amount in body/t is 50% of R_A; when C is 90% of Css ave, Δ Amount in body/t is 10% of R_A. This relationship means that when Δ Amount in body/t is small (i.e., very slow rate of accumulation) for a first-order drug, then C must be close to Css ave.

For capacity-limited drugs, however, clearance (Vm/(Km + C)) is not a constant factor. This expression for clearance is inserted into Equation 10.21 to form Equation 10.22.

$$R_A - \frac{(Vm)}{(Km + C)}(C) = \frac{\Delta \text{ Amount of Drug in Body}}{t} \qquad \text{[Eq. 10.22]}$$

As C exceeds Km, the rate of drug elimination approaches Vm, which is a fixed value (see Phenytoin: Capacity-Limited Metabolism). In such cases, it may be possible to have a rate of elimination that is very close to the rate of drug administration, resulting in a very slow yet prolonged accumulation process.

When R_A is equal to or greater than Vm, accumulation would continue forever or at least until the patient becomes toxic and phenytoin is withheld. Capacity-limited accumulation problems are most dramatic when the plasma concentration greatly exceeds the Km value. In clinical practice this means when either the Km value is low or there is a clinical need to achieve high phenytoin concentrations.

As an example, consider a patient with a Vm of 300 mg/day, a Km of 4 mg/L, and a R_A of 300 mg/day of phenytoin. Under these conditions, in which the rate of phenytoin administration is equal to Vm, the phenytoin concentrations will continue to increase indefinitely. At a phenytoin concentration of 36 mg/L, the rate of elimination should be 270 mg or 90% of the administration rate and the accumulation is only 10% of the maintenance dose.

$$R_A - \frac{(Vm)}{(Km + C)}(C) = \frac{\Delta \text{ Amount of Drug in Body}}{t}$$

$$300 \text{ mg/day} - \frac{(300 \text{ mg/day})}{(4 \text{ mg/L} + 36 \text{ mg/L})}(36 \text{ mg/L}) = \frac{\Delta \text{ Amount of Drug in Body}}{t}$$

$$300 \text{ mg/day} - 270 \text{ mg/day} = 30 \text{ mg/day}$$

If this was a first-order drug, the concentration of 36 mg/L would be 90% of Css ave. However, this is not a first-order drug, and in the example given although R_E is 90% of R_A, at a C of 36 mg/L, the final theoretical Css ave would be infinity because R_A is equal to Vm.

Again, the key point with phenytoin accumulation is that in a patient with relatively stable concentrations over several days or even weeks, the rate of elimination is close to the rate of administration, but the phenytoin concentrations may or may not be at or near steady state.

Time to Reach Steady State

The time required to achieve 90% of steady state can be calculated as follows[53]:

$$t_{90\%} = \frac{(Km)(V)}{[Vm - (S)(F)(Dose/day)]^2}[(2.3\ Vm) - (0.9)(S)(F)(Dose/day)] \quad \text{[Eq. 10.23]}$$

The $t_{90\%}$ is the time required for a patient to achieve 90% of the steady-state plasma concentration on a dosing regimen, given the Km, V, and Vm. The units are mg/L for Km, L for V, and mg/day for Vm and dose.

Equation 10.23 assumes that the initial plasma concentration is zero. If the initial plasma concentration is between zero and the steady-state concentration, 90% of steady state will be achieved sooner than predicted by Equation 10.23. Nevertheless, it is still appropriate to use Equation 10.23 to predict the time to achieve steady-state concentrations even when the initial plasma concentration is greater than zero. When therapy with phenytoin is initiated, at first the drug accumulates rapidly so that initial plasma concentrations do not, in most cases, significantly reduce the time required to achieve 90% of steady state. Equation 10.23 should not be used, however, when the initial plasma concentration is greater than the desired steady-state concentration.

When Does a Phenytoin Concentration Represent a Steady-State Value?

When a phenytoin plasma concentration is measured, there is frequently a question as to whether the concentration represents a steady-state level. This question can be answered by the use of Equation 10.24:

$$90\%\ t = \frac{[115 + (35)(C)][C]}{(S)(F)(Dose/day)} \quad \text{[Eq. 10.24]}$$

C is in mg/L, and the dose/day is in mg/day. This equation is for adults, and the dose/day should be normalized for a 70 kg patient. The 90% t value, which is calculated by this equation, represents the minimum amount of time the patient must have been receiving the maintenance regimen before it can be assumed that the measured C is at steady state. Equation 10.24 is relatively conservative in that in its derivation, a Km value of 2 mg/L has been assumed; therefore, the 90% t value is longer than would be required if the Km value were actually greater than 2 mg/L. Therefore, steady state may already have been achieved in a patient who has been receiving the maintenance regimen for a shorter period than calculated in Equation 10.24. Also note that the C in Equation 10.24 must reflect normal plasma protein binding.

Rate of Decline: Phenytoin Levels

The decline of phenytoin concentration after discontinuation of therapy can be described by Equation 10.25:

$$t = \frac{\left[Km \left(\ln \frac{C_1}{C_2} \right) \right] + (C_1 - C_2)}{\dfrac{Vm}{V}} \qquad \text{[Eq. 10.25]}$$

C_1 is the initial plasma concentration, and C_2 is the plasma concentration at the end of the time interval t. When both C_1 and C_2 are much greater than Km, the rate of metabolism will approach Vm; therefore, the time required to decline from C_1 to C_2 is primarily controlled by the maximum rate of metabolism (Vm) and the apparent volume of distribution (V).

This equation can be used to estimate the Vm value in a patient who has either intentionally or accidentally received excessive phenytoin doses. In this instance, a decline in the phenytoin concentration can be observed over several days. Care should be taken, however, to ensure that no further drug is being administered to the patient. One must also consider that absorption of phenytoin may continue for several days after an acute overdose or following discontinuation of an oral maintenance regimen.[33,54] Given that the usual Vm is in the range of 7 mg/kg/day and V is approximately 0.65 L/kg, the maximum expected decrease in a phenytoin concentration in adults would be approximately 10 mg/L/day.

$$\frac{Vm}{V} = \frac{7 \text{ mg/kg/day}}{0.65 \text{ L/kg}} \approx 10 \text{ mg/L/day}$$

Again this assumes the average value for Vm and V, no additional absorption of phenytoin, and that the beginning (C_1) and ending (C_2) phenytoin concentrations are both well above the patient's Km.

TIME TO SAMPLE

Depending on the disease state being treated and the clinical condition of the patient, the time of sampling for phenytoin can vary greatly. In patients requiring rapid achievement and maintenance of therapeutic phenytoin concentrations, it is usually wise to monitor phenytoin concentrations within 2 to 3 days of therapy initiation. This is to ensure that the patient's metabolism is not remarkably different from that which would be predicted by average literature-derived pharmacokinetic parameters. A second phenytoin concentration would normally be obtained in another 3 to 5 days; subsequent doses of phenytoin can then be adjusted. If the plasma phenytoin concentrations have not changed over a 3- to 5-day period, the monitoring interval can usually be increased to once weekly in the acute clinical setting. In stable patients requiring long-term therapy, phenytoin plasma concentrations are generally monitored at 3- to 12-month intervals.[6,8,55]

The time required to achieve steady state with phenytoin can be prolonged. Therefore, plasma levels of phenytoin should be monitored before steady state to avoid sustained periods of low or high phenytoin concentrations. Nevertheless, these early phenytoin concentrations must be used cautiously in the design of new dosing regimens.

In patients receiving oral phenytoin extended absorption dosage form, especially in divided daily doses, the time of sampling within the dosing interval is not critical, because the slow absorption of phenytoin minimizes the fluctuations between peak and trough concentrations. Trough concentrations are generally recommended, however, for routine monitoring. In patients who are receiving phenytoin doses intravenously, trough concentrations can be adjusted by Equation 10.26 to calculate the average plasma concentration of phenytoin.

$$\text{Css ave} = [\text{Css min}] + \left[(0.5)\frac{(S)(F)(Dose)}{V} \right] \qquad \text{[Eq. 10.26]}$$

Following IV administration, sampling within the first 1 to 2 hours after the end of the infusion should be avoided to ensure complete distribution (see Part 1: Volume of Distribution: Two-Compartment Models). In addition, if fosphenytoin is administered there may be an assay cross-reactivity between fosphenytoin, which is an inactive pro-drug, and the hydrolyzed phenytoin, which is the active drug.[7]

In patients receiving phenytoin orally as an extended absorption dosage form, the average concentration can be approximated by multiplying the change in concentration anticipated with the IV dose by 0.25. This 0.25 factor assumes that the fluctuation in plasma concentrations following oral administration is approximately half of that which would be expected if the drug were administered intravenously. It also assumes that the average concentration lies approximately halfway between the peak and trough concentrations.

$$\text{Css ave} = [\text{Css min}] + \left[(0.25)\frac{(S)(F)(Dose)}{V} \right] \qquad \text{[Eq. 10.27]}$$

Use of Equation 10.27 is most appropriate when patients are receiving single daily doses of > 5 mg/kg and when the phenytoin concentration is < 5 mg/L. In patients with phenytoin concentrations > 5 mg/L or in those receiving their phenytoin in divided daily doses, use of Equation

10.27 is less critical, because the Css peak and Css trough are both close to Css ave.

Question #1. *Calculate the phenytoin loading dose required to achieve a plasma concentration of 20 mg/L in B.F., a 70-kg male. Describe how this loading dose should be administered by both the oral and IV routes.*

Equation 10.28 can be used to estimate the loading dose that will produce a plasma concentration of 20 mg/L. If the volume of distribution for phenytoin is assumed to be 0.65 L/kg (see Key Parameters: Phenytoin), the volume of distribution for B.F. would be 45.5 L (70 kg × 0.65 L/kg). In this case we are assuming that B.F. has not been receiving phenytoin and therefore the $C_{observed}$ or the phenytoin concentration that is present is zero. The salt factor (S) is 0.92 for the oral capsules and injectable phenytoin dosage forms (phenytoin for injection and fosphenytoin) and the bioavailability is 100% (F = 1.0).

$$\text{Loading Dose} = \frac{(V)(C_{desired} - C_{observed})}{(S)(F)} \qquad \text{[Eq. 10.28]}$$

$$\text{Loading Dose} = \frac{(45.5 \text{ L})(20 \text{ mg/L} - 0 \text{ mg/L})}{(0.92)(1)}$$

$$= 989 \text{ mg}$$

This loading dose of 989 mg is reasonably close to the usual, recommended loading dose of 1000 mg or 15 mg/kg.

If this loading dose is administered intravenously as phenytoin for injection, it should be administered slowly to avoid the cardiovascular toxicities associated with the propylene glycol diluent.[3] A maximum rate of 50 mg/min should be used until the entire loading dose is administered or toxicities are encountered.[1] An administration rate of 50 mg/min for the 1000 mg dose would mean that the total dose could be administered over 20 minutes. However, because of the potential for cardiovascular side effects, most clinicians administer 1000 mg loading doses with close monitoring over 45 minutes to 1 hour (i.e., about 15 to 25 mg/min). Also note that this infusion rate is not size adjusted, and children require much slower infusion rates but are generally given the loading dose over about the same time as an adult (i.e., 45 minutes to 1 hour). If the dose were to be given as fosphenytoin, the total dose would be the same with a maximum infusion rate of 150 mg/min. If possible, fosphenytoin would be given at a slower rate (e.g., 75 mg/min) with similar cardiovascular monitoring.

If the 1000 mg loading dose is to be given orally, a 400 mg dose followed by two 300 mg doses (≈5 mg/kg) at 2-hour intervals is recommended so that the entire loading dose is administered over 4 hours. The oral loading dose is divided into three separate doses to decrease the possibility of nausea and vomiting, which may be associated with a single large dose, and to decrease the time to peak concentration.[32,33] When the loading dose is administered orally, slow absorption causes the peak concentration to be delayed and lower than the expected 20 mg/L even if a prompt absorption product is used.[25,32,33] Following oral administration of the extended absorption capsules, the peak concentration is usually about one-half of the value calculated by the IV bolus dose model as predicted by the following:

$$\Delta C = (0.5) \frac{(S)(F)(Dose)}{V} \qquad \text{[Eq. 10.29]}$$

The above equation is based on the slow absorption associated with the phenytoin extended oral products, and the fluctuation in plasma concentration will probably be more than predicted by Equation 10.29 with the prompt absorption products.[25] Although the peak concentration is very likely to be less than 20 mg/L following oral administration, it is uncommon to give larger oral doses to compensate for the delay in absorption. Oral absorption is relatively unpredictable, and increasing the oral dose is not likely to reliably correct the problem. If it were imperative, from a clinical standpoint, to achieve a phenytoin level of 20 mg/L, it would be best to give the phenytoin by the IV route.

Question #2. *S.B. is a 37-year-old, 70-kg man with a seizure disorder that has only partially been controlled with 300 mg/day of phenytoin capsules. His plasma phenytoin concentration has been measured twice over the past year and was 8 mg/L both times. Calculate a maintenance dose to achieve a new steady-state concentration of 15 mg/L.*

To establish the new daily dose, it is necessary to assume a value of Vm or Km for S.B. The usual approach is to rearrange Equation 10.14:

$$(S)(F)(Dose/\tau) = \frac{(Vm)(Css\ ave)}{Km + Css\ ave}$$

and solve for Vm:

$$Vm = \frac{(S)(F)(Dose/\tau)(Km + Css\ ave)}{(Css\ ave)} \qquad \text{[Eq. 10.30]}$$

If Km is assumed to be 4 mg/L, S to be 0.92 (capsules contain the sodium salt), and F to be 1.0, then Vm would be 414 mg/day of acid phenytoin:

$$Vm = \frac{(0.92)(1)(300 \text{ mg/day})(4 \text{ mg/L} + 8 \text{ mg/L})}{(8 \text{ mg/L})}$$

$$Vm = 414 \text{ mg/day of acid phenytoin}$$

To calculate the dose required to achieve a steady-state concentration of 15 mg/L, Equation 10.14:

$$(S)(F)(Dose/\tau) = \frac{(Vm)(Css \text{ ave})}{Km + Css \text{ ave}}$$

can be rearranged as follows:

$$Dose = \frac{(Vm)(Css \text{ ave})(\tau)}{(Km + Css \text{ ave})(S)(F)} \qquad \text{[Eq. 10.31]}$$

Using the assumed Km of 4 mg/L and the calculated Vm of 414 mg/day of acid phenytoin, the daily dose required to achieve a steady-state concentration of 15 mg/L would be:

$$Dose = \frac{(414 \text{ mg/day})(15 \text{ mg/L})(1 \text{ day})}{(4 \text{ mg/L} + 15 \text{ mg/L})(0.92)(1)}$$

$$= 355 \text{ mg of phenytoin sodium}$$

This 18% dosage adjustment should result in a nearly 100% increase in the steady-state plasma level if the assumed Km of 4 mg/L is correct. A daily dose of 355 mg would be difficult to administer; therefore, this initial dosing estimate would probably be rounded off to 350 mg/day and doses of 300 and 400 mg could be prescribed for alternate days. To aid with compliance, it is a common practice to prescribe the 300 mg dose (odd number of capsules) on the odd days of the month and 400 mg (even number of capsules) on the even days of the month. For those months with 31 days, most clinicians tell the patient to simply take the odd number of capsules 2 days in a row.

An alternative approach is illustrated in Figure 10.2. This method allows one to estimate the most probable combination of Km and Vm values for a patient, given the current dosing regimen and measured average steady-state phenytoin concentration.

If the steps outlined in Figure 10.2 are followed, a Km value of 5 mg/L and a Vm value of 6.4 mg/kg/day (448 mg/day for this 70 kg patient) can be determined. When these values are used in Equation 10.31 (or when Figure 10.2 is used), a new dose of ≈350 mg/day is calculated. This method of using the "orbit graph" is perhaps slightly superior to the first in which a Km value of 4 mg/L was assumed. This is because the "orbit"

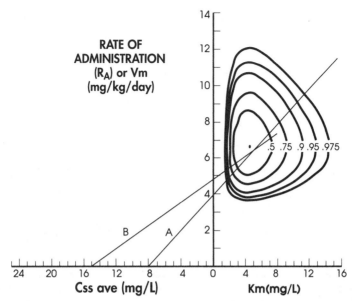

FIGURE 10.2. Orbit graph. The most probable values of Vm and Km for a patient may be estimated using a single steady-state phenytoin concentration and a known dosing regimen. The eccentric circles or "orbits" represent the fraction of the sample patient population whose Km and Vm values are within that orbit. 1) Plot the daily dose of acid phenytoin (mg/kg/day) on the vertical line [Rate of Administration (R_A)]. 2) Plot the steady-state concentration (Css ave) on the horizontal line. 3) Draw a straight line connecting Css ave and daily dose through the orbits (line A). 4) The coordinates of the midpoint of the line crossing the innermost orbit through which line A passes are the most probable values for the patient's Vm and Km. 5) To calculate a new maintenance dose, draw a line from the point determined in Step 4 to the new desired Css ave (line B). The point at which line B crosses the vertical line [(Rate of Administration (R_A)] is the new maintenance dose (mg/kg/day) of acid phenytoin. Line A represents a Css of 8 mg/L on 3.94 mg/kg/day or 276 mg/day of phenytoin acid (0.92 × 300 mg/day of sodium phenytoin) for a 70-kg person. The new steady-state concentration was 15 mg/L. From reference 58, the original figure is modified so that R_A, R_E, and Vm are in mg/kg/day of phenytoin acid. (Reprinted from Applied Pharmacokinetics: Principles of Therapeutic Drug Monitoring. 4th Ed. Baltimore: Lippincott Williams & Wilkins, 2003.)

method attempts to define the most likely set or combination of Km and Vm values for the patient given the dosing history and measured phenytoin concentration.

Figure 10.2 can only be used for adult patients, and the phenytoin concentrations used in plotting lines A and B must represent normal plasma protein binding conditions. Figure 10.2 also requires that the phenytoin concentration be an average steady-state value.

Question #3. *Calculate a loading dose that would rapidly increase S.B.'s plasma phenytoin concentration from 8 to 15 mg/L.*

Equation 10.28 can be used to calculate an incremental loading dose. If the V is 45.5 L (70 kg × 0.65 L/kg), S = 0.92, and F = 1.0, the loading dose required to increase S.B.'s plasma concentration from 8 to 15 mg/L would be:

$$\text{Loading Dose} = \frac{(V)(C_{desired} - C_{observed})}{(S)(F)}$$

$$= \frac{(45.5\ L)(15\ mg/L - 8\ mg/L)}{(0.92)(1)}$$

$$= 346\ mg$$

This loading dose should be given in addition to the new maintenance dose of 350 mg/day so that his total dose today will be approximately 700 mg (a new maintenance dose of 350 mg plus the small loading dose of 350 mg). Administration of the loading dose will result in a more rapid increase of the phenytoin concentration into the desired concentration range while S.B. is receiving the new maintenance dose. If 1 week after the loading dose and starting on the new maintenance dose, the plasma concentration is <10 mg/L, it would suggest that the maintenance dose should again be adjusted. If a loading dose is not given and at the end of 1 week the plasma concentration is <10 mg/L, it would be difficult to determine why the level was low. One possibility would be that the phenytoin level has not yet reached steady state and further accumulation on the new regimen would result in levels near our target of 15 mg/L. A second possibility is that our estimates are incorrect and steady state has been achieved at a lower than expected concentration. In this case an adjustment in the maintenance dose would be appropriate. Administration of the small or incremental loading dose limits the time when the patient has a low phenytoin level and decreases the risk of a seizure. In addition it helps us to determine in a relatively short time (1 to 2 weeks) if we have selected a reasonable maintenance dose for S.B. that, with time, may require at most only minor adjustments as true steady state is achieved.

Question #4. *L.C., a 40-year-old, 80-kg man who has been receiving 300 mg/day of sodium phenytoin for the past 3 weeks (21 days), has a phenytoin level of 14 mg/L. Is this reported level likely to represent a steady-state concentration?*

If phenytoin was eliminated according to first-order pharmacokinetics, 21 days would have been more than enough time for steady state to have been achieved based on a half-life of 15 to 24 hours.

Phenytoin, however, exhibits capacity-limited metabolism; therefore, the time required to achieve steady state is frequently much longer than one would estimate using first-order pharmacokinetic principles. Equation 10.24 should be used to calculate the minimum number of days phenytoin must be administered before it can be safely assumed that the measured concentration represents a steady-state level. First, the daily dose of phenytoin should be normalized to 262.5 mg for a 70-kg individual using a ratio of 300 mg per 80 kg in proportion to $\times$ mg per 70 kg:

$$\left[\frac{300 \text{ mg}}{80 \text{ kg}} \right] [70 \text{ kg}] = 262.5 \text{ mg}$$

When this value is placed into Equation 10.24 along with an assumed F of 1 and an S of 0.92, the 90% t value can be calculated.

$$90\% \text{ t} = \frac{[115 + (35)(C)][C]}{(S)(F)(\text{Dose/day})}$$

$$= \frac{[115 + (35)(14)][14]}{(0.92)(1)(262.5)}$$

$$= 35 \text{ days}$$

The calculated 90% t value of 35 days is longer than the actual duration of therapy (21 days), suggesting that steady state may not yet have been achieved. If an additional loading dose was administered within the first 21 days of therapy, or if the Km value is > 2 mg/L, then the plasma level obtained at 21 days may actually represent a steady-state concentration. Due to this uncertainty, additional phenytoin plasma concentrations should be monitored to detect possible accumulation of phenytoin into a potentially toxic concentration range. While the phenytoin concentration may not yet be at steady state, it is unlikely that the phenytoin concentrations will change rapidly even if it is not yet at steady state. Therefore, some time (e.g., 2 weeks or so) could be allowed before additional levels are obtained. In addition, the patient should be educated about the potential side effects so that if they do occur, their health care provider can be contacted.

Question #5. *A.P., a 52-year-old, 60-kg woman, received a 1000 mg IV loading dose of phenytoin followed by a daily maintenance regimen of 300 mg. Eight days following the initial loading dose, A.P.'s plasma phenytoin level was 11 mg/L. Should her dose be adjusted at this time to achieve the desired phenytoin concentration of 10 to 20 mg/L?*

According to Equation 10.32 below, the 1 gm loading dose administered to A.P. should have resulted in an initial concentration of 23.5 mg/L:

$$C^{\circ} = \frac{(S)(F)(\text{Loading Dose})}{V} \qquad \text{[Eq. 10.32]}$$

$$= \frac{(0.92)(1)(1000 \text{ mg})}{(0.65 \text{ L/kg})(60 \text{ kg})}$$

$$= \frac{920 \text{ mg}}{39 \text{ L}}$$

$$= 23.5 \text{ mg/L}$$

Therefore, the plasma concentration of 11 mg/L 8 days later has declined significantly and, given the non-linearity of phenytoin, it is unlikely to represent steady state. The concentration of 11 mg/L will probably continue to decline if the maintenance regimen remains at 300 mg/day.

The first step in calculating the new maintenance dose would be to estimate the rate at which the body had been eliminating phenytoin as it declined from the initial concentration of 23.5 mg/L to the observed concentration of 11 mg/L. The amount eliminated/time can be calculated by using Equation 10.33, which considers the rate of phenytoin administration $(S)(F)(Dose/\tau)$ and the net change in the amount of phenytoin in the body $([C_2 - C_1]V)/t$.

$$\frac{\text{Amount Eliminated}}{t} = (S)(F)(Dose/\tau) - \left[\frac{(C_2 - C_1)(V)}{t}\right] \quad \text{[Eq. 10.33]}$$

In the above equation, C_1 is the initial phenytoin concentration, which is either predicted or measured, and C_2 is the second phenytoin concentration; "t" is the time interval between C_1 and C_2. It should be pointed out that C_1 and C_2 phenytoin concentrations should represent the same plasma protein binding circumstances as V in Equation 10.32 (i.e., 0.65 L/kg). As suggested in the initial part of the chapter, the author recommends calculating a plasma concentration that represents normal binding conditions rather than correcting the volume of distribution for the altered plasma binding. Assuming the phenytoin levels represent normal plasma binding, the elimination rate for phenytoin during this 8-day interval would be 337 mg/day of acid phenytoin, which corresponds to approximately 366 mg/day of sodium phenytoin.

$$\frac{\text{Amount Eliminated}}{t} = (S)(F)(Dose/\tau) - \left[\frac{(C_2 - C_1)(V)}{t}\right]$$

$$= [(0.92)(1)(300 \text{ mg/day})] - \left[\frac{(11 \text{ mg/L} - 23.5 \text{ mg/L})(39 \text{ L})}{8 \text{ days}}\right]$$

$$= 276 \text{ mg/day} - (-61 \text{ mg/day})$$

$$= 276 \text{ mg/day} + 61 \text{ mg/day}$$

$$= 337 \text{ mg/day of acid phenytoin,}$$

or

$$= 366 \text{ mg/day of sodium phenytoin} \left(\frac{337 \text{ mg/day}}{0.92}\right)$$

This elimination rate represents an average of A.P.'s actual elimination rate (> 366 mg/day when her phenytoin concentration was 23 mg/L and < 366 mg/day when her phenytoin concentration was 11 mg/L). Therefore, a dose of ≈ 360 mg/day should maintain an average phenytoin concentration somewhere between 23 and 11 mg/L.

Question #6. *T.L., a 70-kg patient, initially received a phenytoin loading dose to achieve a concentration of 20 mg/L and then received the usual maintenance dose of 300 mg/day. Ten days later he had CNS symptoms that were consistent with phenytoin toxicity. A level was drawn and reported as 26 mg/L. What would be a new maintenance dose that would eventually achieve a Css ave of approximately 15 mg/L?*

This problem is similar to the previous example. First using a volume of distribution of 45.5 L (0.65 L/kg × 70 kg) and Equation 10.33 we can calculate the average rate of phenytoin elimination as the level rose from 20 to 26 mg/L over the 10 days of treatment.

$$\frac{\text{Amount Eliminated}}{t} = (S)(F)(\text{Dose}/\tau) - \left[\frac{(C_2 - C_1)(V)}{t} \right]$$

$$= [(0.92)(1)(300 \text{ mg/day})] - \left[\frac{(26 \text{ mg/L} - 20 \text{ mg/L})(45.5 \text{ L})}{10 \text{ days}} \right]$$

$$= 276 \text{ mg/day} - (27.3 \text{ mg/day})$$

$$= 248.7 \text{ mg/day of acid phenytoin}$$

If, as in the previous example, we administered 248.7 mg/day of acid phenytoin, the final steady state level would probably be about 23 mg/L or halfway between the initial concentration of 20 mg/L and the level at 10 days of 26 mg/L. In this case the desired steady-state phenytoin concentration is not between C_1 and C_2. Therefore, additional steps are required to estimate the new maintenance dose. Using the amount eliminated per unit of time and the average of C_1 and C_2 in the following equation we can approximate the patient's Vm.

$$\text{Vm} = \frac{\left[\dfrac{\text{Amount Eliminated}}{t} \right] \left[\text{Km} + \left(\dfrac{C_1 + C_2}{2} \right) \right]}{\left(\dfrac{C_1 + C_2}{2} \right)} \qquad \text{[Eq. 10.34]}$$

Assuming a Km value of 4 mg/L, a Vm of 292 mg/day of acid phenytoin is calculated.

$$\text{Vm} = \frac{[248.7 \text{ mg/day}] \left[4 \text{ mg/L} + \left(\dfrac{20 \text{ mg/L} + 26 \text{ mg/L}}{2} \right) \right]}{\left(\dfrac{20 \text{ mg/L} + 26 \text{ mg/L}}{2} \right)}$$

$$= \frac{[248.7 \text{ mg/day}] [27 \text{ mg/L}]}{(23 \text{ mg/L})}$$

$$= 292 \text{ mg/day of acid phenytoin}$$

This new Vm of 292 mg/day of acid phenytoin and the assumed Km value of 4 mg/L would then be used in Equation 10.31 to calculate the new phenytoin maintenance dose of 250 mg/day of phenytoin administered as the sodium salt.

$$\text{Dose} = \frac{(\text{Vm})(\text{Css ave})(\tau)}{(\text{Km} + \text{Css ave})(\text{S})(\text{F})}$$

$$= \frac{(292 \text{ mg/day})(15 \text{ mg/day})(1 \text{ day})}{(4 \text{ mg/L} + 15 \text{ mg/L})(0.92)(1)}$$

$$= 250 \text{ mg/day}$$

This approach is more uncertain than the example in Question 5 for several reasons. In both cases we had to assume a volume of distribution and in both cases there is likely to be some assay error in the reported drug concentrations. However, in this second case we assumed a value for Km and, more importantly, we are extrapolating to a new concentration that is outside the concentrations range we used to estimate the rate of phenytoin elimination. Given the non-linear metabolism of phenytoin, any errors are compounded in the extrapolation to a new steady-state concentration range.

In addition, if the following three rules are not met, Equations 10.33 and 10.34 are less likely to accurately predict the patient's rate of metabolism, Vm, and any subsequent maintenance dose adjustments.

1) The time between C_1 and C_2 should be $\geq$ 3 days.
2) C_2 should be $\leq 2 \times C_1$ if the plasma concentrations are rising. C_2 should be $\geq \frac{1}{2}$ of C_1 if the plasma concentrations are declining.
3) The phenytoin dose, dosage form, and route of administration should be consistent.

If any of the three rules above are broken, Equations 10.33 and 10.34 do not necessarily become invalid, but their accuracy is less than the usual uncertainties associated with phenytoin dose adjustments.

Question #7. *If T.L.'s phenytoin dose was held, what would be the expected time required for T.L. to have his phenytoin level decline to approximately 15 mg/L?*

If T.L.'s dose is held, the decay time can be calculated by Equation 10.25.

$$t = \frac{\left[\text{Km}\left(\ln\frac{C_1}{C_2}\right)\right] + (C_1 - C_2)}{\dfrac{\text{Vm}}{\text{V}}}$$

If we substitute our literature estimates of 45.5 L for volume of distribution (0.65 L/kg $\times$ 70 kg), 4 mg/L for Km, and our patient-specific estimate of Vm, the time required to decline to 15 mg/L would be 2 days.

$$t = \frac{\left[Km\left(\ln\frac{C_1}{C_2}\right)\right] + (C_1 - C_2)}{\frac{Vm}{V}}$$

$$t = \frac{\left[4\text{ mg/L}\left(\ln\frac{26\text{ mg/L}}{15\text{ mg/L}}\right)\right] + (26\text{ mg/L} - 15\text{ mg/L})}{\frac{292\text{ mg/day}}{45.5\text{ L}}}$$

$$t = \frac{[4\text{ mg/L}(0.55)] + (11\text{ mg/L})}{6.4\text{ mg/L/day}}$$

$$= 2\text{ days}$$

Note that because both C_1 and C_2 are well above our estimate of Km (4 mg/L), we could have estimated the daily drop in phenytoin concentration by Vm/V, because at these concentrations the rate of metabolism is relatively fixed at a value approaching Vm. Therefore, this simple method would suggest that if the level fell by 6.4 mg/L in 1 day, in 2 days it would fall by 12.8 mg/L, a value close to our desired decline of 11 mg/L (i.e., 26 mg/L to 15 mg/L). In either case, it is important that, for our estimates to be reasonably correct, the patient does not continue to receive (or absorb from previously administered oral doses) additional phenytoin. In any case the patient should be monitored closely. If after only 1 day the symptoms of phenytoin toxicity have cleared, it might be appropriate to initiate the new maintenance dose at that time (to avoid the risk of seizures). If after holding the dose for 2 days the symptoms are still present, it would be appropriate to obtain another phenytoin level to confirm that the levels are declining as we expected. In addition, if the patient was at "high seizure risk" and the toxicity symptoms were not considered serious, many clinicians might elect to simply reduce the maintenance dose and allow the levels to decline slowly.

Question #8. *R.M., a 32-year-old, 80-kg non-obese man, had been taking 300 mg/day of acid phenytoin; however, his dose was increased to 350 mg/day of acid phenytoin, because his seizures were poorly controlled and because his plasma concentration was only 8 mg/L. Now he complains of minor CNS side effects and his reported plasma phenytoin concentration is 20 mg/L. Renal and hepatic function are normal. Assume that both of the reported plasma concentrations represent steady-state levels and that R.M. has complied with the prescribed dosing regimens. Calculate R.M.'s apparent Vm and Km and a new daily dose of phenytoin that will result in a steady-state level of approximately 15 mg/L.*

The relationship between daily dose and Css can be made linear by plotting daily dose (R_A) versus daily dose divided by Css ave (clearance) for at least two steady-state plasma levels. The graph for R.M. is plotted in

Figure 10.3, in which the rate-in intercept (390 mg/day) is Vm and the slope of the line (−2.5 mg/L) is the negative value of Km.

Using these values, the daily dose of phenytoin that will achieve a steady-state level of 15 mg/L can be calculated using Equation 10.31:

$$\text{Dose} = \frac{(Vm)(Css\ ave)(\tau)}{(Km + Css\ ave)(S)(F)}$$

$$= \frac{(390\ mg/day)(15\ mg/L)(1\ day)}{(2.5\ mg/L + 15\ mg/L)(1)(1)}$$

$$= 334\ mg$$

The most convenient dose for calculated value of 334 mg/day, administered as acid phenytoin, would be 325 mg/day, which could be administered as the suspension. The suspension is available as 125 mg/5mL (25 mg/mL) and therefore the volume to administer would be 13 mL. The suspension should be shaken vigorously and measured accurately to ensure the proper dose is delivered. In addition, the suspension is not recommended to be given on a once daily basis, and the dose should be divided to at least a twice daily regimen (i.e., 6.5 mL twice daily).

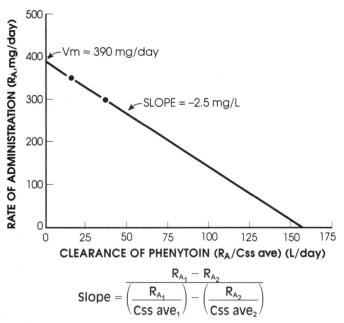

$$\text{Slope} = \frac{R_{A_1} - R_{A_2}}{\left(\dfrac{R_{A_1}}{Css\ ave_1}\right) - \left(\dfrac{R_{A_2}}{Css\ ave_2}\right)}$$

FIGURE 10.3. The rate of administration (R_A) or the daily dose of phenytoin (mg/day) versus the clearance of phenytoin (R_A/Css ave, L/day) is plotted for two or more different daily doses of phenytoin. A straight line of the best fit is drawn through the points plotted. The intercept on the rate of administration axis is Vm (mg/day), and the slope of the line is the negative value of Km.

If, for the convenience of once daily dosing, the acid phenytoin dose were to be converted to a sodium phenytoin extended absorption product, the following equation could be used to calculate an equivalent dose [also see Part 1: Bioavailability (F): Chemical Form (S)]:

$$\frac{\text{Dose of New Dosage Form}}{} = \frac{\text{Amount of Drug Absorbed From Current Dosage Form}}{(S)(F) \text{ of New Dosage Form}} \quad \text{[Eq. 10.35]}$$

Assuming S to be 0.92 and F to be 1 for phenytoin sodium, the equivalent dose would be 363 mg.

$$\frac{\text{Dose of New Dosage Form}}{} = \frac{334 \text{ mg}}{(0.92)(1) \text{ of New Dosage Form}}$$

$$= 363 \text{ mg}$$

This dose might be rounded off to 350 mg/day (300 mg alternating with 400 mg given as 100 mg capsules) or 360 mg/day given as 3 of the 100 mg capsules and 2 of the 30 mg capsules.

If it were decided to round off the dose to the average dose of 350 mg/day, the expected Css ave can be calculated by using Equation 10.15:

$$\text{Css ave} = \frac{(Km)[(S)(F)(\text{Dose}/\tau)]}{Vm - [(S)(F)(\text{Dose}/\tau)]}$$

Using the patient-specific Km value of 2.5 mg/L and the Vm of 390 mg/day of acid phenytoin for R.M., we calculate a Css ave on 350 mg/day of phenytoin sodium of 11.8 mg/L.

$$\text{Css ave} = \frac{(2.5 \text{ mg/L})[(0.92)(1)(350 \text{ mg/1 day})]}{390 \text{ mg/day} - [(0.92)(1)(350 \text{ mg/1 day})]}$$

$$= 11.8 \text{ mg/L}$$

Assuming the concentration of 11.8 mg/L is satisfactory, the patient could be converted from the current acid phenytoin to phenytoin sodium extended absorption. In most cases, the Dilantin Kapseal product would be used, although there are other forms of phenytoin extended absorption available. However, regardless of which product is used, it is important to remember that phenytoin products are not considered to be interchangeable. If a change in dosage form is to be considered, a careful discussion with both the patient and the patient's provider should take place before any changes are made. It is also recommended that follow-up phenytoin levels be obtained to ensure that the conversion from one dosage form to another results in the expected outcome.

An alternate approach to plotting the data for R.M. would be to calculate the negative value of Km by use of Equation 10.36:

$$-Km = \frac{R_1 - R_2}{\left(\dfrac{R_1}{Css_1}\right) - \left(\dfrac{R_2}{Css_2}\right)} \qquad \text{[Eq. 10.36]}$$

where R_1 and R_2 represent the initial and new maintenance doses, respectively. Css_1 and Css_2 represent the steady-state concentrations produced by these doses. Again, assuming S and F to be 1.0, a value of -2.5 mg/L is calculated.

$$-Km = \frac{R_1 - R_2}{\left(\dfrac{R_1}{Css_1}\right) - \left(\dfrac{R_2}{Css_2}\right)}$$

$$= \frac{300 \text{ mg/day} - 350 \text{ mg/day}}{\left(\dfrac{300 \text{ mg/day}}{8 \text{ mg/L}}\right) - \left(\dfrac{350 \text{ mg/day}}{20 \text{ mg/L}}\right)}$$

$$= \frac{-50 \text{ mg/day}}{(37.5 \text{ L/day}) - (17.5 \text{ L/day})}$$

$$= -2.5 \text{ mg/L}$$

The value of 2.5 mg/L can then be used in Equation 10.30 with either of the maintenance doses and the corresponding steady-state levels to calculate the Vm:

$$Vm = \frac{(S)(F)(Dose/\tau)(Km + (Css \text{ ave})}{(Css \text{ ave})}$$

$$= \frac{(1)(1)(300 \text{ mg/day})(2.5 \text{ mg/L} + 8 \text{ mg/L})}{(8 \text{ mg/L})}$$

$$= 393.75 \text{ or} \approx 390 \text{ mg/day}$$

The calculated and graphically determined values for Km and Vm should be exactly the same. Small differences sometimes occur, however, because of differences in mechanical drawing skills or rounding off errors in the calculation.

Question #9. *How long will it take for R.M.'s phenytoin concentration of 20 mg/L to decline to 15 mg/L?*

As with Question #7, the important clinical decision is whether to hold the dose and allow the phenytoin levels to decline as rapidly as possible, or to start a new lower dosing regimen and let the phenytoin concentrations decline slowly with time. The decision would be based on a balance between the severity of the phenytoin side effects and R.M.'s seizure risk. The phenytoin half-life will be of little value in predicting the time required for the plasma concentration to decay because the apparent half-life will change as the plasma concentration changes.

The time required for the phenytoin plasma concentration to fall from an initial concentration (C_1) to a lower concentration (C_2), if we hold the dose, can be calculated using Equation 10.25.

$$t = \frac{\left[Km\left(\ln\frac{C_1}{C_2}\right)\right] + (C_1 - C_2)}{\dfrac{Vm}{V}}$$

For R.M., who has a volume of distribution of 52 L (0.65 1/kg × 80 kg), a Vm of 390 mg/day, and a Km of 2.5 mg/L, the time required for the initial plasma concentration of 20 mg/L to decline to 15 mg/L will be about 0.76 days:

$$t = \frac{\left[Km\left(\ln\frac{C_1}{C_2}\right)\right] + (C_1 - C_2)}{\dfrac{Vm}{V}}$$

$$= \frac{\left[2.5\ mg/L\left(\ln\dfrac{20\ mg/L}{15\ mg/L}\right)\right] + (20\ mg/L - 15\ mg/L)}{\dfrac{390\ mg/day}{52\ L}}$$

$$= 0.76\ days$$

This rate of decline assumes that phenytoin will not continue to be absorbed from the gastrointestinal tract for a significant period following discontinuation of the drug. In the author's experience, however, the initial rate of decline for 1 to 3 days is often less than expected because of prolonged absorption.[33,54]

Question #10. *E.W., a 56-year-old, 60-kg woman, has chronic renal failure and a seizure disorder. She undergoes hemodialysis treatments 3 times a week, has a serum albumin of 3.3 gm/dL, and takes 300 mg/day of phenytoin. Her reported steady-state plasma phenytoin concentration is 5 mg/L. What would be her phenytoin concentration if she had a normal serum albumin concentration and normal renal function? Should her daily phenytoin dose be increased?*

It is critical to carefully evaluate measured phenytoin plasma concentrations in uremic patients because plasma protein binding is altered in these individuals. In patients with normal renal function, about 90% of the measured plasma phenytoin concentration is bound to albumin and 10% is free (fu normal binding = 0.1).[10–12,17] Because binding affinity and albumin concentrations are decreased in uremic patients, the fraction of the total phenytoin concentration that is unbound or free in patients with very poor renal function increases from 0.1 to a range of 0.2 to 0.35[10,13–17] (also see Part I: Figures 3 through 5 and Desired Plasma Concentration).

Since the fraction free (fu) for phenytoin is increased in uremic individuals, lower plasma concentrations will produce pharmacologic effects that are equivalent to those produced by higher levels in non-uremic individuals. E.W.'s case can be used as an illustration.

Using E.W.'s serum albumin of 3.3 gm/dL and her phenytoin concentration of 5 mg/L (Patient's Phenytoin Concentration with Altered Plasma Binding) in Equation 10.3, a phenytoin concentration of 11.9 mg/L is calculated:

$$\frac{\text{Phenytoin Concentration}}{\text{Normal Plasma Binding}} = \frac{\text{Dialysis Patient's Phenytoin Concentration with Altered Plasma Binding}}{\left[(0.9)(0.48)\left(\dfrac{\text{Patient's Serum Albumin}}{4.4\ \text{gm/dL}}\right)\right] + 0.1}$$

$$= \frac{5\ \text{mg/L}}{\left[(0.9)(0.48)\left(\dfrac{3.3\ \text{gm/dL}}{4.4\ \text{gm/dL}}\right)\right] + 0.1}$$

$$= \frac{5\ \text{mg/L}}{0.42}$$

$$= 11.9\ \text{mg/L} \approx 12\ \text{mg/L}$$

Therefore, E.W.'s measured plasma phenytoin concentration of 5 mg/L with altered binding is comparable to a concentration of 12 mg/L in a patient with normal plasma binding. That is, we would expect the reported concentration of 5 mg/L to have the same unbound or free phenytoin concentration as a concentration of 12 mg/L, which represents normal plasma binding. The usually accepted therapeutic range for phenytoin in non-uremic patients with normal binding is 10 to 20 mg/L, and E.W.'s adjusted or normal binding concentration of 12 mg/L would be expected to correspond to the low end of this range. If E.W.'s seizure disorder is well controlled, no adjustment in the maintenance dose is necessary even though the reported concentration of 5 mg/L appears to be well below the usual "therapeutic range." However, if seizures are poorly controlled and phenytoin doses must be adjusted, the comparable plasma concentration for a patient with normal plasma binding (12 mg/L) should be used in all calculations since the values for phenytoin parameters reported in the literature were determined in patients with normal plasma protein binding. Phenytoin is not dialyzed to a significant extent, and dialysis does not change the protein binding characteristics in uremia.[13,14] Therefore, doses should not be adjusted for E.W. on the basis of dialysis. Changes in plasma protein binding occur within a few days after the development of acute renal failure.[56] Conversely, there is some evidence that following a renal transplant, the plasma protein binding of phenytoin increases rapidly over the first 2 to 4 postoperative days and is almost normal 2 weeks after a successful transplant.[15]

Question #11. *I.A. is a 52-year-old, 77-kg man with chronic renal failure who is receiving hemodialysis 3 times a week. Because of a seizure disorder, he has been receiving 300 mg of extended absorption phenytoin sodium each evening for the past year. He has had three seizures over the past year and one in the past month. His phenytoin concentration has been reported to be 3 mg/L on several occasions. His serum albumin is 2.7 gm/dL, and his SCr fluctuates between 3 and 5 mg/dL. Should I.A. have his phenytoin dose increased? What would you recommend?*

Although a Cl_{Cr} of more than 10 mL/min can be calculated using the creatinine clearance equations, it would not be appropriate to use these equations. When a patient is receiving any type of dialysis, the creatinine clearance equations are invalid (see Part I: Creatinine Clearance). Therefore, to calculate I.A.'s phenytoin concentration that represents normal plasma we should use Equation 10.3 as he is a dialysis patient.

$$\frac{\text{Phenytoin Concentration}}{\text{Normal Plasma Binding}} = \frac{\text{Dialysis Patient's Phenytoin Concentration with Altered Plasma Binding}}{\left[(0.9)(0.48)\left(\dfrac{\text{Patient's Serum Albumin}}{4.4 \text{ gm/dL}} \right) \right] + 0.1}$$

$$= \frac{3 \text{ mg/L}}{\left[(0.9)(0.48)\left(\dfrac{2.7 \text{ gm/dL}}{4.4 \text{ gm/dL}} \right) \right] + 0.1}$$

$$= \frac{3 \text{ mg/L}}{[0.265] + 0.1}$$

$$= \frac{3 \text{ mg/L}}{0.365}$$

$$= 8.2 \text{ mg/L or} \approx 8 \text{ mg/L}$$

The normal binding concentration of 8 mg/L is below the usual target concentration range of 10 to 20 mg/L. Assuming I.A. should have his concentration increased to prevent further seizures, we will need to calculate his Vm using an assumed average value of 4 mg/L for Km and the normal binding concentration of 8 mg/L in Equation 10.30 to calculate Vm:

$$Vm = \frac{(S)(F)(Dose/\tau)(Km + Css\ ave)}{(Css\ ave)}$$

$$Vm = \frac{(92)(1)(300\ mg/day)(4\ mg/L + 8\ mg/L)}{(8\ mg/L)}$$

$$= 414\ mg/day\ of\ acid\ phenytoin$$

This revised Vm estimate of 414 mg/day of acid phenytoin, along with our assumed Km, can then be used in Equation 10.31 to calculate a new maintenance dose of 355 mg/day of phenytoin sodium to achieve a target level of 15 mg/L:

$$Dose = \frac{(Vm)(Css\ ave)(\tau)}{(Km + Css\ ave)(S)(F)}$$

$$Dose = \frac{(414\ mg/day)(15\ mg/L)(1\ day)}{(4\ mg/L + 15\ mg/L)(0.92)(1)}$$

$$= 355\ mg$$

Note again in the above equation that the phenytoin concentration normal binding of 8 mg/L is used and not the observed value of 3 mg/L, which represents altered binding.

If the patient is started on this new regimen of 350 mg/day (probably as 300 mg on odd days and 400 mg on even days) it will require some time to accumulate to the new steady-state concentration. To avoid the prolonged period of accumulation toward the new steady state, a small loading dose could be administered. This incremental loading dose can be calculated using Equation 10.28.

$$Loading\ Dose = \frac{(V)(C_{desired} - C_{observed})}{(S)(F)}$$

Again the normal binding concentration of 8 mg/L will be used for $C_{observed}$ and the V represents the usual value of 0.65 L/kg or 50 L for this 77-kg non-obese patient (0.65 L/kg × 77 kg).

$$Loading\ Dose = \frac{(50\ L)(15\ mg/L - 8\ mg/L)}{(0.92)(1)}$$

$$= 380\ mg\ or\ about\ 400\ mg$$

This small loading dose of 400 mg, if given orally, may not increase I.A.'s phenytoin level to 15 mg/L but should increase it to above 10 mg/L and shorten the time required for I.A. to achieve his new steady-state concentration on 350 mg/day. Remember that I.A. should receive both his loading dose and his new maintenance dose so that today he will receive a total of about 700 or 800 mg.

Question #12. *What would you expect the measured or observed phenytoin concentration to be in I.A. when he achieves the new steady-state concentration?*

The value reported by the laboratory can be calculated by placing the targeted normal plasma binding concentration of 15 mg/L in Equation 10.3 and solving for the Patient's Phenytoin Concentration with Altered Plasma Binding.

$$\text{Phenytoin Concentration Normal Plasma Binding} = \frac{\text{Dialysis Patient's Phenytoin Concentration with Altered Plasma Binding}}{\left[(0.9)(0.48)\left(\dfrac{\text{Patient's Serum Albumin}}{4.4 \text{ gm/dL}}\right)\right] + 0.1}$$

$$15 \text{ mg/L} = \frac{\text{Dialysis Patient's Phenytoin Concentration with Altered Plasma Binding}}{\left[(0.9)(0.48)\left(\dfrac{2.7 \text{ gm/dL}}{4.4 \text{ gm/dL}}\right)\right] + 0.1}$$

$$15 \text{ mg/L} = \frac{\text{Dialysis Patient's Phenytoin Concentration with Altered Plasma Binding}}{0.365}$$

$$(15 \text{ mg/L})(0.365) = \text{Dialysis Patient's Phenytoin Concentration with Altered Plasma Binding}$$

$$5.5 \text{ mg/L} = \text{Dialysis Patient's Phenytoin Concentration with Altered Plasma Binding}$$

This phenytoin concentration of 5.5 mg/L for I.A. would be expected to have the same unbound or free phenytoin concentration as a level of 15 mg/L in a patient with normal binding.

It also might be reasonable to provide the clinicians caring for I.A. with a "therapeutic range" that they could use to compare to the assayed or reported phenytoin concentration. Equations 10.6 and 10.7 could be used to calculate a "therapeutic range" for I.A. that is approximately 3.5 to 7 mg/L.

Using Equation 10.6:

Patient's Therapeutic Range With
Low Albumin and on Dialysis that would be Equal to 10 mg/L =

$$10 \text{ mg/L} \times \left[\left(0.9 \times 0.48 \times \frac{\text{Patient's Serum Albumin}}{4.4 \text{ gm/dL}}\right) + 0.1\right]$$

Patient's Therapeutic Range With
Low Albumin and on Dialysis that would be Equal to 10 mg/L =

$$10 \text{ mg/L} \times \left[\left(0.9 \times 0.48 \times \frac{2.7 \text{ gm/dL}}{4.4 \text{ gm/dL}}\right) + 0.1\right]$$

Patient's Therapeutic Range With
Low Albumin and on Dialysis that would be Equal to 10 mg/L =

$$10 \text{ mg/L} \times [0.365]$$

Patient's Therapeutic Range With
Low Albumin and on Dialysis that would be Equal to 10 mg/L $= 3.65 \text{ mg/L}$

And using Equation. 10.7:

Patient's Therapeutic Range With
Low Albumin and on Dialysis that would be Equal to 20 mg/L =

$$20 \text{ mg/L} \times \left[\left(0.9 \times 0.48 \frac{\text{Patient's Serum Albumin}}{4.4 \text{ gm/dL}}\right) + 0.1\right]$$

Patient's Therapeutic Range With
Low Albumin and on Dialysis that would be Equal to 20 mg/L =

$$20 \text{ mg/L} \times \left[\left(0.9 \times 0.48 \times \frac{2.7 \text{ gm/dL}}{4.4 \text{ gm/dL}}\right) + 0.1\right]$$

Patient's Therapeutic Range With
Low Albumin and on Dialysis that would be Equal to 20 mg/L =

$$20 \text{ mg/L} \times [0.365]$$

Patient's Therapeutic Range With
Low Albumin and on Dialysis that would be Equal to 20 mg/L $= 7.3 \text{ mg/L}$

Question #13. *Since phenytoin is bound to plasma protein to a significant extent, will a substantial amount of drug be lost during plasmapheresis or plasma exchange?*

Although 90% of the phenytoin in the serum is bound to albumin, the vascular space represents only a small fraction of the total volume of distribution for phenytoin. Of the total amount of drug in the body, only 5% is within the vascular space. Since most of the phenytoin is actually in the tissue compartments, plasmapheresis or plasma volume exchange should not result in a significant loss of phenytoin from the body. Most studies indicate that somewhere between 5% and 10% of phenytoin is lost from the body during plasmapheresis.[57] Of course, if the procedure was to be repeated many times, the cumulative effect could result in a significant amount of drug loss and the requirement of a replacement dose.

Question #14. *S.T. is a 47-year-old, 60-kg man with glomerular nephritis. His creatinine clearance is reasonably good, but he has a serum albumin concentration of 2.0 gm/dL. S.T. is receiving 300 mg/day of phenytoin and has a steady-state phenytoin concentration of 6 mg/L. What would his phenytoin concentration be if his serum albumin were normal?*

The fraction of a drug concentration that is bound to plasma proteins is a function of the drug's affinity for the binding sites on the plasma protein and the number of binding sites available. The number of binding sites is proportional to the amount or concentration of plasma protein to which the drug is bound. Phenytoin is an acidic drug and appears to be bound primarily to albumin.[11] The relationship between a phenytoin concentration which is observed (Patient's Phenytoin Concentration with Altered Plasma Binding) when a patient has a low serum albumin relative to the phenytoin concentration that would be observed if the serum albumin were normal is described by Equation 10.2 (also see Part I: Desired Plasma Concentration).

$$\frac{\text{Phenytoin Concentration}}{\text{Normal Plasma Binding}} = \frac{\text{Patient's Phenytoin Concentration with Altered Plasma Binding}}{\left[0.9 \times \dfrac{\text{Patient's Serum Albumin}}{4.4 \text{ gm/dL}} \right] + 0.1}$$

The plasma phenytoin concentration that corresponds to a concentration that would be observed if S.T.'s albumin concentration were normal is calculated as follows:

$$\frac{\text{Phenytoin Concentration}}{\text{Normal Plasma Binding}} = \frac{6 \text{ mg/L}}{\left[0.9 \times \dfrac{2.0 \text{ gm/dL}}{4.4 \text{ gm/dL}} \right] + 0.1}$$

$$= \frac{6 \text{ mg/L}}{0.509}$$

$$= 11.8 \text{ mg/L}$$

The Phenytoin Concentration Normal Binding value of 11.8 mg/L should be used when comparing S.T.'s phenytoin concentration to the usual therapeutic range of 10 to 20 mg/L or in any of our calculations.

Question #15. *A.R., a 66-year-old, 60-kg man, was admitted to the hospital because of poor seizure control. He had been receiving 350* *mg/day of phenytoin acid as an outpatient. On admission, he had a phenytoin plasma concentration of 3 mg/L. Noncompliance was suspected, and a dose of 350 mg/day as sodium phenytoin was ordered. Five days after administration a second phenytoin level was reported as 18 mg/L. Has steady state been achieved? Is it reasonable to assume that A.R.'s Vm is close to the average values reported in the literature (i.e., 7 mg/kg/day)?*

The usual guideline of 3 to 4 half-lives as the time required to achieve steady state does not hold true for phenytoin because its metabolism is capacity-limited. The rate of phenytoin accumulation is the difference between the rate of metabolism and the rate of administration. Unlike drugs following first-order elimination, the rate of elimination is not proportionate to the plasma concentration. Therefore, the time required to reach steady state can be prolonged. This will be especially true when the plasma concentrations are much greater than Km. After the daily dose of 350 mg for this 60-kg patient is corrected to 408.3 mg/day for a 70-kg patient:

$$\left[\frac{350 \text{ mg}}{60 \text{ kg}} \right] [70 \text{ kg}] = 408.3 \text{ mg}$$

Equation 10.24 can be used to calculate a 90% t value of 35.7 days.

$$90\% \text{ t} = \frac{[115 + (35)(C)][C]}{(S)(F)(\text{Dose/day})}$$

$$= \frac{[115 + (35)(18)][18]}{(0.92)(1)(408.3)}$$

$$= 35.7 \text{ days}$$

A.R. has been receiving this maintenance regimen for only 5 days; therefore, the plasma concentration of 18 mg/L is very unlikely to represent a steady-state condition. Equation 10.33 can be used to estimate the amount of drug eliminated per day:

$$\frac{\text{Amount Eliminated}}{t} = (S)(F)(\text{Dose}/\tau) - \left[\frac{(C_2 - C_1)(V)}{t} \right]$$

$$= [(0.92)(1)(350 \text{ mg/day})] - \left[\frac{(18 \text{ mg/L} - 3 \text{ mg/L})(0.65 \text{ L/kg} \times 60 \text{ kg})}{5 \text{ days}} \right]$$

$$= 322 \text{ mg/day} - \left(\frac{(15 \text{ mg/L})(39 \text{ L})}{5 \text{ days}} \right)$$

$$= 322 \text{ mg/day} - (117 \text{ mg/day})$$

$$= 205 \text{ mg/day}$$

If a Km of 4 mg/L is assumed, a Vm of about 283 mg/day or 4.7 mg/kg/day is calculated for A.R. using Equation 10.34.

$$Vm = \frac{\left[\dfrac{\text{Amount Eliminated}}{t}\right]\left[Km + \left(\dfrac{C_1 + C_2}{2}\right)\right]}{\left(\dfrac{C_1 + C_2}{2}\right)}$$

$$= \frac{\left[\dfrac{205 \text{ mg}}{1 \text{ day}}\right]\left[4 \text{ mg/L} + \left(\dfrac{3 \text{ mg/L} + 18 \text{ mg/L}}{2}\right)\right]}{\left(\dfrac{3 \text{ mg/L} + 18 \text{ mg/L}}{2}\right)}$$

$$= \frac{\left[\dfrac{205 \text{ mg}}{1 \text{ day}}\right][4 \text{ mg/L} + 10.5 \text{ mg/L}]}{(10.5 \text{ mg/L})}$$

$$= 283 \text{ mg/day}$$

or

$$= \frac{283 \text{ mg/day}}{60 \text{ kg}} = 4.7 \text{ mg/kg/day}$$

This Vm value of approximately 4.7 mg/kg/day day is less than the average value of 7 mg/kg/day but is not unreasonable, and it can be used as a first approximation of a new maintenance dose. Note that even though C_2 was not $\leq 2 \times C_1$ the mass balance approach can be used as an initial adjustment and the estimate of 4.7 mg/kg/day is probably better than the literature average of 7 mg/kg/day for A.R.'s Vm.

Question #16. *Why does changing from oral to intramuscular phenytoin for injection result in a sudden and dramatic decrease in phenytoin levels? Is there a difference between phenytoin for injection and fosphenytoin?*

Phenytoin is a relatively insoluble compound that crystallizes within the muscle following intramuscular (IM) administration.[58] The phenytoin crystals are slowly absorbed and the absorption rate is decreased initially. The subsequent decrease in the plasma concentration of phenytoin will be more than proportional to the reduction in absorption from the IM injection because phenytoin metabolism is capacity-limited. In one study,[59] a change from oral to IM administration resulted in an initial 40% to 60% decrease in the phenytoin plasma level, while the metabolite elimination decreased by only 16% to 20%. Therefore, the IM route of administration for phenytoin should be avoided.

Fosphenytoin for injection is a more soluble ester of phenytoin and has a much more reliable and rapid absorption pattern when administered by the IM route than phenytoin for injection. When administered by the IM route, the majority of patients will achieve plasma concentrations in the therapeutic range within 30 minutes.[6,60] Whereas IM fosphenytoin is more rapidly absorbed than oral phenytoin, most clinicians prefer the IV route when rapid attainment of therapeutic concentrations is required, regardless of whether phenytoin for injection or fosphenytoin is used.

Question #17. *What effect does phenobarbital have on steady-state phenytoin concentrations? What other drugs might interact with phenytoin?*

Clinically, the addition of phenobarbital does not change steady-state phenytoin concentrations.[61] Phenobarbital, however, may induce the metabolism of phenytoin and, thereby, increase the metabolic capacity of phenytoin (i.e., increase Vm). Furthermore, competition between phenobarbital and phenytoin for the same metabolic enzymes could have the effect of increasing Km. If Vm is increased, phenytoin clearance will increase and the phenytoin concentration will decrease. Increasing Km will have the opposite effect; therefore, there may be no consistent effect on the phenytoin concentration. See Equation 10.15:

$$\text{Css ave} = \frac{(Km)[(S)(F)(\text{Dose}/\tau)]}{Vm - [(S)(F)(\text{Dose}/\tau)]}$$

Similar problems exist in evaluating the mechanism for the increased phenytoin concentrations associated with drugs such as isoniazid, chloramphenicol, and cimetidine.[62-64] In the case of isoniazid, animal data suggest that there is noncompetitive inhibition of metabolic enzymes which reduces the Vm.[65] The interaction appears to be more significant in patients who are phenotypically slow acetylators of isoniazid.[65]

Valproic acid, phenylbutazone, and salicylates reportedly displace phenytoin from albumin.[66] This protein displacement would decrease the total phenytoin concentration, but not the free or unbound concentration. Assuming no change in metabolism, the result of the altered binding would be a decreased bound concentration, no change in the free concentration, an increased free fraction, and a decrease in the total concentration, which would be associated with a corresponding and equally offsetting decreased therapeutic range.

The number of drugs reported to interact with phenytoin is large.[67] Many of the drugs are easily recognized as they are commonly reported to either increase (e.g., carbamazepine) or decrease (e.g., amiodarone) the metabolism of other drugs. Phenytoin is a more complex issue in that because of capacity-limited metabolism, even small changes in either absorption or metabolism can result in significant changes in the final steady-state concentration of phenytoin. The potential for even small changes in metabolism to result in substantial changes in the steady-state concentration makes it difficult to predict which drugs will result in clinically significant drug–drug interactions.

REFERENCES

1. Bigger JT, et al. Relationship between the plasma level of diphenylhydantoin sodium and its cardiac antiarrhythmic effects. Circulation 1968;38:363.
2. Pyror FM, et al. Fosphenytoin: pharmacokinetics and tolerance of intramuscular loading doses. Epilepsia 2001;42(2):245–250.
3. Louis S, et al. The cardiocirculatory changes caused by intravenous Dilantin and its solvent. Am Heart J 1967;74:523.
4. Kutt H, et al. Diphenylhydantoin metabolism, blood levels and toxicity. Arch Neurol 1964;11:642.
5. Lund L. Effects of phenytoin in patients with epilepsy in relation to its concentration in plasma. In: David DS, Prichard NBC, eds. Biological Effects of Drugs in Relation to Their Concentration in Plasma. Baltimore: University Park Press, 1972:227.
6. Phenytoin. In: McEvoy GK, ed. American Hospital Formulary Service Drug Information 2002. Bethesda: American Society of Health-System Pharmacists, 2002:2133–2139.
7. Kugler AR, et al. Cross-reactivity of fosphenytoin in two human plasma phenytoin immunoassays. Clin Chem 1998;44:1474–1480.
8. Yukawa E. Optimization of antiepileptic drug therapy. The importance of serum drug concentration monitoring. Clin Pharmacokinet 1996;31:120–130.
9. Lascelles PT, et al. The distribution of plasma phenytoin levels in epileptic patients. J Neurol Neurosurg Psychiatry 1970;33:501.
10. Odar-Cederlof I, et al. Kinetics of diphenylhydantoin in uremic patients: consequence of decreased protein binding. Eur J Clin Pharmacol 1974;7:31.
11. Koch-Weser J, Sellers EM. Binding of drugs to serum albumin. N Engl J Med 1976;294:311.
12. Lund L, et al. Plasma protein binding of diphenylhydantoin in patients with epilepsy. Clin Pharmacol Ther 1972;13:196.
13. Adler DS, et al. Hemodialysis of phenytoin in a uremic patient. Clin Pharmacol Ther 1975;18:65.
14. Reidenberg MM, et al. Protein binding of diphenylhydantoin and desmethylimipramine in plasma from patients with poor renal function. N Engl J Med 1971;285:264.
15. Odar-Cederlof I. Plasma protein binding of phenytoin and warfarin in patients undergoing renal transplantation. Clin Pharmacokinet 1977;2:147.
16. Reidenberg MM. The binding of drugs to plasma proteins and the interpretation of measurements of plasma concentrations of drugs in patients with poor renal function. Am J Med 1977;62:466.
17. Liponi DL, et al. Renal function and therapeutic concentrations of phenytoin. Neurology 1984;34:395.
18. Mattson RH, et al. Valproic acid in epilepsy; clinical and pharmacological effects. Neurology 1978;3:20.
19. Monks A, Richens A. Effect of single dose of sodium valproate on serum phenytoin levels and protein binding in epileptic patients. Clin Pharmacol Ther 1980;27:89.
20. Kerrick JM, Wolff DL, Graves NM. Predicting unbound phenytoin concentrations in patients receiving valproic acid: a comparison of two prediction methods. Ann Pharmacother 1995;29:470–474.
21. Jusko WJ, et al. Nonlinear assessment of phenytoin bioavailability. J Pharmacokinet Biopharm 1976;4:327.

22. Gugler R, et al. Phenytoin: pharmacokinetics and bioavailability. Clin Pharmacol Ther 1976;19:135.

23. Wilder BJ, et al. Effect of food on absorption of Dilantin Kapseals and Myland extended phenytoin sodium capsules. Neurology 2001;57(4):571–573, 582–589.

24. Rosenbaum DH, Rowan AJ, Tuchman L, French JA. Comparative bioavailability of generic phenytoin and Dilantin. Epilepsia 1994;35:656–660.

25. Goff DA, et al. Absorption characteristics of three phenytoin sodium products after administration of oral loading doses. Clin Pharm 1984;3:634–638.

26. Cacek AT. Review of alterations in oral phenytoin bioavailability associated with formulation, antacids, and food. Ther Drug Monit 1986;8:166.

27. Bauer LA. Interference of oral phenytoin absorption by continuous nasogastric feedings. Neurology 1982;32:570.

28. Faraji B, Yu PP. Serum phenytoin levels of patients on gastrostomy tube feeding. J Neuroscience Nurs 1998;30:55–59.

29. Doak KK, et al. Bioavailability of phenytoin acid and phenytoin sodium with enteral feedings. Pharmacotherapy 1998;18:637–645.

30. Carter BL, et al. Effect of antacids on phenytoin bioavailability. Ther Drug Monit 1981;3(4):33–40.

31. Neuvonen PJ. Bioavailability of phenytoin; clinical pharmacokinetic and therapeutic implications. Clin Pharmacokinet 1978;3:20.

32. Wilder BJ, et al. Plasma diphenylhydantoin levels after loading and maintenance doses. Clin Pharmacol Ther 1973;14:797.

33. Jung D, et al. Effect of dose on phenytoin absorption. Clin Pharm Ther 1980;28:479.

34. Havidberg E, Dam M. Clinical pharmacokinetics of anticonvulsants. Clin Pharmacokinet 1976;1:151.

35. Glazko AJ, et al. Metabolic disposition of diphenylhydantoin in normal human subjects following intravenous administration. Clin Pharmacol Ther 1969;10:498.

36. Abernathy DR, Greenblatt DJ. Phenytoin disposition in obesity: determination of loading dose. Arch Neurol 1985;42:568–571.

37. Bochner F, et al. Effects of dosage increments on blood phenytoin concentrations. J Neurol Neurosurg Psychiatry 1972;35:873.

38. Arnold K, et al. The rate of decline of diphenylhydantoin in human plasma. Clin Pharmacol Ther 1970;11:121.

39. Houghton GW, Richens A. Rate of elimination of tracer doses of phenytoin at different steady state serum phenytoin concentrations in epileptic patients. Br J Clin Pharmacol 1974;1:155.

40. Lund L, et al. Pharmacokinetics of single and multiple doses of phenytoin in man. Eur J Clin Pharmacol 1974;7:81.

41. Mawer GE, et al. Phenytoin dose adjustments in epileptic patients. Br J Clin Pharmacol 1974;1:163.

42. Lambie DG, et al. Therapeutic and pharmacokinetic effects of increasing phenytoin in chronic epileptics on multiple drug therapy. Lancet 1976;2:386.

43. Richens A. A study of the pharmacokinetics of phenytoin (diphenylhydantoin) in epileptic patients, and the development of a nomogram for making dose increments. Epilepsia 1975;16:627.

44. Ludden TM, et al. Individualization of phenytoin dosage regimens. Clin Pharmacol Ther 1977;21:287.

45. Martin E, et al. The clinical pharmacokinetics of phenytoin. J Pharmacokinet Biopharm 1977;5:579.

46. Mullen PW. Optimal phenytoin therapy: a new technique for individualizing dosage. Clin Pharmacol Ther 1978;23:228.

47. Privitera MD. Clinical rules for phenytoin dosing. Ann Pharmacother 1993;27:1169–1173.

48. Atkinson AJ, Shaw JM. Pharmacokinetic study of a patient with diphenylhydantoin toxicity. Clin Pharmacol Ther 1973;14:521.

49. Bauer LA, Blouin RA. Phenytoin Michaelis-Menten pharmacokinetics in caucasian pediatric patients. Clin Pharmacokinet 1983;8:545.

50. Grasela TH, et al. Steady state pharmacokinetics of phenytoin from routinely collected patient data. Clin Pharmacokinet 1983;8:355.

51. Dodson WE. Nonlinear kinetics of phenytoin in children. Neurology 1982;32:42–48.

52. Chiba K, et al. Michaelis-Menten pharmacokinetics of diphenylhydantoin: an application in the pediatric age patient. J Pediatr 1980;96:479.

53. Tozer TN, Winter ME. Phenytoin. In: Evans WE, et al., eds. Applied Pharmacokinetics: Principles of Therapeutic Drug Monitoring. 3rd Ed. Vancouver: Applied Therapeutics, 1992:1.

54. Wilder BJ, et al. Correlation of acute diphenylhydantoin intoxication with plasma levels and metabolite excretion. Neurology 1973;23:1329.

55. Warner A, Privitera M, Bates D. Standards of laboratory practice: antiepileptic drug monitoring. Clin Chem 1998;44:1085–1095.

56. Andreasen F, Jakobsen P. Determination of furosemide in blood and its binding to proteins in normal plasma and in plasma from patients with acute renal failure. Acta Pharmacol Toxicol (Copenh)1974;35:49.

57. Matzke GR. Does plasma exchange alter drug therapy? [Editorial] Clin Pharm 1984;3:421.

58. Wilensky AJ, et al. Inadequate serum levels after intramuscular administration of diphenylhydantoin. Neurology 1973;23:318.

59. Wilder BJ, et al. A method for shifting from oral to intramuscular diphenylhydantoin administration. Clin Pharmacol Ther 1974;16:507.

60. Uthman BM, Wilder BJ, Ramsay RE. Intramuscular use of fosphenytoin: an overview. Neurology 1996;46(6 Suppl1) S24–S28.

61. Morselli PL, et al. Interaction between phenobarbital and DPH in animals and epileptic patients. Ann NY Acad Sci 1971;169:88.

62. Kutt H, et al. Depression of parahydroxylation of diphenylhydantoin by antituberculosis chemotherapy. Neurology 1966;16:594.

63. Rose JQ, et al. Intoxication caused by interaction of chloramphenicol and phenytoin. JAMA 1977;237:2630.

64. Bartle WR, et al. Dose-dependent effect of cimetidine on phenytoin kinetics. Clin Pharmacol Ther 1983;33:649.

65. Kutt H, et al. Inhibition of diphenylhydantoin metabolism in rats and in rat liver microsomes by antitubercular drugs. Neurology 1968;18:706.

66. Richens A, Dunlop A. Serum phenytoin levels in the management of epilepsy. Lancet 1975;2:247.

67. Drug Facts and Comparison. 56th Ed. St. Louis: Facts and Comparison, 2002.

11

PROCAINAMIDE

Maureen S. Boro and Michael E. Winter

Procainamide is used to treat ventricular and atrial tachyarrhythmias. It can be administered orally, intramuscularly, or intravenously. A loading dose of ≈1000 mg (15 mg/kg) is generally followed by a constant intravenous infusion or an oral maintenance dose. The short plasma half-life of procainamide dictates the use of 3- to 4-hour dosing intervals unless sustained-release drug products are used. Sustained-release procainamide formulations are designed to be administered every 6 hours (various manufacturers)[1-3] and every 12 hours (Procanbid).[4] To enhance patient adherence, less frequent dosing is ideal. An exception would be in patients who cannot take solid dosage forms (e.g., patients fed via nasogastric tubes).

KEY PARAMETERS: **Procainamide**	
Therapeutic Plasma Concentration	4–8 mg/L
F	0.85
S	0.87
V^a	2 L/kg
Cl^b Cl_{renal} $Cl_{acetylation}$ (Average) $Cl_{acetylation}$ (Fast) $Cl_{acetylation}$ (Slow) Cl_{other}	 $[3][Cl_{Cr}]^c$ 0.13 L/kg/hr 0.19 L/kg/hr 0.07 L/kg/hr 0.1 L/kg/hr
$t^{1/2}$ α β^d	 5 min 3 hr

[a]Decreased by 25% in patients with low cardiac output.
[b]Decreased by 25% to 50% in patients with low cardiac output. Cl is the total of the renal, acetylation, and other metabolic clearance routes for procainamide.
[c]Units of Cl_{Cr} must be consistent when Cl_{renal} is added to $Cl_{acetylation}$ and Cl_{other} (i.e., L/hr or L/kg/hr).
[d]Half-life increases in patients with renal and/or cardiac dysfunction.

Pharmacokinetic predictions are complicated because procainamide is cleared renally and metabolically. Procainamide is metabolized to an active metabolite, N-acetylprocainamide (NAPA), which is an antiarrhythmic agent in its own right. The activity of the NAPA metabolite is uncertain and probably variable. Monitoring NAPA plasma concentrations may be appropriate in patients with diminished renal function because NAPA is eliminated primarily by the kidneys. Understanding the metabolite will allow the clinician to anticipate which patients are "at risk" and to perhaps recognize drug effects of the "unseen" metabolite.

THERAPEUTIC AND TOXIC PLASMA CONCENTRATIONS

Procainamide plasma concentrations of 4 to 8 mg/L are usually considered therapeutic.[5,6] Minor toxicities such as gastrointestinal disturbances, weakness, mild hypotension, and changes in the electrocardiogram (10% to 30% prolongation of the PR, QT, or QRS intervals) usually do not occur at plasma concentrations < 8 mg/L. Toxicities may develop in as many as 30% of patients when plasma concentrations exceed 12 to 13 mg/L.[6] Although not concentration dependent, long-term procainamide administration has been associated with immunologic reactions (systemic lupus erythematosus).[7] Plasma concentrations in the range of 15 to 20 mg/L, however, have been appropriate in some patients.[8-10] Patients in whom unusually high target procainamide concentrations were needed suffered from severe arrhythmias that were difficult to control with conventional therapy. With the availability of newer cardiac agents, the tendency is to maintain procainamide levels within the usual therapeutic range of 4 to 8 mg/L.

BIOAVAILABILITY (F)

The bioavailability of orally administered procainamide is approximately 85% (F = 0.85).[11] Absorption is usually rapid, and plasma concentrations peak 1 to 2 hours after administration of non–sustained-release dosage forms. Considerable variation in absorption can occur,[11] and absorption can be very slow and possibly incomplete in patients with congestive heart failure (CHF).[5]

There are two types of long acting procainamide products available: procainamide *sustained-release* tablets (Pronestyl-SR and generic manufacturers) and Procanbid extended-release tablets. Although difficult to determine from the data available, the sustained-release procainamide products appear to be completely absorbed over approximately 3 to 4 hours.[1-3,12] This absorption period limits the dosing interval for the sustained-release products to 6 hours in the majority of patients. Only in patients with a low clearance and prolonged elimination half-life can the dosing interval be extended beyond 6 hours. Care should be taken when changing sustained-release products by evaluating the extent and pattern of absorption.[12,13]

Also available are Procanbid extended-release tablets. The exact model for absorption of Procanbid extended-release tablets is not well documented. However, it appears from clinical studies that the absorption pattern is sufficiently long so that a continuous infusion model is an appropriate pharmacokinetic approach when Procanbid extended-release tablets are administered to most patients on an every 12 hour basis.[4] Although there have been reports of intact sustained-release tablets in the stool, these actually represent the inert matrix which remains after complete absorption of the drug.[1,14]

For the purposes of consistency in this chapter, procainamide sustained-release products refer to Pronestyl-SR and the generic products which have an absorption duration of approximately 4 hours. When Procanbid extended-release is used, this is referring to a product with a longer duration of absorption permitting use of a continuous infusion model when administered every 12 hours. Procainamide products should not be automatically considered as interchangeable. In clinical practice, it is imperative to evaluate the absorption characteristics for the product that your patient is receiving.

VOLUME OF DISTRIBUTION (V)

The volume of distribution of procainamide is ≈ 2 L/kg.[6,15] This volume is unchanged by renal failure[15] but is decreased by approximately 25% in patients with decreased cardiac output.[6] In obese patients, the volume of distribution appears to correlate best with ideal body weight (IBW).[16]

Like lidocaine, procainamide distributes into an initial volume of distribution (Vi).[5,6,17] Since the myocardium responds as though it were located in the initial volume of distribution, loading doses (which are calculated based on a volume of distribution of 2 L/kg) should be given at a rate slow enough to avoid excessive plasma concentrations in Vi (see Question #2).

CLEARANCE (Cl)

The clearance of procainamide in an average 70-kg patient with good renal and cardiac function is ≈ 550 mL/min. In these patients, about one-half of the dose is cleared by metabolism, and the other one-half is cleared renally.[5] The clearance of procainamide can be broken down into three primary components:[5,11,18,19] a renal clearance (Cl_{renal}) which is approximately 3 times creatinine clearance; acetylation clearance ($Cl_{acetylation}$) which is based on acetylation phenotype; and a non-renal, non-acetylated metabolic clearance which will be referred to as clearance "other" (Cl_{other}). Clearance by acetylation is approximately 0.19 L/kg/hr in fast acetylators and 0.07 L/kg/hr in slow acetylators. When uncertain as to fast or slow acetylator, it is common clinical practice to use an average $Cl_{acetylation}$ of 0.13 L/kg/hr. Cl_{other} is ≈ 0.1 L/kg/hr. The acetylation pathway results in the production of NAPA, a metabolite with pharmacologic activity. The clearance "other" pathway metabolites appear to be inactive cardiovascularly.

Although subjects with excellent renal function and cardiac output may have procainamide clearances > 30 L/hr,[11,17,18] clearances of one-half this value are common in patients with diminished renal function or cardiac output.[6,8] It is difficult to know the degree to which each of the clearance pathways is affected by CHF. One approach that is recommended in patients with CHF is to decrease the total calculated clearance (which is based on renal function, metabolic function, and body weight) to approximately 50% of the original value. Even if there is just a hint of CHF, it is common practice to decrease the total procainamide clearance by half to avoid clearance values that are too large which result in expected dosage regimens and steady-state procainamide concentrations that are excessive.

The clearance of procainamide in obese subjects is increased relative to their ideal body weight.[16] This appears to be due to increased renal clearance. Therefore, in obese subjects the renal clearance of procainamide should be based on total body weight (TBW) and the metabolic clearance on the patient's ideal body weight (see Question #9).

Increased procainamide concentrations resulting from decreased clearance of procainamide have been reported with concurrent administration of procainamide and cimetidine.[20,21] Also cited is an increase in NAPA concentrations.[20] Ranitidine appears less likely to interact with procainamide.[21,22] Other interactions suggesting potential increase in procainamide concentrations have been reported with ofloxacin[23] and trimethoprim.[24] Interactions with procainamide and amiodarone[25,26] have been cited but it is uncommon to use these agents in combination. If used together it is important to realize that the interactions are pharmacodynamic in nature but may also be pharmacokinetic. With the long half-life of amiodarone, the window of the interaction might be prolonged. In the clinical setting it is important to be aware of the potential for these and other drug–drug interactions and the effects on both procainamide and NAPA. Significant changes in clearance should be considered when designing therapeutic dosage regimens.

HALF -LIFE (t½)

The apparent distribution half-life (α t½) is about 5 minutes.[6,11,17] The elimination half-life (β t½) of procainamide is a function of its volume of distribution and clearance. For a 70 kg patient with an average volume of distribution of 2 L/kg (140 L) and a clearance of 33 L/hr, the calculated elimination half-life (using Equation 11.1) is approximately 3 hours.

$$t_{1/2} = \frac{(0.693)(V)}{Cl} \qquad \text{[Eq. 11.1]}$$

$$= \frac{(0.693)(140\ L)}{33\ L/hr}$$

$$= 3\ hr$$

This half-life is short, and frequent dosing will be necessary unless a continuous intravenous infusion or a sustained-release oral product is used. For the immediate-release procainamide oral product, to stay in the therapeutic range of 4 to 8 mg/L, tau will need to be less than or equal to the half-life.

With the exception of Procanbid, the absorption time for the sustained-release procainamide drug products is somewhat short and is approximately 4 hours. This suggests that depending on the patient's procainamide half-life and the dosing interval chosen for the sustained-release drug product, the intermittent infusion model (Equation 11.2) is most appropriate for calculating procainamide trough concentrations.

$$Css_2 = \frac{\frac{(S)(F)(Dose/t_{in})}{Cl}(1 - e^{-K\,t_{in}})}{(1 - e^{-K\tau})}(e^{-Kt_2}) \qquad \text{[Eq. 11.2]}$$

Note that for the trough concentration, t_2 is the time interval (in hours) from the end of absorption to the next procainamide dose (i.e., $\tau - t_{in}$). This is the time over which the procainamide concentration will decay. As previously discussed in Part I, if t_2 or the time of decay is $\leq 1/3\ t_{1/2}$, a continuous infusion model (Equation 11.3) can be used.

$$Css\ ave = \frac{(S)(F)(Dose/\tau)}{Cl} \qquad \text{[Eq. 11.3]}$$

For most patients receiving sustained-release procainamide products every 6 hours or Procanbid extended-release tablets every 12 hours, Equation 11.3 is probably reasonable, even if one suspects that the value of t_2 is longer than one-third of the half-life. This is because there is some variation in both the onset and the duration of absorption from sustained-release products. Therefore, the complexity of Equation 11.2 is probably not warranted in clinical practice unless the procainamide dosing intervals are 8 or 12 hours for the sustained-release product or longer than 12 hours for Procanbid extended-release and the procainamide half-life is short.

N-ACETYLPROCAINAMIDE (NAPA)

Therapeutic and Toxic Plasma Concentrations

Although it is clear that NAPA has antiarrhythmic activity, the exact relationship between plasma N-acetylprocainamide concentrations and its antiarrhythmic activity has not been clearly established. Some researchers have observed that NAPA's activity is similar to that of procainamide when equal plasma concentrations are compared;[27-29] however, others have found that plasma concentrations of approximately 10 to 20 mg/L are required for partial suppression of ventricular contractions.[30,31] Little additional antiarrhythmic benefits are observed when NAPA concentrations exceed 30 mg/L.[31]

Interestingly, when the therapeutic levels of 4 to 8 mg/L were established for procainamide,[5,6] NAPA concentrations were not considered, even though plasma NAPA concentrations are approximately equal to procainamide concentrations in many patients.[32,33] Although the activity of NAPA as an antiarrhythmic is in question, therapeutic and/or toxic effects are possible in some patients.[34] This may be related to elevated NAPA concentrations or an unusual patient sensitivity to NAPA. Therefore, monitoring plasma NAPA concentrations may be useful, although in the majority of patients, knowledge of the plasma NAPA concentration does not alter the course of procainamide therapy. However, understanding the pharmacokinetics of procainamide and NAPA will help clinicians to anticipate which patients will be at risk for high NAPA concentrations and when to proceed with caution.

Animal studies suggest that NAPA may be less toxic than procainamide. Although significant cardiac toxicity has not been observed with NAPA concentrations as high as 40 mg/L,[31,35] NAPA may have resulted in serious cardiac toxicity in isolated individuals when NAPA levels exceeded 30 mg/L.[34] In addition, systemic lupus erythematosus may be less likely to be associated with NAPA than with procainamide.[29]

NAPA Production

The rate of NAPA production depends on the plasma concentration of procainamide and its clearance by acetylation, which is genetically determined. Approximately 50% of Blacks and Whites are rapid acetylators. Asians and especially Northern Asians (e.g., Japanese) tend to be predominately fast acetylators (80 to 90%). Rapid acetylators convert ≈30% of an administered dose of procainamide to NAPA, whereas slow acetylators convert ≈15%.[36] This percentage conversion is based on the acetylation clearance, which is approximately 0.19 L/kg/hr for a rapid acetylator and 0.07 L/kg/hr for a slow acetylator. The percentage conversion increases in patients with diminished renal function because a greater percentage of procainamide is cleared by the acetylation pathway.[15,19] This is illustrated by Equation 11.4.

$$\text{Fraction of Procainamide Converted to NAPA} = \frac{Cl_{acetylation}}{Cl_{renal} + Cl_{acetylation} + Cl_{other}} \qquad \text{[Eq. 11.4]}$$

Volume of Distribution (V)

The volume of distribution for NAPA appears to be about 1.5 L/kg.[37,38]

Clearance (Cl)

NAPA has a renal clearance that is approximately 1.6 times creatinine clearance and a metabolic or non-renal clearance that is ≈ 0.025 L/kg/hr.[37]

Half-Life (t½)

The usual half-life of NAPA in patients with normal renal function is approximately 6 hours. However, the half-life may increase to 30 hours or more in patients with poor renal function.[15,18]

TIME TO SAMPLE (PROCAINAMIDE AND NAPA)

Because procainamide has a relatively short half-life (3 hours), steady-state concentrations are achieved within 12 to 24 hours after therapy has begun. Although steady state is achieved quickly, the sampling time must be selected carefully within the dosing interval. When standard non–sustained-release dosage forms of procainamide are administered on a regular, intermittent basis, trough plasma concentrations are probably more reproducible than peak concentrations. With sustained-release procainamide, however, the sampling time becomes relatively less important. Nevertheless, when dosing intervals exceed 6 hours for procainamide sustained-released or 12 hours for Procanbid extended-release, significant peak to trough variations may occur in patients with short procainamide half-lives. Therefore, for procainamide immediate-release and long acting procainamide products, trough levels are usually recommended.[39]

Procainamide concentrations are most appropriately monitored within the first 24 to 48 hours of therapy, although additional plasma concentrations may be required if significant changes in the patient's clinical status are observed. The half-life for NAPA is twice as long as that for procainamide, and steady state will not be achieved for at least 24 hours in patients with good renal function; as long as 1 week may be required for patients with significantly decreased renal function.

Question #1. *A.L., a 62-year-old, 70-kg man, was admitted to the coronary care unit with a diagnosis of acute myocardial infarction.*

A.L. has a history of mild CHF and a creatinine clearance of ≈50 mL/min. A.L. developed premature ventricular contractions (PVCs), which were unresponsive to lidocaine. Calculate a parenteral loading dose of procainamide designed to achieve a plasma concentration of ≈8 mg/L.

To calculate the loading dose required to achieve a procainamide plasma concentration of 8 mg/L, the volume of distribution must be estimated. Because A.L. has mild CHF, the expected volume of distribution would be 1.5 L/kg (25% reduction from normal)[6] or 105 L (1.5 L/kg × 70 kg). Using Equation 11.5 and assuming F to be 1.0 for parenteral administration and S to be 0.87 for the hydrochloride salt, the loading dose of procainamide would be:

$$\text{Loading Dose} = \frac{(V)(C)}{(S)(F)} \qquad \text{[Eq. 11.5]}$$

$$= \frac{(105\ L)(8\ mg/L)}{(0.87)(1)}$$

$$= 965.5\ mg\ or \approx 1000\ mg$$

This calculated loading dose of 1000 mg is a standard procainamide loading dose.[40] A reasonable target for the loading dose is to achieve a procainamide concentration of 6 to 8 mg/L.

Question #2. *If the loading dose of 1000 mg is to be given intravenously, how should it be administered?*

Because procainamide is administered into an initial volume of distribution (Vi)[5,6,17] and the myocardium responds as though it were located in this initial volume,[6,17,40] procainamide should be administered as a slow infusion to avoid high distribution phase concentrations.[18] If the entire loading dose is given as a single rapid bolus, the initial plasma concentration will greatly exceed the desired 8 mg/L and toxicities are likely.

The apparent initial volume of distribution is approximately one-third of the total V, and the apparent distribution half-life is about 5 minutes.[6,17] Initially it was recommended that 100 mg be given every 5 minutes (avoiding accumulation in Vi) until the arrhythmia is abolished, toxicities are observed, or the total loading dose is administered.[40] Although the maximum recommended infusion rate is 50 mg/min, in most clinical settings when procainamide loading doses are administered they are given as a controlled infusion at a rate of ≈20 mg/min to achieve therapeutic concentrations rapidly while avoiding excessive accumulation in the first compartment. In A.L. this would suggest the 1000 mg loading dose would be infused over about 45 minutes to an hour.

While the loading dose is infusing, the patient should be monitored for side effects, such as hypotension and rhythm disturbances, which may be related to excessive concentrations of procainamide.

Question #3. *Calculate an infusion rate in mg/min that will maintain an average plasma procainamide concentration of 6 mg/L for A.L, the patient described in Question #1.*

Because the maintenance dose is determined by the patient's clearance, this parameter must be estimated before the infusion rate can be calculated. Using A.L.'s creatinine clearance (Cl_{cr}) of 3 L/hr (50 mL/min), an average acetylation clearance of 0.13 L/kg/hr and a Cl_{other} of 0.1 L/kg/hr, a total clearance of ≈ 25 L/hr is calculated.

$$Cl_{total} = Cl_{renal} + Cl_{acetylation} + Cl_{other} \qquad \text{[Eq. 11.6]}$$

$$Cl_{renal} = (3)(Cl_{cr})$$

$$= (3)(3 \text{ L/hr})$$

$$= 9 \text{ L/hr}$$

$$Cl_{acetylation} \text{(Average)} = (0.13 \text{ L/kg/hr})(70 \text{ kg})$$

$$= 9.1 \text{ L/hr}$$

$$Cl_{other} = (0.1 \text{ L/kg/hr})(70 \text{ kg})$$

$$= 7 \text{ L/hr}$$

$$Cl_{total} = Cl_{renal} + Cl_{acetylation} + Cl_{other}$$

$$= 9 \text{ L/hr} + 9.1 \text{ L/hr} + 7 \text{ L/hr}$$

$$= 25.1 \text{ L/hr}$$

Because A.L. has mild CHF, this clearance value should probably be decreased by half. Therefore, his expected clearance would be 12.5 L/hr (25.1 L/hr $\times$ 0.5 for CHF).

Using this clearance value of 12.5 L/hr and assuming S to be 0.87 and F to be 1.0, Equation 11.7 can be used to calculate a maintenance infusion.

$$\text{Maintenance Dose} = \frac{(Cl)(Css \text{ ave})(\tau)}{(S)(F)} \qquad \text{[Eq. 11.7]}$$

$$= \frac{(12.5 \text{ L/hr})(6 \text{ mg/L})(1 \text{ hr})}{(0.87)(1)}$$

$$= 86 \text{ mg/hr or} \approx 90 \text{ mg/hr}$$

This infusion rate of 90 mg/hr (1.5 mg/min) is within the usual guidelines for procainamide infusions of 1 to 4 mg/min. In clinical practice, patients similar to A.L. are usually started on infusions of 1 to 2 mg/min and infusion rate adjustments are dictated by the patient's response and measured procainamide concentrations.

Question #4. *A.L. received the 1000 mg procainamide loading dose at 7:00 p.m. (infused over 1 hour). At 8:00 p.m. the maintenance dose of 90 mg/hr was started. What would you expect A.L.'s procainamide concentration to be at 6:00 a.m. the following morning?*

By using Equation 11.1 to calculate A.L.'s half-life, it can be determined if the level at 6:00 a.m. was drawn at steady state.

$$t\frac{1}{2} = \frac{(0.693)(V)}{Cl}$$

$$= \frac{(0.693)(105 \text{ L})}{12.5 \text{ L/hr}}$$

$$= 5.8 \text{ hr}$$

Since A.L. has only been receiving the maintenance infusion for 10 hours (8:00 p.m. to 6:00 a.m.) and his $t\frac{1}{2}$ is 5.8 hours, he is not yet expected to be at steady state.

Two non-steady-state equations need to be used to calculate the procainamide level. These equations will require that the elimination rate constant (K) be calculated. It can be determined from the half-life using Equation 11.8:

$$K = \frac{0.693}{t\frac{1}{2}} \qquad \text{[Eq. 11.8]}$$

$$= \frac{0.693}{5.8 \text{ hr}}$$

$$= 0.119 \text{ hr}^{-1}$$

Equation 11.9 will determine the amount of the loading dose remaining that is contributing to the drug concentration. In Equation 11.9, the t_1 refers to the time (in hours) from the start of the loading dose infusion to when the drug level is drawn.

$$C_{t_1} = \frac{(S)(F)(Dose)}{V}(e^{-Kt_1}) \qquad \text{[Eq. 11.9]}$$

$$C_{t_1} = \frac{(0.87)(1)(1000 \text{ mg})}{105 \text{ L}}(e^{-(0.119 \text{ hr}^{-1})(11 \text{ hr})})$$

$$= 8.3 \text{ mg/L } (0.27)$$

$$= 2.2 \text{ mg/L}$$

Equation 11.10 can be used to determine the contribution of the maintenance dose to the drug level. In this equation, t_2 refers to the time (in hours) that the maintenance dose is infusing; in this case it is the time from when the maintenance dose was started until the level was drawn.

$$C_{t_2} = \frac{(S)(F)(Dose/\tau)}{Cl}(1 - e^{-Kt_2}) \qquad \text{[Eq. 11.10]}$$

$$C_{t_2} = \frac{(0.87)(1)(90 \text{ mg/hr})}{12.5 \text{ L/hr}}(1 - e^{-(0.119 \text{ hr}^{-1})(10 \text{ hr})})$$

$$= 6.3 \text{ mg/L } (1 - 0.30)$$

$$= 4.4 \text{ mg/L}$$

A.L.'s procainamide concentration at 6:00 a.m. would be the sum of Equation 11.9 and Equation 11.10 or 6.6 mg/L (2.2 mg/L + 4.4 mg/L). If A.L.'s procainamide concentration was much different than 6.6 mg/L, then an iterative search holding volume constant and solving for clearance to fit the measured procainamide concentration would have been done with Equations 11.9 and 11.10 as displayed below:

$$C = \frac{(0.87)(1)(1000 \text{ mg})}{105 \text{ L}}\left(e^{-\left(\frac{Cl}{105 \text{ L}}\right)(11 \text{ hr})}\right) + \frac{(0.87)(1)(90 \text{ mg/hr})}{Cl}\left(1 - e^{-\left(\frac{Cl}{105 \text{ L}}\right)(10 \text{ hr})}\right)$$

Question #5. *B.D., a 70-kg man with a Cl_{Cr} of 30 mL/min, has been receiving a constant procainamide infusion of 100 mg/hr ($\approx$1.7 mg/min). This infusion rate has resulted in a steady-state plasma procainamide concentration of 5 mg/L. Calculate an oral immediate-release dosing regimen that will maintain his plasma procainamide concentrations between 4 and 8 mg/L.*

Trough concentrations of procainamide should not be less than one-half of the peak concentrations; thus, the dosing interval should not exceed the half-life. The half-life of procainamide for B.D. can be estimated if the volume of distribution and clearance are known. If B.D. does not have significant CHF, the average volume of distribution (140 L based on 2 L/kg) can be used. His procainamide clearance can be determined by use of Equation 11.11 because a steady-state procainamide plasma concentration resulting from a given maintenance infusion dose is known. An S of 0.87 and an F of 1.0 can be assumed:

$$Cl = \frac{(S)(F)(Dose/\tau)}{Css\ ave} \qquad [Eq.\ 11.11]$$

$$= \frac{(0.87)(1)(100\ mg/hr)}{5\ mg/L}$$

$$= 17.4\ L/hr$$

Using this clearance (17.4 L/hr) and the expected volume of distribution of 140 L, Equation 11.1 can be used to calculate B.D.'s half-life.

$$t\frac{1}{2} = \frac{(0.693)(V)}{Cl}$$

$$= \frac{(0.693)(140\ L)}{17.4\ L/hr}$$

$$= 5.6\ hr$$

Based on this half-life and assuming that a non–sustained-release dosage form is administered, a dosing interval of 4 to 6 hours should be used.

The oral maintenance dose can be calculated in a number of ways. One method is to first select a dosing interval. Then, using the steady-state equation, a maintenance dose, which will achieve an average concentration halfway between the desired peak and trough levels, can be calculated. For example, using a desired average steady-state concentration of 6 mg/L, a dosing interval of 4 hours, the calculated clearance of 17.4 L/hr, an S of 0.87, and an F of 0.85, a maintenance dose of ≈565 mg every 4 hours is calculated using Equation 11.7.

$$Maintenance\ Dose = \frac{(Cl)(Css\ ave)(\tau)}{(S)(F)}$$

$$= \frac{(17.4\ L/hr)(6\ mg/L)(4\ hr)}{(0.87)(0.85)}$$

$$= 565\ mg\ every\ 4\ hr$$

As a general rule, the dosing interval should be equal to or less than the drug's half-life when the desired peak is less than or equal to twice the trough concentration. Immediate-release procainamide is available in 250, 375, and 500 mg dosage forms; therefore, a dose of 500 mg every 4 hours might be selected. The peak and trough concentrations from this dose can be calculated using Equations 11.12 and 11.13, respectively.

$$Css\ max = \frac{\dfrac{(S)(F)(Dose)}{V}}{1 - e^{-KT}} \qquad [Eq.\ 11.12]$$

$$Css\ min = Css\ max\ (e^{-KT}) \qquad [Eq.\ 11.13]$$

To solve the above equations, the elimination rate constant (K) must first be calculated using Equation 11.8:

$$K = \frac{0.693}{t\frac{1}{2}}$$

$$= \frac{0.693}{5.6\ hr}$$

$$= 0.124\ hr^{-1}$$

Then, a Css max of 6.8 mg/L can be calculated:

$$Css\ max = \frac{\dfrac{(S)(F)(Dose)}{V}}{1 - e^{-KT}}$$

$$= \frac{\dfrac{(0.87)(0.85)(500\ mg)}{140\ L}}{1 - e^{-(0.124\ hr^{-1})(4\ hr)}}$$

$$= \frac{2.64\ mg/L}{1 - 0.61}$$

$$= \frac{2.64\ mg/L}{0.39}$$

$$= 6.8\ mg/L$$

Once Css max is known, a Css min of 4.1 mg/L can also be calculated:

$$Css\ min = Css\ max\ (e^{-KT})$$

$$= 6.8\ mg/L\ (e^{-(0.124\ hr^{-1})(4\ hr)})$$

$$= 6.8\ mg/L\ (0.61)$$

$$= 4.1\ mg/L$$

The predicted peak and trough plasma concentrations of 6.8 mg/L and 4.1 mg/L, respectively, were based on the assumption that absorption occurs rapidly. The dampening effect of absorption will produce peak concentrations that are slightly lower and trough concentrations that are slightly higher than predicted by the IV bolus model. One should recall that absorption rates vary considerably among patients,[11] especially those with CHF.[5]

If a sustained-release procainamide were to be used, one could first determine the daily dose of the infusion using Equation 11.14.

$$\text{Amount of Drug Absorbed or Amount Reaching the Systemic Circulation} = (S)(F)(Dose) \qquad \text{[Eq. 11.14]}$$

$$= (0.87)(1)(100\ mg/hr)(24\ hr/day)$$

$$= 2088\ mg/day$$

Then, Equation 11.15 could be used to adjust for the difference in oral bioavailability.

$$\frac{\text{Dose of New}}{\text{Dosage Form}} = \frac{\text{Amount of Drug Absorbed From Current Dosage Form}}{(S)(F)\ \text{of New Dosage Form}} \qquad \text{[Eq. 11.15]}$$

$$= \frac{2088\ mg/day}{(0.87)(0.85)}$$

$$= 2824\ mg/day$$

If this new dose were to be given every 6 hours (4 times daily), then the individual doses given every 6 hours would be essentially equivalent to B.D.'s IV infusion rate of 100 mg/hr.

$$\frac{2824\ mg}{4} = 706\ mg\ every\ 6\ hours$$

Because the sustained-release procainamide products are available as 250, 500, and 750 mg tablets, the dosage form closest to the calculated dose is 750 mg. To confirm that procainamide sustained-release 750 mg every 6 hours will produce a concentration similar to that achieved with the 100 mg/hr infusion, Equation 11.3 can be used to estimate the steady-state procainamide concentration.

$$\text{Css ave} = \frac{(S)(F)(Dose/\tau)}{Cl}$$

$$= \frac{(0.87)(0.85)(750 \text{ mg/6 hr})}{17.4 \text{ L/hr}}$$

$$= \frac{92 \text{ mg/hr}}{17.4 \text{ L/hr}}$$

$$= 5.3 \text{ mg/L}$$

Procanbid extended-release are available as 500 mg and 1000 mg tablets. Since they are dosed every 12 hours, taking the total daily dose and dividing by 2 (2824 mg/2 = 1412 mg every 12 hours), a dose of 1500 mg every 12 hours would be appropriate. Because the dosing rate (Dose/τ) is the same, the Css ave will be the same for procainamide sustained-release 750 mg every 6 hours as Procanbid extended-release 1500 mg every 12 hours as displayed below using Equation 11.3:

$$\text{Css ave} = \frac{(S)(F)(Dose/\tau)}{Cl}$$

$$= \frac{(0.87)(0.85)(1500 \text{ mg/12 hr})}{17.4 \text{ L/hr}}$$

$$= \frac{92 \text{ mg/hr}}{17.4 \text{ L/hr}}$$

$$= 5.3 \text{ mg/L}$$

As discussed earlier, using a continuous infusion model for sustained-release procainamide products administered every 6 hours or Procanbid extended-release tablets every 12 hours is probably reasonable given the minimal fluctuation in plasma concentration anticipated within the dosing interval. If a longer dosing interval had been chosen in either case, the continuous infusion model would be a little more problematic given the expected half-life of 5.6 hours. The decay time might result in significant fluctuations of the plasma concentration within the dosing interval (see Question #6).

Question #6. *Using B.D.'s pharmacokinetic parameters, calculate the expected peak and trough concentrations from a sustained-release procainamide product when dosed 1000 mg every 8 hours.*

To calculate the steady-state peak and trough concentrations produced by a sustained-release drug product, one of two models can be used. In the first model, an average steady-state concentration is calculated on the assumption that procainamide plasma concentrations will fluctuate minimally during a dosing interval because absorption is prolonged. Using Equation 11.3 to make this calculation, an average concentration of 5.3 mg/L is predicted.

$$\text{Css ave} = \frac{(S)(F)(Dose/\tau)}{Cl}$$

$$= \frac{(0.87)(0.85)(1000 \text{ mg/8 hr})}{17.4 \text{ L/hr}}$$

$$= \frac{92 \text{ mg/hr}}{17.4 \text{ L/hr}}$$

$$= 5.3 \text{ mg/L}$$

As an alternative, Equation 11.2, which describes an intermittent steady-state infusion model, can be used. The term t_2 is the time interval between the end of the infusion and the time at which the concentration is measured (see Part I: Selecting the Appropriate Equation). When calculating the peak concentration with a dosing interval of 8 hours, for procainamide sustained-release t_{in} is assumed to be 4 hours and t_2 to be zero hours. When calculating the trough concentration, t_2 in Equation 11.2 is assumed to be 4 hours $(\tau - t_{in})$. Using the previously calculated parameters for clearance, elimination rate constant, S, and F, a peak concentration of 6.6 mg/L and a trough concentration of 4 mg/L can be calculated as shown below.

$$Css_2 = \frac{\dfrac{(S)(F)(Dose/t_{in})}{Cl}}{(1 - e^{-K\tau})}(1 - e^{-K t_{in}})(e^{-Kt_2})$$

$$= \frac{\dfrac{(0.87)(0.85)(1000 \text{ mg/4 hr})}{17.4 \text{ L/hr}}}{(1 - e^{-(0.124 \text{ hr}^{-1})(8 \text{ hr})})}(1 - e^{-(0.124 \text{ hr}^{-1})(4 \text{ hr})})(e^{-(0.124 \text{ hr}^{-1})(0 \text{ hr})})$$

$$= \frac{10.6 \text{ mg/L}(1 - 0.61)}{(1 - 0.37)}(1)$$

$$= 6.6 \text{ mg/L}$$

$$Css_2 \text{ (Trough)} = (6.6 \text{ mg/L})(e^{-Kt_2})$$

$$= (6.6 \text{ mg/L})(e^{-(0.124 \text{ h}^{-1})(4 \text{ hr})})$$

$$= (6.6 \text{ mg/L})(0.61)$$

$$= 4 \text{ mg/L}$$

If the absorption time for a sustained-release dosage form is substantially different than 4 hours, t_{in} should be adjusted accordingly. The intermittent infusion model should be used to determine the fluctuations in the concentrations that will occur during the dosing interval when $\tau - t_{in}$ is greater than one-third of the $t_{1/2}$.

Question #7. *G.Y. is a 55-year-old Asian man taking Procanbid 1500 mg orally every 12 hours along with digoxin for his atrial fibrillation. He weighs 70 kg and has an estimated Cl_{Cr} of 30 mL/min. G.Y.'s steady-state procainamide concentration is 5 mg/L. Estimate his plasma NAPA concentration.*

The steady-state NAPA concentration (Css ave) can be determined from Equation 11.3 once the necessary parameters are derived. In this case it can be assumed that S and F are 1.0, since NAPA is produced directly from plasma procainamide. The rate of NAPA production (Dose/τ) can be calculated by multiplying the average steady-state procainamide concentration by the acetylation clearance of procainamide. Assuming G.Y. is phenotypically a rapid acetylator (Asian ethnicity), the clearance to NAPA would be 0.19 L/kg/hr or 13.3 L/hr (0.19 L/kg/hr × 70 kg).

Using this clearance value of 13.3 L/hr and G.Y.'s average procainamide concentration of 5 mg/L, the hourly NAPA production rate is 66.5 mg.

$$\text{Rate of Conversion to NAPA} = \left(\frac{\text{Css ave}}{\text{(Procainamide)}}\right)\left(Cl_{\text{acetylation}}\right) \quad \text{[Eq. 11.16]}$$

$$= (5 \text{ mg/L})(13.3 \text{ L/hr})$$

$$= 66.5 \text{ mg/hr}$$

This approach assumes that the molecular weight of procainamide and NAPA are not substantially different and that each milligram of procainamide converted to NAPA represents a milligram of NAPA. Once the rate of NAPA production (which is essentially the infusion rate of NAPA) and the clearance for NAPA are known, the average steady-state plasma concentration can be calculated from Equation 11.3, in which the rate of conversion to NAPA equals (S)(F)(Dose/τ). If G.Y. has a creatinine clearance of 1.8 L/hr (30 mL/min), his expected NAPA clearance would be 4.63 L/hr as shown below.

$$\text{NAPA } Cl_{\text{total}} = (1.6)(Cl_{Cr} \text{ in L/hr}) + (0.025 \text{ L/kg/hr})(\text{Weight in kg}) \quad \text{[Eq. 11.17]}$$

$$= (1.6)(1.8 \text{ L/hr}) + (0.025 \text{ L/kg/hr})(70 \text{ kg})$$

$$= 2.88 \text{ L/hr} + 1.75 \text{ L/hr}$$

$$= 4.63 \text{ L/hr}$$

For this NAPA clearance, the 2.88 L/hr represents NAPA Cl_{renal} and 1.75 L/hr represents the NAPA $Cl_{\text{metabolic}}$.

Using the NAPA clearance of 4.63 L/hr and the expected rate of conversion to NAPA of 66.5 mg/hr, a steady-state NAPA concentration of 14.4 mg/L can be calculated with Equation 11.3.

$$\text{Css ave} = \frac{(S)(F)(Dose/\tau)}{Cl}$$

$$= \frac{66.5 \text{ mg/hr}}{4.63 \text{ L/hr}}$$

$$= 14.4 \text{ mg/L}$$

Question #8. *What is the clinical significance of plasma NAPA concentrations? How might they alter the clinical use of procainamide and the interpretation of plasma procainamide concentrations?*

Therapeutic plasma concentrations of procainamide were established before it was known that NAPA could be contributing to the therapeutic and, possibly, toxic effects of procainamide. The ratio of NAPA to procainamide concentrations is primarily a function of acetylation phenotype and renal function. Patients with poor renal function who are rapid acetylators will have the highest ratios of NAPA to procainamide concentrations.

Patients with high NAPA to procainamide ratios may experience therapeutic effects even when average or trough concentrations of procainamide are below those usually associated with antiarrhythmic efficacy. The longer half-life of NAPA may also explain why many patients, especially those with renal failure, are well controlled with procainamide at dosing intervals not expected to be effective based on the procainamide half-life. Although the procainamide levels may be fluctuating, the NAPA levels tend to change relatively little, providing antiarrhythmic benefit for the patient.

If NAPA is contributing to the antiarrhythmic effect, the full efficacy of a procainamide dosing regimen cannot be evaluated until NAPA concentrations have reached steady state. In patients with renal failure who have a NAPA half-life of 30 hours or longer, 5 days or more may be required before steady-state NAPA concentrations are achieved and maximal antiarrhythmic effects are observed. A similar situation will be encountered when procainamide is discontinued in patients with poor renal function. Within 24 to 36 hours after discontinuing the drug, procainamide levels will be undetectable. However, one cannot ascertain whether the patient can be maintained without procainamide until several more days have elapsed and NAPA levels have declined substantially.

The ratio of NAPA to procainamide concentrations could be evaluated to establish whether a patient is a rapid or slow acetylator. Since the rate of NAPA production equals the rate of NAPA elimination at steady state, the ratio of the average procainamide concentration to the average

NAPA concentration at steady state should equal the total clearance of NAPA divided by procainamide's clearance by acetylation.

$$\text{Rate of NAPA Production} = \text{Rate of NAPA Elimination}$$

$$\left(\frac{\text{Css ave}}{\text{Procainamide}}\right)\left(\text{Procainamide Cl}_{\text{acetylation}}\right) = \left(\frac{\text{Css ave}}{\text{NAPA}}\right)(\text{NAPA Cl}_{\text{renal}} + \text{NAPA Cl}_{\text{metabolic}})$$

or

$$\frac{\text{Css ave Procainamide}}{\text{Css ave NAPA}} = \frac{\text{NAPA Cl}_{\text{renal}} + \text{NAPA Cl}_{\text{metabolic}}}{\text{Procainamide Cl}_{\text{acetylation}}}$$

This concept was applied to the development of Figure 11.1, which can be used as an aid to estimate whether a patient is a rapid or slow acetylator. To use this graph, measured NAPA and procainamide concentrations must be sampled under steady-state conditions and should approximate average concentrations within the dosing interval. The creatinine clearance is expressed in mL/min for a 70-kg individual; therefore, if a patient's weight varies significantly from 70 kg, the creatinine clearance should be normalized to the 70-kg weight.

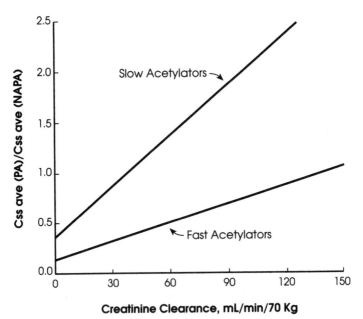

FIGURE 11.1. Graphic representation of the expected procainamide to NAPA ratios at Css ave versus renal function for fast and slow acetylators. This graph was derived using average clearance values for rapid and slow acetylators and by adjusting NAPA clearance to renal function. Ratios of procainamide to NAPA concentrations, which lie between the lines for fast and slow acetylators, would be assigned to the closest adjacent line. Phenotype status is uncertain for patients with procainamide to NAPA concentration ratios that are intermediate.

Question #9. *I.C., a 45-year-old, 100-kg, 5 foot 9 inch man with a serum creatinine of 1.5 mg/dL, has severe CHF and ventricular arrhythmias, which are to be treated with oral procainamide. Recommend a dose of procainamide for this obese patient to achieve an average procainamide concentration of 5 mg/L.*

Because I.C. is obese, one would first estimate his ideal body weight (IBW) using Equation 11.18.

$$\text{Ideal Body Weight for males in kg} = 50 + (2.3)(\text{Height in Inches} > 60) \qquad \text{[Eq. 11.18]}$$

$$= 50 + (2.3)(9)$$

$$= 70.7 \text{ kg}$$

To calculate I.C.'s procainamide clearance, his renal, acetylation, and other clearance values would need to be calculated. One could use Equation 11.20 and calculate his creatinine clearance in mL/kg/min by removing the weight component of Equation 11.19.

$$\frac{\text{Cl}_{cr} \text{ for males}}{\text{(mL/min)}} = \frac{(140 - \text{Age})(\text{Weight})}{(72)(\text{SCr}_{ss})} \qquad \text{[Eq. 11.19]}$$

$$\frac{\text{Cl}_{cr} \text{ for males}}{\text{(mL/kg/min)}} = \frac{(140 - \text{Age})}{(72)(\text{SCr}_{ss})} \qquad \text{[Eq. 11.20]}$$

$$= \frac{(140 - 45)}{(72)(1.5 \text{ mg/dL})}$$

$$= 0.88 \text{ mL/kg/min}$$

$$\frac{\text{Cl}_{cr}}{\text{(L/kg/hr)}} = \left(\frac{\text{Cl}_{cr}}{\text{(mL/kg/min)}}\right)\left(\frac{60 \text{ min/hr}}{1000 \text{ mL/L}}\right)$$

$$= (0.88 \text{ mL/kg/min})\left(\frac{60 \text{ min/hr}}{1000 \text{ mL/L}}\right)$$

$$= 0.0528 \text{ L/kg/hr}$$

Using this creatinine clearance of 0.0528 L/kg/hr, I.C.'s renal clearance of procainamide (based on total body weight in this obese patient[16]) is 15.84 L/hr.

$$\text{Cl}_{renal} = (3)(\text{Cl}_{cr})$$

$$= (3)(0.0528 \text{ L/kg/hr})(100 \text{ kg})$$

$$= 15.84 \text{ L/hr}$$

I.C.'s metabolic clearance can be estimated by using I.C.'s ideal body weight and assuming the average value for $Cl_{acetylation}$ and the standard value for Cl_{other}. Ideal body weight was used here because procainamide's metabolic clearance appears to correlate more closely to non-obese weight.[16]

$$Cl_{acetylation} = (0.13 \text{ L/kg/hr})(\text{Weight in kg})$$

$$= (0.13 \text{ L/kg/hr})(70.7 \text{ kg})$$

$$= 9.19 \text{ L/hr}$$

$$Cl_{other} = (0.1 \text{ L/kg/hr})(\text{Weight in kg})$$

$$= (0.1 \text{ L/kg/hr})(70.7 \text{ kg})$$

$$= 7.07 \text{ L/hr}$$

Combining the three clearance factors, I.C.'s total procainamide clearance can be calculated using Equation 11.6. Because I.C. has CHF, his total clearance (≈ 32 L/hr) should be reduced by approximately 50% to ≈ 16 L/hr.

$$Cl_{total} = Cl_{renal} + Cl_{acetylation} + Cl_{other}$$

$$= 15.84 \text{ L/hr} + 9.19 \text{ L/hr} + 7.07 \text{ L/hr}$$

$$= 32.1 \text{ L/hr}$$

Reducing the total clearance by 0.5 for CHF:

$$= (32.1 \text{ L/hr})(0.5)$$

$$= 16.05 \text{ L/hr}$$

To estimate I.C.'s elimination rate constant and half-life, his V must be calculated. Using ideal body weight[16] and considering that CHF reduces the volume of distribution from about 2 L/kg to 1.5 L/kg, I.C.'s half-life (using Equation 11.1) is estimated to be ≈ 4.5 hours.

$$V = (1.5 \text{ L/kg})(70.7 \text{ kg})$$

$$= 106 \text{ L}$$

$$t_{1/2} = \frac{(0.693)(V)}{Cl}$$

$$= \frac{(0.693)(106 \text{ L})}{16 \text{ L/hr}}$$

$$= 4.59 \text{ hr}$$

Using Equation 11.7, a maintenance dose of approximately 650 mg every 6 hours is calculated.

$$\text{Maintenance Dose} = \frac{(Cl)(Css\ ave)(\tau)}{(S)(F)}$$

$$= \frac{(16\ L/hr)(5\ mg/L)(6\ hr)}{(0.87)(0.85)}$$

$$= 649\ mg\ (every\ 6\ hours)$$

Assuming I.C.'s procainamide is to be given as a sustained-release drug product, one could choose to administer either 500 or 750 mg every 6 hours. Using Equation 11.3, average steady-state concentrations of approximately 3.9 and 5.8 mg/L can be calculated for each of these doses, respectively.

$$Css\ ave = \frac{(S)(F)(Dose/\tau)}{Cl}$$

$$= \frac{(0.87)(0.85)(500\ mg/6\ hr)}{16\ L/hr}$$

$$= 3.85\ mg/L$$

or

$$= \frac{(0.87)(0.85)(750\ mg/6\ hr)}{16\ L/hr}$$

$$= 5.8\ mg/L$$

Procanbid extended-release tablets could also have been used. With Procanbid, Equation 11.7 would have predicted a maintenance dose of approximately 1300 mg every 12 hours:

$$\text{Maintenance Dose} = \frac{(Cl)(Css\ ave)(\tau)}{(S)(F)}$$

$$= \frac{(16\ L/hr)(5\ mg/L)(12\ hr)}{(0.87)(0.85)}$$

$$= 1298\ mg\ (every\ 12\ hours)$$

In this example either Procanbid extended-release 1000 mg or 1500 mg every 12 hours could be suggested. Because the dosing rate (Dose/τ) is the same for the Procanbid extended-release 1000 mg every 12 hours as for the procainamide sustained-release 500 mg every 6 hours, the Css ave would be $\approx$3.9 mg/L (using Equation 11.3). The same is true for Procanbid extended-release tablets of 1500 mg every 12 hours and procainamide sustained-release 750 mg every 6 hours (expecting Css ave of $\approx$5.8 mg/L using Equation 11.3).

Because of the uncertainty in initial parameter estimates, I.C. should be observed carefully for both lack of efficacy and procainamide toxicity. Although the clinical outcome is clearly the therapeutic goal, plasma concentrations may help to determine the optimal dose for I.C. that will control his arrhythmia while minimizing the possibility of adverse effects.

REFERENCES

1. Flanagan AD. Pharmacokinetics of a sustained release procainamide preparation. Angiology 1982;33:71–77.
2. Smith TC, Kinkel AW. Plasma levels of procainamide after administration of conventional and sustained-release preparations. Curr Ther Res 1980;27:217.
3. Vlasses PH, et al. Immediate release and sustained-release procainamide: bioavailability at steady-state in cardiac patients. Ann Intern Med 1983;89:613.
4. Yang BB, et al. Pharmacokinetic and pharmacodynamic comparisons of twice daily and four times daily formulations of procainamide in patients with frequent ventricular premature depolarization. J Clin Pharmacol 1996;36:623–633.
5. Koch-Weser J. Pharmacokinetics of procainamide in man. Ann NY Acad Sci 1971;169:370.
6. Koch-Weser J, Klein SW. Procainamide dosage schedules, plasma concentrations and clinical effects. JAMA 1971;215:1454.
7. Woosley RL, et al. Effect of acetylator phenotype on the rate at which procainamide induces antinuclear antibodies and the lupus syndrome. N Engl J Med 1978;298:1157.
8. Engel TR, et al. Modification of ventricular tachycardia by procainamide in patients with coronary artery disease. Am J Cardiol 1980;46:1033.
9. Giardina EV, et al. Efficacy, plasma concentrations and adverse effects of a new sustained release procainamide preparation. Am J Cardiol 1980;46:855.
10. Greenspan AM, et al. Large dose procainamide therapy for ventricular tachyarrhythmia. Am J Cardiol 1980;46:453.
11. Manion CV, et al. Absorption kinetics of procainamide in humans. J Pharm Sci 1977;66:981.
12. Hilleman DE, et al. Comparative bioequivalence and efficacy of two sustained-release procainamide formulations in patients with cardiac arrhythmias. Drug Intell Clin Pharm 1988;22:554–558.
13. Reiffel JA. Issues in the use of generic antiarrhythmic drugs. Curr Opin Cardiol 2001;16:23–29.
14. Job ML, et al. Carcass of a pill: no cause for alarm. N Engl J Med 1981;305:231.
15. Gibson TP, et al. Kinetics of procainamide and N-acetylprocainamide in renal failure. Kidney Int 1977;12:422.
16. Christoff PV, et al. Procainamide disposition in obesity. Drug Intell Clin Pharm 1983;17:516.
17. Galeazzi RL, et al. Relationship between the pharmacokinetics and pharmacodynamics of procainamide. Clin Pharmacol Ther 1976;20:278.
18. Lima JJ, et al. Pharmacokinetic approach to intravenous procainamide therapy. Eur J Clin Pharmacol 1978;13:303.
19. Lima JJ, et al. Clinical pharmacokinetics of procainamide infusions in relation to acetylator phenotype. J Pharmacokinet Biopharm 1979;7:69.

20. Bauer LA, Black D, Gensler A. Procainamide-cimetidine drug interaction in elderly male patients. J Am Geriatr Soc 1990;38:467–469.

21. Rodvold KA, et al. Interaction of steady-state procainamide with H2-receptor antagonists cimetidine and ranitidine. Ther Drug Monit 1987;9:378–383.

22. Rocci ML Jr, et al. Ranitidine-induced changes in the renal and hepatic clearances of procainamide are correlated. J Pharmacol Exp Ther 1989;248:923–928.

23. Martin DE, et al. Effects of ofloxacin on the pharmacokinetics and pharmacodynamics of procainamide. J Clin Pharmacol 1996;36:85–91.

24. Vlasses PH, et al. Trimethoprim inhibition of the renal clearance of procainamide and N-acetylprocainamide. Arch Intern Med 1989;149:1350–1353.

25. Windle J, et al. Pharmacokinetic and electrophysiologic interactions of amiodarone and procainamide. Clin Pharmacol Ther 1987;41:603–610.

26. Marchlinski FE, et al. Comparison of individual and combined effects of procainamide and amiodarone in patients with sustained ventricular tachyarrhythmias. Circulation 1988;78:583–591.

27. Elson J, et al. Antiarrhythmic potency on N-acetylprocainamide. Clin Pharmacol Ther 1975;17:134.

28. Bagwell EE, et al. Correlation of the electrophysiological and antiarrhythmic properties of the N-acetyl metabolite of procainamide with plasma and tissue drug concentration in the dog. J Pharmacol Exp Ther 1976;197:38.

29. Drayer DE, et al. N-acetylprocainamide: an active metabolite of procainamide. Proc Soc Exp Biol Med 1974;146:358.

30. Lee WK, et al. Antiarrhythmic efficacy of N-acetylprocainamide in patients with premature ventricular contractions. Clin Pharmacol Ther 1976;19:508.

31. Atkinson AJ Jr, et al. Dose ranging trial of N-acetylprocainamide in patients with premature ventricular contractions. Clin Pharmacol Ther 1977;21:575.

32. Karlsson E, et al. Acetylation of procainamide in man studied with a new gas chromatographic method. Br J Pharmacol 1974;1:467.

33. Reidenburg MM, et al. Polymorphic acetylation of procainamide in man. Clin Pharmacol Ther 1975;17:722.

34. Vlasses PH, et al. Lethal accumulations of procainamide metabolite in renal insufficiency [Abstract]. Drug Intell Clin Pharm 1984;18:493.

35. Bottorff MB, et al. High-dose procainamide in chronic renal failure. Drug Intell Clin Pharm 1983;17:279.

36. Gibson TP. Acetylation of procainamide in man and its relationship to isonicotinic acid-hydrazide acetylation phenotype. Clin Pharmacol Ther 1975;17:395.

37. Strong JM, et al. Pharmacokinetics in man of the N-acetylated metabolite of procainamide. J Pharmacokinet Biopharm 1975;3:223.

38. Strong JM, et al. Absolute bioavailability in man of N-acetylprocainamide determined by a novel stable isotope method. Clin Pharmacol Ther 1975;18:613.

39. Valdes R Jr, Jortani SA, Gheorghiade M. Standards of laboratory practice: cardiac drug monitoring. Clin Chem 1998;44:1096–1109.

40. Giardina EV, Heissenbuttel RH. Intermittent intravenous procainamide to treat ventricular arrhythmias. Ann Intern Med 1973;78:183.

12

THEOPHYLLINE

Amir Aminimanizani and Michael E. Winter

Theophylline is a bronchial smooth muscle relaxant and is widely used to treat bronchial asthma and other respiratory diseases. Although theophylline is currently relegated to a third-line agent in the treatment of asthma, knowledge of its pharmacokinetics can help to ensure that the drug is used safely in those patients in whom its use is appropriate. Theophylline is poorly soluble in water (about 1%) and in the past was usually administered intravenously as the more soluble ethylenediamine salt of theophylline, aminophylline. Currently, dilute solutions of theophylline in concentrations ranging from 0.4 to 4 mg/mL are more commonly used for intravenous (IV) administration. There are numerous oral preparations of theophylline, aminophylline, and other theophylline salts. In addition, aminophylline and other theophylline salts are sometimes administered rectally as suppositories. Following rectal administration, theophylline is absorbed slowly and erratically.

Doses vary widely and should be based on pharmacokinetic considerations and plasma theophylline concentrations. Aminophylline is the most widely used salt of theophylline. An aminophylline loading dose of 300 to 500 mg for an average 70-kg patient (5 to 6 mg/kg) usually is administered by slow IV injection. Typically, the loading dose is followed by IV aminophylline infused at a rate of approximately 30 to 50 mg/hr (0.5 mg/kg/hr). The usual oral maintenance dose of theophylline non–sustained-release dosage forms is 200 to 300 mg 3 to 4 times a day or 200 to 400 mg twice daily for sustained release products.

THERAPEUTIC AND TOXIC PLASMA CONCENTRATIONS

The historic therapeutic plasma concentration range for theophylline is 10 to 20 mg/L[1-3]; however, improvement in respiratory function can be observed with plasma concentrations as low as 5 mg/L.[1] For this reason most clinicians target theophylline concentrations of approximately 10 mg/L or lower. In addition, desired levels will vary depending on the disease state in question. For use in chronic obstructive pulmonary disease (COPD), serum theophylline concentrations ranging from 8 to 15 mg/L have been shown to improve pulmonary symptoms while minimizing serious adverse effects.[4,5] Treatment for children with apnea of prematurity (AOP) requires theophylline concentrations of at least 5 mg/L, with 10 mg/L generally accepted as therapeutic.[6,7]

Nausea and vomiting are the most common side effects of theophylline. Although these effects can occur at concentrations as low as 13 to 15 mg/L, they are observed more frequently at plasma concentrations exceeding 20 mg/L.[3,8] Cardiac symptoms such as tachycardia are usually minor within the therapeutic range[9]; premature atrial and ventricular contractions are less predictable but are usually associated with theophylline levels exceeding 40 mg/L.[10] Insomnia and nervousness are side effects that occur over a wide range of concentrations. More severe central nervous system (CNS) manifestations such as seizures usually occur at plasma concentrations exceeding 50 mg/L[10,11] but have been observed in patients with theophylline concentrations less than 30 mg/L.[11,12]

Side effects such as nausea and vomiting that usually occur at lower plasma concentrations cannot be used as reliable indicators of excessive theophylline concentrations. These less severe toxic effects are not always observed, even at high plasma concentrations. In a series of eight patients who suffered from theophylline-induced seizures, only one patient had premonitory signs such as nausea, vomiting, tachycardia, or nervousness which were recognized as signs of toxicity.[11]

The bronchodilating effects of theophylline are proportional to the log of the theophylline concentration. This means that as the theophylline concentration increases, there will be a less than proportional increase in bronchodilation.[10] For this reason, many patients with theophylline concentrations greater than 20 mg/L will experience about the same thera-

KEY PARAMETERS	
Therapeutic Plasma Concentration[a]	5–20 mg/L
F	100%
S[b]	See Table 12.1
V[c]	0.5 L/kg
Cl[d]	0.04 L/kg/hr
t½	8 hours

[a]Usual target concentrations are approximately 10 mg/L.
[b]See Table 12.1
[c]The use of total body versus ideal body weight in obese patients is uncertain. See
    Theophylline Volume of Distribution (V) and Half-life (t½) sections.
[d]See Tables 12.2 and 12.3 and Theophylline Clearance (Cl) section.

peutic benefit as that associated with concentrations less than 20 mg/L. The patients with higher concentrations, however, will be at much higher risk for theophylline toxicity. Patients should always be maintained at the lowest possible theophylline plasma concentration that produces a satisfactory therapeutic endpoint. Given the limited bronchodilating effects of theophylline and its potential for toxicity , most clinicians choose an initial target concentration of ≈10 mg/L. Many patients, however, have their conditions well controlled with theophylline concentrations in the range of 5 to 10 mg/L and do not require dose adjustments of their theophylline therapy. To optimize the bronchodilating effects of theophylline in acute asthma attacks, it is almost always used in conjunction with inhaled beta-antagonists, which generally produce more rapid and significant bronchodilating effects than theophylline.

BIOAVAILABILITY (F)

Nonsustained-Release Dosage Forms

The absorption of theophylline and theophylline derivatives, when administered as either liquid or nonsustained-release oral dosage forms, appears to be rapid and complete. Plasma theophylline concentrations peak about 1 to 2 hours after oral administration.[13] Selection of these oral theophylline dosage forms that do not have sustained-release characteristics should be based primarily on cost and convenience if the quality of product can be assured. Theophylline products are available in a large number of salt forms, examples of which are listed in Table 12.1. When changing from one theophylline salt to another, care should be taken to administer an equivalent theophylline dose.

Sustained-Release (SR) Dosage Forms

A large number of sustained-release dosage forms of theophylline have been marketed. These products are designed to release theophylline slowly so that patients who metabolize the drug rapidly (e.g., children and smokers) can maintain theophylline plasma concentrations within the therapeutic range when usual dosing intervals of 6 to 12 hours are used. Most of these drug products are completely absorbed[13,14]; however, there are major differences between these products with regard to duration of absorption. Some of these dosage forms are absorbed over 3 to 4 hours, whereas others appear to be absorbed over 8 to 12 hours.[13,14] For those products that have a longer duration of absorption, administration every 8 to 12 hours is usually acceptable. Nevertheless, as the duration of absorption increases, the possibility of incomplete bioavailability increases because the duration of absorption begins to exceed the gastrointestinal transit time.[13]

Dosage forms that can be administered once daily are available; however, the need for these has been questioned.[15,16] The primary concern with

TABLE 12.1 **Selected Theophylline Dosage Forms and Their Salt Factors**

Dosage Form	S
Non–sustained-release	
Aminophylline (generic)	0.8–0.84
Elixophyllin (generic)	1
Slo-Phyllin	1
Theophylline (generic)	1
Coated and sustained-release	
Choledyl SA	0.64
Respbid	1
Slo-bid Gyrocaps	1
Theo-24	1
Theobid Duracaps	1
Theolair-SR	1
Uni-Dur	1
Uniphyl	1

S = Fraction of labeled dose which is theophylline.

the once daily dosing products is the rate and extent of absorption. For example, there is evidence that concurrent administration of Theo-24 with a high-fat meal can accelerate its absorption and thereby produce a "dose-dumping" effect.[17] Although no "dose dumping" was observed after the ingestion of Uniphyl with a high-fat meal, a change in the rate of absorption was apparent.[18]

    In addition to the problems associated with the once daily dosage forms, the variability in absorption among products designed to be administered every 6 to 12 hours may be greater than originally suspected.[19] Most clinicians are reluctant to use once daily products because of the possibility that absorption may be variable.

VOLUME OF DISTRIBUTION (V)

The volume of distribution for theophylline is $\approx$0.5 L/kg,[10,20,21] and distribution follows a two-compartment model [see Part I: Volume of Distribution (V)]. The bronchioles behave as though they are located in the second or tissue compartment; however, toxic effects are associated with high concentrations in the initial volume of distribution. Therefore, theophylline toxicity may be experienced when theophylline is administered too rapidly or when theophylline accumulates in the first compartment.

The volume of distribution in premature newborns is $\approx$0.7 L/kg.[22] After 1 year of age, however, the volume of distribution is $\approx$0.5 L/kg.[23,24] The volume of distribution for theophylline is increased to $\approx$0.6 L/kg in patients with cystic fibrosis.[25,26]

The volume of distribution for theophylline in obese subjects is somewhat controversial. The Food and Drug Administration (FDA) and one author recommend that the ideal or non-obese weight be used to calculate the loading dose or volume of distribution,[27,28] whereas others have suggested that the use of total body weight may be more appropriate.[29,30] Because the disposition of theophylline in obese subjects is uncertain, the non-obese or ideal body weight should be used when calculating theophylline loading doses. This may result in a smaller volume of distribution and a conservative loading dose. This approach may not be appropriate when calculating theophylline half-lives [see Theophylline Half-Life $(t\frac{1}{2})$]. The primary concern here is that if the true volume of distribution is larger than calculated using ideal body weight, the true $t\frac{1}{2}$ will be longer than calculated. This error may lead to incorrect assumptions about the time required to achieve steady state.

CLEARANCE (Cl)

The average theophylline clearance is 0.04 L/kg/hr, based on lean or ideal body weight.[10,27,30,31] A number of clinical factors influence theophylline clearance (Table 12.2).

TABLE 12.2 **Disease States That Affect Theophylline Clearance**

Disease	Factor[a]	References
Smoking history	1.6	20, 34
Congestive heart failure	0.5[b]	20, 35, 36
Cystic fibrosis	1.5	25, 26, 57
Acute pulmonary edema	0.5	37
Acute viral illness	0.5	58
Hepatic cirrhosis	0.5	38
Severe obstructive pulmonary disease	0.8	20
Obesity	IBW[c]	29

[a]Indicates the estimate for clearance adjustments. The product of all the factors which are present (also see Table 12.3) should be multiplied by the average clearance value (0.04 L/kg/hr). Multiple factors increase the uncertainty in clearance prediction.
[b]The effect of CHF on theophylline clearance is variable depending on the severity of the cardiac failure.
[c]IBW = ideal body weight should be used.

Obesity

Obese subjects have a theophylline clearance that is most accurately estimated by using non-obese weight.[27,29,30,32] As a general guideline, the ideal body weight can be estimated using previously discussed equations [see Part I: Creatinine Clearance (Cl_{Cr}): Estimating Creatinine Clearance from Steady-State Serum Creatinine Concentrations: Adjusting to Body Size and Weight].

Smoking

Cigarette smokers have a theophylline clearance about 1.5 to 2 times that of non-smokers.[20,33,34] The effects of smoking (one pack of cigarettes per day) appear to last several months after the cigarettes have been discontinued.[34] Therefore, patients admitted to the hospital with a recent history of smoking should be considered smokers throughout their hospitalization even if they refrain from smoking during hospitalization.

Diseases

Congestive heart failure (CHF), in contrast to cigarette smoking, reduces theophylline clearance to about 50% of normal.[20,31,35,36] Pulmonary edema has also been reported to reduce theophylline clearance,[37] although this effect may be secondary to the associated CHF. Severe pulmonary disease reduces theophylline clearance to approximately 80% of the average value.[20] Hepatic cirrhosis also can significantly reduce theophylline clearance.[20,38] Premature newborns have a theophylline clearance that is very low even when adjusted for weight or body surface area.[39]

Diet

Diet also influences the metabolism of theophylline. Patients ingesting high-protein, low-carbohydrate diets generally metabolize theophylline more rapidly, presumably because the diet induces hepatic enzymes.[40] Dietary intake of other methylxanthines, such as caffeine, can decrease the rate of theophylline metabolism to a limited extent.[41] Although the effects of diet have been well documented, they usually produce relatively minor changes in theophylline therapy if the patient's diet remains reasonably consistent.

Drug Interactions

Many drug interactions with theophylline have been documented,[31,42] but only the most common of these will be presented here (Table 12.3). Macrolide antibiotics, such as triacetyloleandomycin and erythromycin, reduce theophylline clearance by as much as 25% to 50%;[42-44] however, the interaction with erythromycin has been disputed.[44] Ciprofloxacin has been shown to reduce theophylline clearance by as much as 30%.[45] Unlike ciprofloxacin, the newer fluoroquinolones (levofloxacin, gatifloxacin, and moxifloxacin) show negligible or no effect on theophylline metabolism.[46-48]

Phenobarbital increases theophylline metabolism in some individuals by as much as 30%,[49] but this induction of theophylline metabolism has not been observed by all investigators.[50] Phenytoin (Dilantin) increases theophylline clearance by a factor of ≈ 1.6.[42]

Cimetidine (Tagamet) appears to reduce theophylline metabolism by about 40%. In these patients, the theophylline clearance should be multiplied by 0.6.[42] Similar effects on theophylline clearance were not observed when ranitidine (Zantac) was administered at doses 10 times greater than those generally prescribed.[51] In addition, no significant drug interactions were observed when famotidine (Pepcid) was administered to COPD patients receiving theophylline.[52] Rifampin can increase theophylline metabolism; however, the increase in clearance is only about 20% to 25%.[42] Intravenous isoproterenol (Isuprel) has also been shown to increase the clearance of theophylline by about 20%.[53] Unfortunately, the predictability of clearance changes secondary to the addition of these drugs is poor, indicating that while some change may be expected, patients need to be evaluated individually. This concept applies to disease states as well.

When multiple factors influencing theophylline clearance are present, the prediction of theophylline drug levels is uncertain; therefore, plasma levels should be monitored.

HALF -LIFE (t½)

The usual theophylline half-life in adult patients is approximately 8 hours; however, it is quite variable. For example, the theophylline half-life can be as short as 3 to 4 hours in patients who smoke or in those receiving drugs known to induce theophylline metabolism. In contrast, the theophylline

TABLE 12.3 **Selected Drugs That Affect Theophylline Clearance**

Drug	Factor[a]
Cimetidine	0.6
Ciprofloxacin	0.7
Erythromycin	0.75
Influenza vaccine	0.5
Phenobarbital	1.3
Phenytoin	1.6
Propranolol	0.6
Rifampin	1.3

[a]Adapted from references 32, 60–63. The product of all factors that are present (also see Table 12.2) should be multiplied by the average clearance value (0.04 L/kg/hr). Multiple factors increase the uncertainty in clearance prediction.

half-life can be as long as 18 to 24 hours in patients with severe CHF or in those receiving drugs that inhibit theophylline metabolism.

The theophylline half-life in obese subjects is frequently longer than 8 hours. When attempting to estimate whether steady state has been achieved in obese subjects, it may be wise to use total body weight instead of ideal body weight in calculating the volume of distribution. This will ensure that the longest possible half-life is being used.

TIME TO SAMPLE

Because the average theophylline half-life is approximately 8 hours, routine monitoring of theophylline plasma concentrations can usually begin approximately 24 hours after the initiation of therapy or a change in the maintenance regimen. Plasma samples obtained earlier, especially those obtained within the first 18 hours of therapy, should be interpreted cautiously because steady state may not have been achieved. Patients admitted to acute care centers frequently have been taking sustained-release theophylline products as outpatients. For these individuals, plasma samples obtained within the first 12 to 24 hours after admission may represent an unknown rate of theophylline absorption from doses taken before admission.

In patients receiving nonsustained-release or liquid dosage forms of theophylline, routine monitoring of theophylline plasma concentrations is probably most reliable when trough levels are obtained. Some patients may have relatively short theophylline half-lives; peak theophylline plasma concentrations should be estimated by adding the increase in theophylline concentration expected from a single dose to the trough concentration, as in Equation 12.1:

$$\text{Css max} = [\text{Css min}] + \left[\frac{(S)(F)(\text{Dose})}{V} \right] \qquad [\text{Eq. 12.1}]$$

This equation is only applicable to rapidly absorbed dosage forms, because the change in concentration following the administration of a sustained-release theophylline product is much less than the value calculated by Equation 12.1. In patients receiving sustained-release theophylline products, the time of sampling is less critical. Whereas trough concentrations are recommended, samples obtained at the midpoint of the dosing interval may also be acceptable.

Question #1. *K.M., who is receiving a theophylline infusion, has a plasma theophylline concentration of 30 mg/L. If the theophylline infusion rate is decreased to one-third, so that the new plasma theophylline concentration is 10 mg/L, will the pharmacologic (bronchodilating) effect also be reduced to one-third?*

No. The bronchodilating effect of theophylline is proportional to the log of the theophylline concentration.[1] A 67% reduction in the plasma theophylline concentration in K.M. may be well tolerated, since the bronchodilating effect will be decreased by much less than 67%. Before any alteration in the theophylline plasma concentration is considered, the clinical status of the patient must be assessed. In some cases, a change in dosage may have serious consequences: toxicity may appear if an increase in plasma concentration is attempted, or bronchospasm may be exacerbated if the concentration is reduced. However, based on the assumption that the theophylline concentration is not an error, almost all clinicians would want to reduce the theophylline concentration to less than 20 mg/L, if not to 10 mg/L.

Question #2. *R.J., an 80-kg, 50-year-old man, is seen in the emergency department with asthma that is unresponsive to epinephrine. Estimate a loading dose of aminophylline that will produce a plasma theophylline concentration of 10 mg/L.*

Assuming R.J. has received no recent aminophylline doses, Equation 12.2 can be used to determine the loading dose:

$$\text{Loading Dose} = \frac{(V)(C)}{(S)(F)} \qquad \text{[Eq. 12.2]}$$

The salt form (S) of aminophylline is either 0.80 or 0.84 depending on whether the hydrous (0.80) or anhydrous (0.84) form was used to compound the drug product. The usual volume of distribution for theophylline is approximately 0.4 to 0.5 L/kg.[3,20,21] If 0.5 L/kg is used,[20] R.J.'s volume of distribution is 40 L.

$$\text{Theophylline V(L)} = (0.5 \text{ L/kg})(\text{Weight})$$
$$= (0.5 \text{ L/kg})(80 \text{ kg})$$
$$= 40 \text{ L}$$

The calculated loading dose of aminophylline would be 500 mg.

$$\text{Loading Dose} = \frac{(V)(C)}{(S)(F)}$$
$$= \frac{(40 \text{ L})(10 \text{ mg/L})}{(0.8)(1)}$$
$$= \frac{400 \text{ mg}}{0.8}$$
$$= 500 \text{ mg}$$

This aminophylline dose is within the usual 300 to 500 mg loading dose range and is consistent with standard values of 5 to 6 mg/kg that are used clinically. If a target concentration greater than or less than 10 mg/L was the goal, correspondingly larger or smaller doses would have been calculated. In most clinical situations, loading doses larger than 500 mg would not be administered regardless of the patient size or the pharmacokinetic calculations performed.

Question #3. *What would be a reasonable loading dose for R.J. if he is obese and has an estimated ideal body weight of 60 kg?*

The Food and Drug Administration (FDA) recommends that ideal body weight be used to calculate the loading dose.[27] Others have argued that the volume of distribution (which is the major determinant of loading dose) correlates best with total body weight rather than lean or ideal body weight.[29,30] Because there is uncertainty with regard to the relationship between ideal or total body weight and the apparent volume of distribution for theophylline, some care should be taken when calculating loading doses for obese patients. In general, it is sufficient to calculate a theophylline loading dose that will produce a theophylline concentration below the usual target level of 10 mg/L. This should not be a problem as long as a theophylline concentration of at least 5 mg/L is achieved. If a target level > 10 mg/L is desired, one should ensure that the upper end of the therapeutic range (20 mg/L) is not exceeded.

For obese patients whose ideal body weight is less than one-half their total body weight, the calculated loading dose of theophylline will be substantially different when the calculation is based on ideal body weight. In these individuals, it may be more appropriate to use a value somewhere between the ideal and total body weights to calculate the volume of distribution. In any case, theophylline plasma concentrations should be monitored and the loading dose limited to no more than 500 mg. A theophylline level taken approximately 1 to 2 hours after the initial loading dose will help establish the approximate volume of distribution for obese subjects.

Question #4. What factors will influence the theophylline loading dose?

A major factor (other than obesity) known to influence the loading dose of theophylline is the presence of theophylline in the plasma. The preexisting theophylline concentration can be accounted for in the calculation of a theophylline loading dose by use of Equation 12.3:

$$\text{Incremental Loading Dose} = \frac{(V)(C_{desired} - C_{initial})}{(S)(F)} \quad \text{[Eq. 12.3]}$$

Because STAT theophylline levels are not widely available, it is common clinical practice to obtain a plasma sample and administer an empiric loading dose of 3 mg/kg of aminophylline (2.5 mg/kg of theophylline) if the patient has taken theophylline within the past 12 to 24 hours but is not believed to have taken the drug on a regular basis. This reduced (one-half) loading dose increases the plasma theophylline concentration by about 5 mg/L, which will produce some bronchodilation if the initial plasma theophylline concentration is zero. It is hoped that this increment of 5 mg/L will not result in toxicity if the patient's initial theophylline concentration is elevated.

If the patient is believed to have been compliant with the outpatient theophylline dosing regimen, the loading dose should be omitted and the patient should be started on a maintenance regimen. Care should be taken, however, to obtain an accurate outpatient medication history because many patients receiving sustained-release theophylline products will continue to absorb the drug for 8 to 24 hours after admission. This will depend on the time of the last outpatient dose and the type of product prescribed.

Question #5. *How rapidly should the aminophylline/theophylline loading dose be administered if it is given intravenously?*

Theophylline displays two-compartment pharmacokinetics in which the therapeutic or bronchodilating effects correlate more closely with concentrations in the second or tissue compartment.[54] Since the toxic effects of theophylline correlate with high concentrations in the initial volume of distribution, the loading dose is usually infused over 30 minutes to minimize accumulation within the first compartment and to avoid toxicity.[1,21,54]

Question #6. *R.J., the patient described in Question #2, received the 500 mg loading dose of aminophylline; a theophylline plasma concentration of 10 mg/L was achieved. What aminophylline infusion rate will maintain an average steady-state level of 10 mg/L?*

Because this problem involves a constant infusion that will be given to maintain a steady-state plasma concentration, Equation 12.4 can be used:

$$\text{Maintenance Dose} = \frac{(Cl)(Css\ ave)(\tau)}{(S)(F)} \qquad [\text{Eq. 12.4}]$$

Using an average theophylline clearance of 0.04 L/kg/hr (3.2 L/hr for R.J. who weighs 80 kg),[20] a salt factor (S) of 0.8, and a bioavailability (F) of 100% (F = 1), the maintenance infusion rate would be 40 mg/hr of aminophylline based on the following calculation:

$$\begin{aligned}
\text{Maintenance Dose} &= \frac{(Cl)(Css\ ave)(\tau)}{(S)(F)} \\[6pt]
&= \frac{(3.2\ \text{L/hr})(10\ \text{mg/L})(1\ \text{hr})}{(0.8)(1)} \\[6pt]
&= \frac{32\ \text{mg}}{0.8} \\[6pt]
&= 40\ \text{mg of aminophylline per hour}
\end{aligned}$$

Question #7. *Calculate a maintenance dose for R.J. if he had been an obese individual with a total body weight of 80 kg and an ideal body weight of 60 kg.*

The clearance of theophylline appears to correlate best with ideal body weight in obese patients.[27,29,30] If R.J.'s ideal body weight is 60 kg, the assumed clearance would be 2.4 L/hr (0.04 L/kg/hr × 60 kg) and the maintenance dose would be 30 mg/hr of aminophylline according to the calculations below.

$$\text{Maintenance Dose} = \frac{(Cl)(Css\ ave)(\tau)}{(S)(F)}$$

$$= \frac{(2.4\ \text{L/hr})(10\ \text{mg/L})(1\ \text{hr})}{(0.8)(1)}$$

$$= \frac{24\ \text{mg}}{0.8}$$

$$= 30\ \text{mg of aminophylline per hour}$$

Question #8. *Assume that R.J. (80 kg non-obese weight) has severe obstructive pulmonary disease, CHF, and smokes more than 1 pack of cigarettes per day. Calculate a maintenance dose of aminophylline that will maintain the average steady-state theophylline plasma concentration at 10 mg/L.*

If none of the factors known to alter theophylline clearance were present, R.J.'s expected theophylline clearance would be 3.2 L/hr (0.04 L/kg/hr × 80 kg). However, smoking, severe obstructive pulmonary disease, and CHF alter theophylline clearance by factors of 1.6, 0.8, and 0.5, respectively (see Table 12.2). The product of these factors is 0.64.

$$(1.6)(0.8)(0.5) = 0.64$$

The average theophylline clearance value should be multiplied by this factor of 0.64 to estimate R.J.'s theophylline clearance.

$$(3.2\ \text{L/hr})(0.64) = 2\ \text{L/hr}$$

This clearance could then be used in Equation 12.4 (see below) to calculate a maintenance dose of 25 mg/hr of aminophylline.

$$\text{Maintenance Dose} = \frac{(Cl)(Css\ ave)(\tau)}{(S)(F)}$$

$$= \frac{(2\ \text{L/hr})(10\ \text{mg/L})(1\ \text{hr})}{(0.8)(1)}$$

$$= \frac{20\ \text{mg}}{0.8}$$

$$= 25\ \text{mg of aminophylline per hour}$$

When multiple factors are known to alter theophylline clearance in a patient, the ability to accurately predict theophylline clearance diminishes. In these situations, initial doses may be adjusted based on literature estimates; however, theophylline plasma concentrations should be monitored to ensure that the patient does not develop excessive or subtherapeutic theophylline plasma concentrations. Even though R.J. will probably discontinue smoking during the acute exacerbation of his respiratory disease, the smoking factor should still be used when estimating theophylline clearance. Most clinicians assume the induction of theophylline metabolism continues for at least 3 months and perhaps for as long as 1 year after a patient has stopped smoking.

Question #9. *Approximate R.J.'s theophylline half-life, assuming the clearance is 2 L/hr (as calculated in Question #8) and the volume of distribution is 40 L (as calculated in Question #2).*

The half-life is a function of clearance and volume of distribution and can be calculated using Equation 12.5 as shown below.

$$t_{1/2} = \frac{(0.693)(V)}{Cl} \qquad \text{[Eq. 12.5]}$$

$$= \frac{(0.693)(40 \text{ L})}{2 \text{ L/hr}}$$

$$= \frac{27.7 \text{ L}}{2 \text{ L/hr}}$$

$$= 13.85 \text{ hr}$$

This half-life is considerably longer than the average value of 6 to 10 hours because R.J. has multiple factors that are known to alter, in this case reduce, theophylline clearance.

Question #10. *How long should the aminophylline infusion be continued before a plasma sample is obtained to monitor the plasma theophylline concentration for R.J.?*

The earliest time to sample plasma for a theophylline concentration is usually 14 to 20 hours after starting the maintenance infusion (approximately 2 times the usual half-life). Although the expected theophylline half-life for R.J. is approximately 14 hours, obtaining a sample early minimizes the time during which plasma concentrations are low (if the clearance is greater than expected) and prevents excessive accumulation (if the clearance is less than expected). Plasma theophylline concentrations obtained within 2 half-lives cannot be reliably used to calculate R.J.'s clearance or to predict the steady-state concentration. This is because the revised clearance and therefore the projected steady-state concentration is very sensitive to small errors in the assayed drug concentration and/or volume of distribution estimates.

If the theophylline concentration at 14 to 20 hours is significantly higher than expected (clearance is less than expected), the infusion rate should be reduced at that time. A second plasma concentration should then be obtained the following day to reevaluate R.J.'s clearance and predicted steady-state concentration.

If the theophylline concentration is much lower than expected, then an incremental loading dose might be calculated to increase the concentration from the observed level to a desired concentration by use of Equation 12.3.

$$\text{Incremental Loading Dose} = \frac{(V)(C_{desired} - C_{initial})}{(S)(F)}$$

Increasing the infusion rate at this time should be undertaken with extreme caution because the low theophylline concentrations may be due in part to a larger than expected volume of distribution rather than a higher than expected clearance.

Question #11. *M.K., a 58-year-old, 60-kg woman, was admitted to the hospital in status asthmaticus. She received an IV aminophylline loading dose of 375 mg at 9:00 p.m., followed by a constant aminophylline infusion of 60 mg/hr. The next morning at 7:00 a.m. (10 hours after the bolus and initiation of the infusion), a plasma sample was obtained and the reported theophylline concentration was 18 mg/L. Calculate the apparent clearance and half-life of theophylline in M.K.*

The reported plasma concentration of 18 mg/L probably does not represent a steady-state concentration because the sample was obtained only 10 hours after the infusion was begun. The plasma concentration-versus-time curve (which describes a bolus followed by a constant infusion) and the plasma concentration (which is produced by this mode of administration) are depicted in Part I: Selecting the Appropriate Equation: Loading Dose Followed by Infusion.

The reported plasma concentration of 18 mg/L is the sum of the plasma concentration produced by the loading dose (Equation 12.6) and that produced by the infusion (Equation 12.7):

Loading Dose and Decay Equation:

$$C_{t_1} = \left[\frac{(S)(F)(\text{Loading Dose})}{V} (e^{-Kt_1}) \right] \qquad \text{[Eq. 12.6]}$$

Nonsteady-State Infusion Equation:

$$C_{t_1} = \left[\frac{(S)(F)(Dose/\tau)}{Cl} (1 - e^{-Kt_1}) \right] \qquad \text{[Eq. 12.7]}$$

$$C_1 = \left[\begin{array}{c} \text{Loading Dose and} \\ \text{Decay Equation} \end{array} \right] + \left[\begin{array}{c} \text{Nonsteady-State} \\ \text{Infusion Equation} \end{array} \right]$$

$$18 \text{ mg/L} = \left[\frac{(S)(F)(\text{Loading Dose})}{V} (e^{-Kt_1}) \right] + \left[\frac{(S)(F)(Dose/\tau)}{Cl} (1 - e^{-Kt_1}) \right]$$

By replacing K with Cl/V:

$$K = \frac{Cl}{V} \qquad \text{[Eq. 12.8]}$$

and assuming the following: S is 0.8, F is 1, t_1 is 10 hours, the loading dose is 375 mg; the maintenance dose infusion is 60 mg/hr; and V is 0.5 L/kg (30 L for this 60 kg patient), the above equation can be reduced to the following:

$$18 \text{ mg/L} = \left[\frac{(0.8)(1)(375 \text{ mg})}{V} \left(e^{-\left(\frac{Cl}{V}\right)(10 \text{ hr})} \right) \right] + \left[\frac{(0.8)(1)(60 \text{ mg/hr})}{Cl} \left(1 - e^{-\left(\frac{Cl}{V}\right)(10 \text{ hr})} \right) \right]$$

$$= \left[(10 \text{ mg/L}) \left(e^{-\left(\frac{Cl}{30 \text{ L}}\right)(10 \text{ hr})} \right) \right] + \left[\frac{(48 \text{ mg/hr})}{Cl} \left(1 - e^{-\left(\frac{Cl}{30 \text{ L}}\right)(10 \text{ hr})} \right) \right]$$

Unfortunately, clearance cannot be solved for directly but must be determined through trial and error by finding a value resulting in a theophylline concentration of 18 mg/L. If one has a good clinical history, the factors known to alter clearance should aid in making the initial estimate for clearance. In this case, no history is provided, so a clearance of 0.04 L/kg/hr could be tried in the above equation.

$$\text{Theophylline Clearance} = (0.04 \text{ L/kg/hr})(\text{Weight})$$

$$= (0.04 \text{ L/kg/hr})(60 \text{ kg})$$

$$= 2.4 \text{ L/hr}$$

Substitution of this clearance value in Equation 12.9 would result in a final steady-state theophylline concentration of only 20 mg/L as shown below.

$$\text{Css ave} = \frac{(S)(F)(\text{Dose}/\tau)}{Cl} \qquad \text{[Eq. 12.9]}$$

$$= \frac{(0.8)(1)(60 \text{ mg}/1 \text{ hr})}{2.4 \text{ L/hr}}$$

$$= 20 \text{ mg/L}$$

Following the initial loading dose, the expected concentration was 10 mg/L. The theophylline concentration then rose in 10 hours to 18 mg/L. It is unlikely that a theophylline concentration that has increased from 10 to 18 mg/L in only 10 hours will plateau at the predicted steady state value of 20 mg/L. Therefore, M.K.'s clearance is likely to be less than 2.4 L/hr. Furthermore, if a clearance of 2.4 L/hr is inserted into the previous equation, the predicted theophylline concentration at 10 hours would only be 15 mg/L. If a new clearance estimate of 2.0 L/hr is used, the calculated theophylline concentration at 10 hours is 17 mg/L as seen below.

$$C_{10 \text{ hr}} = \left[(10 \text{ mg/L}) \left(e^{-\left(\frac{2 \text{ L/hr}}{30 \text{ L}} \right)(10 \text{ hr})} \right) \right] + \left[\frac{(0.8)(60 \text{ mg/hr})}{2 \text{ L/hr}} \left(1 - e^{-\left(\frac{2 \text{ L/hr}}{30 \text{ L}} \right)(10 \text{ hr})} \right) \right]$$

$$= [(10 \text{ mg/L})(e^{-(0.0667 \text{ hr}^{-1})(10 \text{ hr})})] + [(24 \text{ mg/L})(1 - e^{-(0.0667 \text{ hr}^{-1})(10 \text{ hr})})]$$

$$= [(10 \text{ mg/L})(0.51)] + [(24 \text{ mg/L})(1 - 0.51)]$$

$$= 5.1 \text{ mg/L} + 11.8 \text{ mg/L}$$

$$= 16.9 \text{ mg/L or} \approx 17 \text{ mg/L}$$

Since this predicted plasma theophylline concentration is also less than that which was observed, the clearance must be less than 2.0 L/hr. Further trials would demonstrate that a clearance value of 1.65 L/hr results in a predicted theophylline level of 18 mg/L.

Using this clearance estimate of 1.65 L/hr and the assumed volume of distribution of 30 L, the calculated theophylline half-life would be 12.6 hours (Equation 12.5).

$$t\frac{1}{2} = \frac{(0.693)(V)}{Cl}$$

$$= \frac{(0.693)(30 \text{ L})}{1.65 \text{ L/hr}}$$

$$= 12.6 \text{ hr}$$

Because the time interval between the initial plasma concentration of 10 mg/L and the observed 18 mg/L was less than 1 revised half-life, the accuracy of this revised clearance is questionable. Remember that a single drug sample obtained within 2 half-lives of starting a drug regimen contains little information about clearance and the eventual Css ave (see Part 1: Interpretation of Plasma Drug Concentrations: Revising Pharmacokinetic Parameters). This drug level does suggest, however, that M.K.'s theophylline clearance is substantially less than the average literature value of 2.4 L/hr and that some downward adjustment in dose at this point is appropriate.

Question #12. *Assuming that the desired steady-state plasma theophylline concentration for M.K. is less than 20 mg/L, determine whether the maintenance dose needs to be adjusted.*

Because clearance is the primary determinant of the steady-state plasma concentration, this adjusted value (1.65 L/hr) can be used to estimate the plasma theophylline concentration produced by an aminophylline infusion of 60 mg/hr (Equation 12.9).

$$\text{Css ave} = \frac{(S)(F)(Dose/\tau)}{Cl}$$

$$= \frac{(0.8)(1)(60 \text{ mg}/1 \text{ hr})}{1.65 \text{ L/hr}}$$

$$= \frac{48 \text{ mg/hr}}{1.65 \text{ L/hr}}$$

$$= 29 \text{ mg/L}$$

The infusion rate should be adjusted because the predicted steady-state plasma theophylline concentration of 29 mg/L exceeds 20 mg/L. The new infusion rate can be calculated from Equation 12.4 by inserting the desired steady-state plasma concentration and using the clearance estimate of 1.65 L/hr. If a steady-state plasma concentration of 15 mg/L is desired, the new maintenance infusion will be approximately 30 mg/hr of aminophylline.

$$\text{Maintenance Dose} = \frac{(Cl)(Css \text{ ave})(\tau)}{(S)(F)}$$

$$= \frac{(1.65 \text{ L/hr})(15 \text{ mg/L})(1 \text{ hr})}{(0.8)(1)}$$

$$= \frac{24.75 \text{ mg}}{(0.8)}$$

$$= 30.9 \text{ mg or} \approx 30 \text{ mg of aminophylline per hour}$$

Another plasma theophylline concentration should be measured the following morning after the infusion rate has been reduced to ensure that the clearance estimate used (1.65 L/hr) is reasonably close to M.K.'s actual value.

Question #13. *O.P., a 72-kg male, became nauseated after receiving 68 mg/hr of IV theophylline for several days. A plasma sample for theophylline was obtained and the infusion was discontinued. Twelve hours later, a second plasma sample was obtained. The reported plasma theophylline concentrations were 32 mg/L and 16 mg/L, respectively. Estimate the hourly dose of theophylline required to maintain the plasma theophylline concentration at 15 mg/L.*

In this case, there are two ways to calculate a new maintenance dose. One method entails using Equation 12.10 to estimate the elimination rate constant based on the established theophylline decay pattern in O.P.

$$K = \frac{\ln\left(\dfrac{C_1}{C_2}\right)}{t} \qquad \text{[Eq. 12.10]}$$

In this example, C_1 is 32 mg/L, C_2 is 16 mg/L, and t is the 12 hours between the two plasma concentrations.

$$K = \frac{\ln\left(\dfrac{32}{16}\right)}{12 \text{ hr}}$$

$$= \frac{\ln(2)}{12 \text{ hr}}$$

$$= \frac{0.693}{12 \text{ hr}}$$

$$= 0.058 \text{ hr}^{-1}$$

The estimated K is then used with an assumed volume of distribution to calculate clearance. Once clearance is known, the new maintenance dose can be calculated. If the volume of distribution is assumed to be 0.5 L/kg or 36 L (0.5 L/kg × 72 kg), a clearance of 2.1 L/hr can be estimated from Equation 12.11 as shown below.

$$Cl = (K)(V) \qquad \text{[Eq. 12.11]}$$

$$= (0.058 \text{ hr}^{-1})(36 \text{ L})$$

$$= 2.1 \text{ L/hr}$$

Now, using Equation 12.4, the maintenance dose can be calculated. Assuming S, F, and τ are 1, 1, and 1 hour, respectively:

$$\text{Maintenance Dose} = \frac{(Cl)(Css\ ave)(\tau)}{(S)(F)}$$

$$= \frac{(2.1\ L/hr)(15\ mg/L)(1\ hr)}{(1)(1)}$$

$$= 31.5\ mg\ of\ theophylline\ per\ hour$$

Thus, a theophylline infusion of 30 mg/hr should result in a steady-state plasma theophylline concentration of approximately 15 mg/L.

A second method to calculate the new maintenance dose assumes that the plasma concentration of 32 mg/L represents a steady-state level. Then, the apparent theophylline clearance can be calculated directly by Equation 12.12 as follows:

$$Cl = \frac{(S)(F)(Dose/\tau)}{Css\ ave} \qquad \text{[Eq. 12.12]}$$

$$= \frac{(1)(1)(68\ mg/1\ hr)}{32\ mg/L}$$

$$= \frac{68\ mg/hr}{32\ mg/L}$$

$$= 2.1\ L/hr$$

In this particular case, both methods of calculation resulted in identical estimates of theophylline clearance for O.P. The first method should be used if steady state has not been achieved or if the dosing history is unreliable. This method, however, requires a reasonable time interval (one half-life or more) between plasma samples C_1 and C_2 and a reliable estimate of the volume of distribution. The second method is preferred when the volume of distribution estimate is questionable or when the elimination rate constant cannot be estimated accurately. However, it does require an accurate dosing history and steady-state conditions.

Question #14. *E.C., a 56-year-old, 50-kg woman receiving 20 mg/hr of theophylline, has a steady-state theophylline level of 12 mg/L. She is to start taking cimetidine. How should her theophylline infusion be adjusted?*

Cimetidine reduces theophylline clearance[13,31,51] by about 40%, although this percentage is highly variable. E.C.'s theophylline clearance, therefore, should be about 60% of her current clearance after cimetidine is initiated. One approach to adjusting the theophylline infusion rate is to calculate E.C.'s theophylline clearance before cimetidine therapy using Equation 12.12 and to multiply this clearance value by a factor of 0.6.

$$Cl = \frac{(S)(F)(Dose/\tau)}{Css\ ave}$$

$$= \frac{(1)(1)(20\ mg/1\ hr)}{12\ mg/L}$$

$$= 1.67\ L/hr$$

Clearance (after cimetidine) = (Clearance before cimetidine)(0.6)

$$= [1.67\ L/hr][0.6]$$

$$= 1\ L/hr$$

Cimetidine inhibition of theophylline metabolism should be observed as soon as reasonable cimetidine plasma concentrations are achieved. Therefore, the theophylline infusion rate should be reduced at the time, or shortly after, cimetidine therapy is initiated. Using the clearance value of 1 L/hr in Equation 12.4, the new infusion rate would be 12 mg/hr, assuming the target concentration is still 12 mg/L.

$$Maintenance\ Dose = \frac{(Cl)(Css\ ave)(\tau)}{(S)(F)}$$

$$= \frac{(1\ L/hr)(12\ mg/L)(1\ hr)}{(1)(1)}$$

$$= 12\ mg\ of\ theophylline\ per\ hour$$

Not all patients receiving concomitant cimetidine therapy experience a reduction in theophylline clearance or a reduction to the degree that was assumed in this example.[55,56] Therefore, one may elect not to change the infusion rate at the time cimetidine is initiated. Instead, one could monitor theophylline plasma concentrations to ensure that they do not rise to excessive levels. This second approach is most appropriate for patients who are poorly controlled with theophylline and in whom a reduced plasma concentration of theophylline may seriously compromise their respiratory status. This latter approach also may be more reasonable when the initial theophylline concentrations are in the lower therapeutic range (i.e., < 12 mg/L). When plasma theophylline concentrations are less than 12 mg/L, a cimetidine-induced reduction in the theophylline clearance by 40% is unlikely to result in a new steady-state theophylline concentration greater than 20 mg/L.

Question #15. *S.R., a 70-kg, 40-year-old man, has been receiving an IV aminophylline infusion at a rate of 35 mg/hr. His steady-state plasma theophylline concentration is 15 mg/L. Calculate an appropriate oral* *dosing regimen and estimate the peak and trough levels that would be produced by this regimen.*

One method used to convert an IV dose to an equivalent oral dose is to multiply the hourly IV dose by the dosing interval to be used for oral therapy. For example, if theophylline is dosed at 6-hour intervals for S.R., the equivalent oral dose would be 210 mg of aminophylline every 6 hours (35 mg/hr × 6 hours = 210 mg). It is assumed here that the same salt form (aminophylline) will be used and the bioavailability of the oral form is 100% (F = 1) (see Key Parameters and Table 12.1). The usual aminophylline dosage form of 200 mg is reasonably close to the calculated dose of 210 mg and would probably be prescribed.

The peak and trough plasma concentrations produced by intermittent dosing will be higher and lower, respectively, than the average concentration achieved during the infusion. There are two methods that can be used to estimate Css max and Css min.

Method I. A quick way to estimate the peak and trough plasma concentrations when the same average dose is given on an intermittent schedule is to first calculate the expected difference between the peak and trough concentrations by dividing the dose by the volume of distribution. Then, by adding one-half of this value to the average plasma concentration, the peak concentration can be estimated. Similarly, by subtracting one-half of this value from the average plasma concentration, the trough concentration can be estimated.

The plasma concentration after a dose is administered is the sum of the existing plasma concentration before the dose (trough concentration) and the change in plasma concentration (ΔC) produced by that dose. If absorption is assumed to be rapid, the maximum difference between peak and trough plasma concentrations (ΔC) can be estimated by use of Equation 12.13.

$$\Delta C = \frac{(S)(F)(Dose)}{V} \qquad \text{[Eq. 12.13]}$$

Assuming S is 0.8, F is 1, and V is 0.5 L/kg, each 200 mg dose of aminophylline should produce a 4.6 mg/L increment in plasma theophylline concentration.

$$\Delta C = \frac{(S)(F)(Dose)}{V}$$

$$= \frac{(0.8)(1)(200 \text{ mg})}{(0.5 \text{ L/kg})(70 \text{ kg})}$$

$$= \frac{160 \text{ mg}}{35 \text{ L}}$$

$$= 4.6 \text{ mg/L}$$

One-half of this change in plasma concentration is 2.3 mg/L. Therefore, the peak and trough concentrations produced by the prescribed regimen should be approximately 17.3 mg/L and 12.7 mg/L, respectively, as shown below using Equations 12.14 and 12.15:

$$\text{Css max} = [\text{Css ave}] + \left[(0.5)\frac{(S)(F)(\text{Dose})}{V}\right] \qquad \text{[Eq. 12.14]}$$

$$= 15\ \text{mg/L} + 2.3\ \text{mg/L}$$

$$= 17.3\ \text{mg/L}$$

$$\text{Css min} = [\text{Css ave}] - \left[(0.5)\frac{(S)(F)(\text{Dose})}{V}\right] \qquad \text{[Eq. 12.15]}$$

$$= 15\ \text{mg/L} - 2.3\ \text{mg/L}$$

$$= 12.7\ \text{mg/L}$$

This approach (i.e., Method I) assumes that 1) the oral dose will produce the same average plasma concentration as the IV infusion, 2) the oral dosage form will be absorbed rapidly and completely, and 3) the dosing interval is equal to or less than the theophylline half-life. If the dosing interval is greater than one half-life, the exponential decay results in a Css ave below the arithmetic average of the peak and trough concentrations.

Method II. A second method to calculate the peak and trough plasma concentrations is to estimate the clearance, volume of distribution, and elimination rate constant in S.R. and then to use Equations 12.16 and 12.17 to estimate the maximum and minimum plasma concentrations:

$$\text{Css max} = \frac{\frac{(S)(F)(\text{Dose})}{V}}{(1 - e^{-K\tau})} \qquad \text{[Eq. 12.16]}$$

$$\text{Css min} = (\text{Css max})(e^{-K\tau}) \qquad \text{[Eq. 12.17]}$$

To use these equations, the elimination rate constant (K) must first be estimated. The theophylline K for S.R. is a function of his theophylline clearance and volume of distribution. The clearance can be calculated from the observed steady-state plasma theophylline concentration using Equation 12.12:

$$CI = \frac{(S)(F)(Dose/\tau)}{Css\ ave}$$

$$= \frac{(0.8)(1)(35\ mg/1\ hr)}{15\ mg/L}$$

$$= \frac{28\ mg/hr}{15\ mg/L}$$

$$= 1.87\ L/hr$$

If the volume of distribution is assumed to be 35 L (0.5 L/kg × 70 kg), the elimination rate constant can be calculated from Equation 12.8.

$$K = \frac{CI}{V}$$

$$= \frac{1.87\ L/hr}{35\ L}$$

$$= 0.053\ hr^{-1}$$

Based on this K of 0.053 hr^{-1}, a V of 35L, and a τ of 6 hours, using Equation 12.16, the calculated maximum plasma theophylline concentration after each 200 mg aminophylline dose is 16.9 mg/L.

$$Css\ max = \frac{\dfrac{(S)(F)(Dose)}{V}}{(1 - e^{-K\tau})}$$

$$= \frac{\dfrac{(0.8)(1)(200\ mg)}{35\ L}}{(1 - e^{-(0.053hr^{-1})(6\ hr)})}$$

$$= \frac{\dfrac{160\ mg}{35\ L}}{(1 - e^{-0.32})}$$

$$= \frac{4.57\ mg/L}{0.27}$$

$$= 16.9\ mg/L$$

The minimum plasma concentration before each dose would be 12.3 mg/L (Equation 12.17).

$$Css\ min = (Css\ max)(e^{-K\tau})$$

$$= (16.9\ mg/L)(e^{-(0.053\ hr^{-1})(6\ hr)})$$

$$= (16.9\ mg/L)(e^{-(0.32)})$$

$$= 12.3\ mg/L$$

These estimates are reasonably close to those calculated by Method I and differ primarily because the average steady-state theophylline concentration from the oral regimen will be slightly lower than the assumed level of 15 mg/L. This is in part because the oral dose is 200 mg rather than the calculated dose of 210 mg (35 mg/hr × 6 hours) given by IV infusion. Also, the true "average" concentration is a little closer to the trough than the peak concentration owing to the exponential decay curve.

Question #16. *What types of patients are likely to experience wide fluctuations in their plasma theophylline concentrations when taking oral doses every 6 hours?*

Patients with a short theophylline half-life (i.e., less than 6 hours) will tend to have higher peak plasma concentrations and lower trough concentrations when the dosing interval is 6 hours or more. Because the volume of distribution of theophylline is reasonably constant, patients who have a large theophylline clearance will have a short theophylline half-life (Equation 12.5).

$$t\frac{1}{2} = \frac{(0.693)(V)}{Cl}$$

In general, pediatric patients tend to have higher theophylline clearances and shorter theophylline half-lives than the average adult.[57-59] Adults who smoke but do not have other disease states (e.g., CHF) also tend to have theophylline half-lives shorter than 6 hours.[33,34] Wide fluctuations in the plasma theophylline concentration can be minimized in these cases by shortening the dosing interval or by prescribing a sustained-release preparation.

Question #17. *When should plasma samples for theophylline concentrations be obtained for a patient who is on an oral regimen with a constant dosing interval?*

Plasma samples should be obtained immediately before a scheduled dose because trough concentrations are more predictable than peak concentrations. Peak plasma concentrations can be delayed by slow absorption, resulting in substantial error (see Part I: Interpretation of Plasma Drug Concentrations: Plasma Sampling Time).

Since the theophylline half-life is short in many patients, the difference between the trough and peak concentrations can be substantial. Theophylline toxicity frequently occurs when the dose is increased to bring trough concentrations into the usually accepted therapeutic range of 10 to 20 mg/L. Such toxicity may be prevented by first estimating the peak plasma concentration. Adding the increment in plasma concentration that will be produced by each dose to the observed trough concentration will usually give a reasonable approximation of the peak plasma concentration. This principle is illustrated in the following question.

Question #18. *M.G., who weighs 31 kg, has been receiving 200 mg of aminophylline every 6 hours for several days. A plasma theophylline sample drawn immediately before a scheduled dose was 5.0 mg/L. Estimate the peak plasma concentration after each dose and the expected $t^1/_2$ based on this observed trough concentration.*

The reported plasma theophylline concentration of 5.0 mg/L is a trough concentration. The peak plasma concentration will be the sum of this trough plasma concentration and the expected change in theophylline concentration resulting from each dose. The change in theophylline concentration can be calculated by use of Equation 12.13 (see Question #15).

$$\Delta C = \frac{(S)(F)(Dose)}{V}$$

If the average V of 0.5 L/kg is assumed, M.G.'s V would be 15.5 L (0.5 L/kg $\times$ 31 kg). Therefore,

$$\Delta C = \frac{(S)(F)(Dose)}{V}$$

$$= \frac{(0.8)(1)(200 \text{ mg})}{15.5 \text{ L}}$$

$$= 10.3 \text{ mg/L}$$

Thus, each 200 mg dose of aminophylline will increase the trough theophylline concentration by ≈ 10 mg/L, so the peak plasma concentration will be 15.3 mg/L (Equation 12.1).

$$\text{Css max} = [\text{Css min}] + \left[\frac{(S)(F)(Dose)}{V} \right]$$

$$= 5 \text{ mg/L} + 10.3 \text{ mg/L}$$

$$= 15.3 \text{ mg/L}$$

The actual peak concentration will be somewhat lower because oral absorption is not instantaneous and some of the dose will be eliminated during the absorption phase.

To calculate the expected half-life, first use Equation 12.10 to estimate the elimination rate constant. Note that in Equation 12.10 below, t is the entire dosing interval of 6 hours. This is because absorption, in the bolus model, is assumed to be instantaneous. Therefore, the peak concentration is assumed to occur directly over the trough. This results in a decay time from peak to trough (C_1 to C_2) that is equal to the dosing interval (see Part I: Interpretation of Plasma Drug Concentrations: Choosing a Model to Revise or Estimate a Patient's Clearance at Steady State).

$$K = \frac{\ln\left(\frac{C_1}{C_2}\right)}{t}$$

$$= \frac{\ln\left(\frac{15.3 \text{ mg/L}}{5 \text{ mg/L}}\right)}{6 \text{ hr}}$$

$$= \frac{\ln(3.06)}{6 \text{ hr}}$$

$$= \frac{1.12}{6 \text{ hr}}$$

$$= 0.187 \text{ hr}^{-1}$$

We can then use Equation 12.18 to estimate the half-life.

$$t\frac{1}{2} = \frac{0.693}{K} \qquad \text{[Eq. 12.18]}$$

$$= \frac{0.693}{0.187 \text{ hr}^{-1}}$$

$$= 3.7 \text{ hr}$$

If the dosing interval of 6 hours is maintained and the dose doubled, all concentrations within the dosing interval would be expected to double. Therefore, if the dose were doubled, the new steady-state trough and peak concentrations for M.G. would be 10 and 30 mg/L, respectively. Clearly, peak concentrations of 30 mg/L are above the usual accepted therapeutic range. Given the patient's estimated theophylline half-life of ≈3.7 hours, one may have to be satisfied with relatively low trough concentrations, which may be appropriate. If higher theophylline concentrations are desired, a sustained-release drug product should be used, because intervals shorter than 6 hours would make it very difficult for a patient to maintain compliance.

Question #19. *E.L. is a 48-kg female receiving an aminophylline infusion of 50 mg/hr; her steady-state plasma theophylline concentration is 15 mg/L. Parenteral aminophylline is discontinued and oral aminophylline is prescribed (300 mg at 9:00 a.m., 1:00 p.m., 5:00 p.m., and 9:00 p.m.). What problems would you anticipate with this dosing regimen?*

Since the average daily administration rate is the same (1200 mg/day) for both regimens, the average steady-state level will be the same. However, because the interval between doses is irregular (every 4 hours between 9:00 a.m. and 9:00 p.m. followed by an interval of 12 hours between 9:00 p.m. and 9:00 a.m.), the plasma theophylline concentration will be increasing above the Css ave during the day and declining below the Css ave during the night and early morning hours (see Figure 12.1).

The two plasma levels of most interest are the peak concentration just after the 9:00 p.m. dose and the trough concentration just before the 9:00 a.m. dose. These plasma levels should represent the highest and lowest levels produced by this dosing regimen.

Because the dosing interval is irregular, the usual steady-state Css max and Css min equations cannot be used. Instead, the plasma level at any given time must be thought of as the sum of that produced by four separate doses, each of which is given every 24 hours (i.e., each 9:00 a.m. dose is given every 24 hours, each 1:00 p.m. dose is given every 24 hours, etc.). As illustrated by Equation 12.19, the plasma level produced by any *one* of the four regimens is the Css max for that dose multiplied by the fraction of drug remaining at that point in time.

$$C_1 = (\text{Css max})(\text{Fraction remaining}) \qquad \text{[Eq. 12.19]}$$

$$\text{Css}_1 = \frac{\dfrac{(S)(F)(\text{Dose})}{V}}{(1 - e^{-K\tau})}(e^{-Kt_1})$$

The actual plasma level at any given time will be the sum of the levels produced by each of the four regimens. Since each regimen is given every 24 hours, τ is 24 hours.

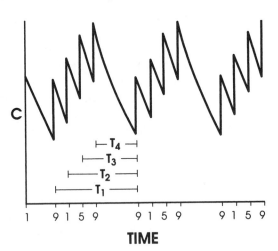

TIME

FIGURE 12.1. Plasma level time curve for a dosing regimen of 300 mg aminophylline at 9:00 a.m., 1:00 p.m., 5:00 p.m., and 9:00 p.m. Note that plasma concentrations are lowest just before the 9:00 a.m. dose and highest just after the 9:00 p.m. dose. Even though the interval between doses is irregular, each dose is given every 24 hours, at 9:00 a.m., 1:00 p.m., 5:00 p.m., and 9:00 p.m., respectively (see Equation 12.20)

$$C = \left[\frac{\dfrac{(S)(F)(Dose)}{V}}{[1 - e^{-(K)(\tau)}]} (e^{-Kt_1}) \right] + \left[\frac{\dfrac{(S)(F)(Dose)}{V}}{[1 - e^{-(K)(\tau)}]} (e^{-Kt_2}) \right] + \cdots$$

Or, more simply stated:

$$C = \frac{\dfrac{(S)(F)(Dose)}{V}}{[1 - e^{-(K)(\tau)}]} (e^{-Kt_1} + e^{-Kt_2} + e^{-Kt_3} + e^{-Kt_4}) \qquad \text{[Eq. 12.20]}$$

where t_1, t_2, t_3, and t_4 represent the time intervals between the time of administration for each dose and the time at which one wishes to predict the plasma theophylline level.

To solve the above equation for C, first calculate K, which can be derived from the clearance and volume of distribution. Since a steady-state level (15 mg/L) and dose (50 mg/hr) are known, clearance can be calculated through the use of Equation 12.12.

$$Cl = \frac{(S)(F)(Dose/\tau)}{Css\ ave}$$

$$= \frac{(0.8)(1)(50\ mg/1\ hr)}{15\ mg/L}$$

$$= 2.67\ L/hr$$

If the volume of distribution is assumed to be 24 L (0.5 L/kg × 48 kg), the elimination rate constant can be calculated using Equation 12.8.

$$K = \frac{Cl}{V}$$

$$= \frac{2.67\ L/hr}{24\ L}$$

$$= 0.11\ hr^{-1}$$

The plasma level after the 9:00 p.m. dose can now be determined by considering t_1 through t_4 as the number of hours since the last 9:00 a.m., 1:00 p.m., 5:00 p.m., and 9:00 p.m. doses were administered. Therefore, t_1 through t_4 would be 12, 8, 4, and 0 hours, respectively. This assumes that the 9:00 p.m. dose was rapidly absorbed so that the bolus model can be used.

$$C \text{ at 9 p.m.} = \frac{\dfrac{(0.8)(1.0)(300 \text{ mg})}{24 \text{ L}}}{[1 - e^{-(0.11)(24 \text{ hr})}]} (e^{-(0.11)(12 \text{ hr})} + e^{-(0.11)(8 \text{ hr})} + e^{-(0.11)(4 \text{ hr})} + e^{-(0.11)(0 \text{ hr})})$$

$$= \frac{10 \text{ mg/L}}{[1 - e^{-(2.64)}]} (e^{-(1.32)} + e^{-(0.88)} + e^{-(0.44)} + e^{-0})$$

$$= \left[\frac{10 \text{ mg/L}}{1 - 0.071} \right] [0.27 + 0.41 + 0.64 + 1]$$

$$= \left[\frac{10 \text{ mg/L}}{0.929} \right] [2.32]$$

$$= 25 \text{ mg/L}$$

The plasma concentration just before the 9:00 a.m. dose could be calculated using Equation 12.20 and the appropriate time intervals. In this case, the time intervals since the last 9:00 a.m., 1:00 p.m., 5:00 p.m., and 9:00 p.m. dose would be 24 hours, 20 hours, 16 hours, and 12 hours, respectively.

Another method, which could be used to determine the level just before the morning dose, would be to multiply the peak concentration of 25 mg/L by the fraction remaining after 12 hours (Equation 12.21).

$$C_2 = (C_1)(e^{-Kt}) \hspace{3cm} \text{[Eq. 12.21]}$$

$$= (25 \text{ mg/L})(e^{-(0.11 \text{ hr}^{-1})(12 \text{ hr})})$$

$$= (25 \text{ mg/L})(0.27)$$

$$= 6.7 \text{ mg/L (Immediately Prior to 9 a.m. Dose)}$$

In summary, while it is possible that E.L. could be well controlled clinically on this irregular dosing schedule, a regular dosing interval of 6 hours, though much less convenient, would result in lower peaks and higher trough concentrations (20.8 mg/L and 10.8 mg/L, respectively). Thus, toxicity would be minimized and the therapeutic response maximized (Equations 12.16 and 12.17).

$$\text{Css max} = \frac{\frac{(S)(F)(\text{Dose})}{V}}{(1 - e^{-K\tau})}$$

$$= \frac{\frac{(0.8)(1.0)(300 \text{ mg})}{24 \text{ L}}}{(1 - e^{-(0.11 \text{ hr}^{-1})(6 \text{ hr})})}$$

$$= \frac{10 \text{ mg/L}}{(1 - e^{-0.66})}$$

$$= \frac{10 \text{ mg/L}}{(1 - 0.52)}$$

$$= \frac{10 \text{ mg/L}}{(0.48)}$$

$$= 20.8 \text{ mg/L}$$

$$\text{Css min} = (\text{Css max})(e^{-K\tau})$$

$$= (20.8 \text{ mg/L})(e^{-(0.11 \text{ hr}^{-1})(6 \text{ hr})})$$

$$= (20.8 \text{ mg/L})(e^{-(0.66)})$$

$$= (20.8 \text{ mg/L})(0.52)$$

$$= 10.8 \text{ mg/L}$$

An alternative to the 6-hour dosing interval is the use of a sustained-release product, which can be administered less frequently. Such a product would minimize the fluctuation in the theophylline plasma concentrations between dosing intervals and would thus decrease the possibility of toxic peak levels and subtherapeutic trough levels in a patient who requires a high Css ave for clinical control.

Question #20. *If E.L. was prescribed 600 mg of a sustained-release dosage form of theophylline every 12 hours, how would one calculate the expected theophylline concentrations?*

Assuming that the theophylline product has slow-release characteristics over approximately 12 hours, the plasma concentrations of theophylline should not change very much with a dosing interval of 12 hours. The administration of this oral form could thus be treated as an infusion described by Equation 12.9.

$$\text{Css ave} = \frac{(S)(F)(\text{Dose}/\tau)}{Cl}$$

In this case, we are assuming S and F are 1.

$$\text{Css ave} = \frac{(1)(1)(600 \text{ mg}/12 \text{ hr})}{2.67 \text{ L/hr}}$$

$$= \frac{50 \text{ mg/hr}}{2.67 \text{ L/hr}}$$

$$= 18.7 \text{ mg/L}$$

Calculation of peak and trough levels using Equations 12.16 and 12.17 would be inappropriate since the levels should fluctuate relatively little within the dosing interval.

As an alternative, an intermittent infusion model could be used to calculate the "peak" theophylline concentration, which should occur at the end of the absorption time. The subsequent trough concentration will occur t_2 hours after the end of the absorption process and just before the next dose (Equation 12.22) (also see Part I: Selecting the Appropriate Equation: Sustained-Release Dosage Forms).

$$\text{Css}_2 = \frac{\dfrac{(S)(F)(\text{Dose}/t_{in})}{Cl}(1 - e^{-Kt_{in}})}{(1 - e^{-KT})}(e^{-kt_2}) \qquad \text{[Eq. 12.22]}$$

For most sustained-release theophylline products, the t_{in} or duration of absorption is estimated to be between 8 and 12 hours. If a t_{in} of 12 hours is selected, it can be seen that E.L.'s theophylline concentration would be essentially a continuous infusion, as calculated previously. If the shorter duration of 8 hours is selected, then the peak concentration would be expected to occur approximately 8 hours after the administration of the dose, and the trough concentration would occur approximately 4 hours after that, or just before the next dose. Using an 8-hour duration of absorption, the expected peak concentration would be 22 mg/L.

$$\text{Css}_2 = \left[\frac{\dfrac{(1)(1)(600 \text{ mg}/8 \text{ hr})}{2.67 \text{ L/hr}}(1 - e^{-(0.11 \text{ hr}^{-1})(8 \text{ hr})})}{(1 - e^{-(0.11 \text{ hr}^{-1})(12 \text{ hr})})}\right]\left[e^{-(0.11 \text{ hr}^{-1})(0 \text{ hr})}\right]$$

$$= \frac{(28 \text{ mg/L})(0.58)}{(0.73)}(1)$$

$$= 22 \text{ mg/L}$$

The corresponding trough concentration 4 hours later would be 14 mg/L (Equation 12.21).

$$C_2 = (C_1)(e^{-Kt})$$

$$= [22\ \text{mg/L}][e^{-(0.11\ \text{hr}^{-1})(4\ \text{hr})}]$$

$$= 14\ \text{mg/L}$$

Because of the potentially elevated peak concentrations and the uncertainty regarding the actual rate of the absorption from sustained-release drug products, a reduction in dose might be warranted. In addition, because the half-life for E.L. is relatively short, a dosing interval of 8 hours might be more appropriate. The shorter dosing interval would diminish the possibility of excessive peak and lower trough concentrations to some extent. If the intermittent infusion model is used and if shorter dosing intervals are selected, the duration of absorption (t_{in}) in Equation 12.22 should always be equal to or less than the dosing interval (τ). If the expected duration of absorption is longer than the dosing interval, one normally would use a continuous infusion model (Equation 12.9 for Css ave) because the overlapping infusions would tend to minimize the fluctuation in plasma concentrations.

$$\text{Css ave} = \frac{(S)(F)(\text{Dose}/\tau)}{Cl}$$

When treatment is converted from IV to oral theophylline therapy, it should be considered a change in the dosing regimen even if the patient is receiving approximately the same amount of theophylline per day. This is because theophylline concentrations obtained soon after changing the route of administration may be very sensitive to the specific model selected for predicting the drug concentration (i.e., bolus versus infusion; short versus long t_{in}) rather than the patient's pharmacokinetic parameters (i.e., clearance and volume of distribution). For this reason, theophylline levels should normally be obtained no sooner than 1 day (approximately 3 to 4 half-lives) after the route of administration has been changed.

REFERENCES

1. Mitenko PA, Ogilvie RI. Rational intravenous doses of theophylline. N Engl J Med 1973;289:600.
2. Bierman CW, et al. Acute and chronic therapy in exercise induced bronchospasm. Pediatrics 1977;60:845.
3. Jenne JW. Pharmacokinetics of theophylline: application to adjustment of the clinical dose of aminophylline. Clin Pharmacol Ther 1972;13:349.
4. Murciano D, et al. A randomized, controlled trial of theophylline in patients with severe chronic obstructive pulmonary disease. N. Engl J Med 1989;320:1521–1525.
5. Ferguson GT, Cherniack RM. Management of chronic obstructive pulmonary disease. N Engl J Med 1993;328:1017–1022.
6. Aranda JV, Turmen T. Methylxanthines in apnea of prematurity. Clin Perinatol 1979; 6:87–108.

7. Kriter KE, Blanchard J. Management of apnea in infants. Clin Pharmacy 1989;8:577–587.

8. Jacobs MH, et al. Clinical experience with theophylline: relationships between dosage, serum concentration and toxicity. JAMA 1976;235:1983.

9. Ogilvie R, et al. Cardiovascular response to increasing theophylline concentrations. Eur Clin Pharmacol 1977;12:409.

10. Piafsky KM, Ogilvie RI. Dosage of theophylline in bronchial asthma. N Engl J Med 1975;292:1218.

11. Zillich CW, et al. Theophylline-induced seizures in adults. Ann Intern Med 1975;82:784.

12. Yarnell PR, Chu NS. Focal seizures and aminophylline. Neurology 1975;25:819.

13. Hendeles L, et al. A clinical and pharmacokinetic basis for the selection and use of slow-release theophylline products. Clin Pharmacokinet 1984;9:95.

14. Upton RA, et al. Evaluation of the absorption from some commercial sustained-release theophylline products. J Pharmacokinet Biopharm 1980;8:131.

15. Barr WH. The once-daily theophylline controversy. [Editorial] Pharmacotherapy 1984;4:167.

16. Weinberger MM. Theophylline: QID, TID, BID, and now QD? Pharmacotherapy 1984; 4:181.

17. Hendeles L, et al. Food-induced dose-dumping from a "once-a-day" theophylline product as a cause of theophylline toxicity. Chest 1984;87:758.

18. Karim A, et al. Food-induced changes in theophylline absorption from controlled-release formulations. Part I: substantial increased and decreased absorption with Uniphyl tablets and Theo-Dur sprinkle. Clin Pharmacol Ther 1985;38:77.

19. Dietrich R, et al. Intra-subject variation and sustained-release theophylline absorption. J Allergy Clin Immunol 1981;67:465.

20. Powell JR, et al. Theophylline disposition in acutely ill hospitalized patients. Am Rev Respir Dis 1978;118:229.

21. Mitenko PA, Ogilvie RI. Pharmacokinetics of intravenous theophylline. Clin Pharmacol Ther 1972;14:509.

22. Aranda J, et al. Pharmacokinetic aspects of theophylline in premature infants. N Engl J Med 1976;295:413.

23. Loughnan PM, et al. Pharmacokinetic analysis of the disposition of intravenous theophylline in young children. J Pediatr 1976;88:874.

24. Rosen JP, et al. Theophylline pharmacokinetics in the young infant. Pediatrics 1979; 64:248.

25. Isles A, et al. Theophylline disposition in cystic fibrosis. Am Rev Respir Dis 1983;127:417.

26. Larsen GI, et al. Intravenous aminophylline in patients with cystic fibrosis. Am J Dis Child 1980;134:1143.

27. FDA Drug Bulletin. IV guidelines for theophylline products. 1980(Feb);10:4–6.

28. Zahorska-Markiewicz B, Waluga M, Zielinski M, Klin M. Pharmacokinetics of theophylline in obesity. Int J Clin Pharmacol Ther 1996;34(9):393–395.

29. Gal P, et al. Theophylline disposition in obesity. Clin Pharmacol Ther 1978;24:438.

30. Koup JR, Vawter TK. Theophylline pharmacokinetics in an extremely obese patient. Clin Pharm 1983;2:181.

31. Hendeles L, Weinberger M. Theophylline: a "state of the art" review. Pharmacotherapy 1983;3:2.

32. Edwards DJ, et al. Theophylline. In: Evans WE et al., eds. Applied Pharmacokinetics: Principles of Therapeutic Drug Monitoring. 3rd Ed. Vancouver: Applied Therapeutics 1992;13:1–38.

33. Powell JR, et al. The influence of cigarette smoking and sex on theophylline disposition. Am Rev Respir Dis 1977;116:17.

34. Hunt SN, et al. Effects of smoking on theophylline disposition. Clin Pharmacol Ther 1976;19:546.

35. Jenne JW, et al. Apparent theophylline half-life fluctuations during treatment of acute left ventricular failure. Am J Hosp Pharm 1977;34:408.

36. Jusko WJ, et al. Intravenous theophylline therapy: nomogram guideline. Ann Intern Med 1977;86:400.

37. Piafsky KM, et al. Theophylline kinetics in acute pulmonary edema. Clin Pharmacol Ther 1977;21:310.

38. Piafsky KM, et al. Theophylline disposition in patients with hepatic cirrhosis. N Engl J Med 1977;296:1495.

39. Aranda JV, et al. Pharmacokinetic aspects of theophylline in premature newborns. N Engl J Med 1976;295:413.

40. Kappas A, et al. Influence of dietary protein and carbohydrate on antipyrine and theophylline metabolism in man. Clin Pharmacol Ther 1976;20:643.

41. Monks T, et al. The effect of increased caffeine intake on the metabolism and pharmacokinetics of theophylline in man. Biopharm Drug Dispos 1981;2:31.

42. Jonkman JHG, Upton RA. Pharmacokinetic drug interactions with theophylline. Clin Pharmacokinet 1984;9:309.

43. Weinberger M, et al. Inhibition of theophylline clearance by triacetyloleandomycin. J Allergy Clin Immunol 1977;59:228.

44. Pfeifer HJ, et al. Effects of three antibiotics on theophylline kinetics. Clin Pharmacol Ther 1979;26:36.

45. Schwartz J, Jauregui L, Lettieri J, Bachmann, K. Impact of ciprofloxacin on theophylline clearance and steady-state concentrations in serum. Antimicrob Agents Chemother 1988;32(1):75–77.

46. Stahlberg H, et al. Effects of gatifloxacin on the pharmacokinetics of theophylline in healthy young volunteers. [Abstract] J Antimicrob Chemother 1999;44(Suppl A):136.

47. Stass H, Kubitza D. Lack of pharmacokinetic interaction between moxifloxacin, a novel 8-methoxyfluoroquinolone, and theophylline. Clin Pharmacokinet 2001;40(Suppl 1):63–70.

48. Gisclon LG, Curtin CR, Fowler CL, et al. Absence of pharmacokinetic interaction between intravenous theophylline and orally administered levofloxacin. J Clin Pharmacol 1997;37:744–750.

49. Landay RA. Effect of phenobarbital on theophylline disposition. J Allergy Clin Immunol 1978;62:27.

50. Piafsky KM, et al. Effect of phenobarbital on the disposition of intravenous theophylline. Clin Pharmacol Ther 1977;22:336.

51. Kelly HW, et al. Ranitidine at very large doses does not inhibit theophylline elimination. Clin Pharmacol Ther 1986;39:577.

52. Bachmann K, et al. Controlled study of the putative interaction between famotidine and theophylline in patients with chronic obstructive pulmonary disease. J Clin Pharm 1995;35(5):529–535.

53. Hemstreet MP, et al. Effect of intravenous isoproterenol on theophylline kinetics. J Allergy Clin Immunol 1982;69:360.

54. Mitenko PA, Ogilvie RI. Rapidly achieved plasma concentrations plateaus, with observation on theophylline kinetics. Clin Pharmacol Ther 1972;13:329.

55. Ambrose PJ, Harralson AF. Lack of effect of cimetidine on theophylline clearance. Drug Intell Clin Pharm 1981;15:389.

56. Bauman JH, Kimmelblatt BJ. Cimetidine as an inhibitor of drug metabolism: therapeutic implications and drug review of the literature. Drug Intell Clin Pharm 1982;16:380.

57. Levy G, et al. Pharmacokinetic analysis of the effect of theophylline on pulmonary function in asthmatic children. J Pediatr 1978;86:789.

58. Maselli R, et al. Pharmacologic effect of intravenously administered aminophylline in asthmatic children. J Pediatr 1970;76:777.

59. Wyatt R, et al. Oral theophylline dosage for the management of chronic asthma. J Pediatr 1978;92:125.

60. Knoppert DC, et al. Cystic fibrosis: enhanced theophylline metabolism may be linked to the disease. Clin Pharmacol Ther 1988;44:254–264.

61. Chang K, et al. Altered theophylline pharmacokinetics during acute respiratory viral illness. Lancet 1978;1:1132.

62. Upton RA. Pharmacokinetic interactions between theophylline and other medications (part I). Clin Pharmacokinet 1991;20:66–80.

63. Upton RA. Pharmacokinetic interactions between theophylline and other medications (part II). Clin Pharmacokinet 1991;20:135–150.

13

TRICYCLIC ANTIDEPRESSANTS: AMITRIPTYLINE, DESIPRAMINE, IMIPRAMINE, AND NORTRIPTYLINE

Mark D. Watanabe and Michael E. Winter

Tricyclic antidepressants (TCAs) have been used clinically for approximately 40 years. This chapter focuses on amitriptyline, desipramine, imipramine, and nortriptyline because assay procedures for these agents are widely available and therapeutic ranges have been established. For many other antidepressants, the reported "therapeutic ranges" primarily represent the usual plasma concentrations produced by standard doses. Most clinicians adjust TCA doses by monitoring the drug's efficacy and side effects; plasma levels are monitored only in specific situations (see Tricyclic Antidepressants: Time to Sample). When TCAs are used for clinical indications other than depression [e.g., enuresis, attention deficit disorder (ADD), and other mood disorders], dose adjustments are based primarily on clinical observations. Because very little data are available on target plasma concentrations for these alternate therapeutic uses, most clinicians tend to use the therapeutic range established for depression.

A number of factors make plasma level monitoring of TCAs difficult. One major problem lies in the inability to establish a clearly defined therapeutic end-point. Also, active metabolites and altered plasma protein binding can complicate the ability to relate measured plasma concentrations to a therapeutic response. The wide variability in the dose to plasma concentration ratio stimulated investigators to establish a therapeutic range.[1] To a great extent, the variability in plasma concentrations can be attributed to a high first-pass hepatic clearance of the TCAs which results in a relative low and variable bioavailability. Genetically determined interindividual differences in the rates of metabolic biotransformation and elimination of TCAs may also contribute to this variance. Although some of these agents are available in parenteral dosage forms, they are not commonly administered by this route. In addition, the maximum therapeutic effect is usually not apparent for several weeks following the initiation of TCAs even though steady-state plasma concentrations are usually achieved within 1 week.[2-4]

With the introduction of newer antidepressants having more tolerable side effect profiles and lower risks for overdose (e.g., the selective serotonin reuptake inhibitors, selective norepinephrine reuptake inhibitors, and other novel agents influencing a variety of brain neurotransmitters), emerging practice standards in the treatment of depression have relegated TCAs to a less significant role as common first-line agents. However, their longstanding use as antidepressants have resulted in a wealth of clinical knowledge that can still be applied to cases in which they might be indicated as the pharmacotherapy of choice.

KEY PARAMETERS: Tricyclic Antidepressants

Therapeutic Range	
Amitriptyline	120–250 µg/L[a]
Desipramine	100–250 µg/L
Imipramine	180–350 µg/L[b]
Nortriptyline	50–150 µg/L
Free fraction (α)[c]	
Amitriptyline, Desipramine, Imipramine, Nortriptyline	<0.1
F	
Amitriptyline, Desipramine, Imipramine	0.4
Nortriptyline	0.5
S	
Amitriptyline, Desipramine, Imipramine, Nortriptyline	1.0
Vd[d]	
Amitriptyline	15 L/kg
Desipramine, Imipramine, Nortriptyline	20 L/kg
Cl[d]	
Amitriptyline	0.7 L/kg/hr
Desipramine	0.6 L/kg/hr
Imipramine	0.9 L/kg/hr
Nortriptyline	0.4 L/kg/hr
$t\frac{1}{2}$[d]	
Amitriptyline, Desipramine, Imipramine	20 hours
Nortriptyline	30 hours

[a]Therapeutic range includes sum of amitriptyline + nortriptyline.
[b]Therapeutic range includes sum of imipramine + desipramine.
[c]Free fraction is variable with significant plasma protein binding to serum proteins other than albumin.
[d]These values represent average estimates from the literature and, therefore, use of any two to extract a third parameter may not result in the reported average value.

THERAPEUTIC AND TOXIC PLASMA CONCENTRATIONS

The therapeutic range for the TCAs is not as well established as it is for many of the other drugs described in this text. Plasma protein-binding to various blood elements accounts for some of the difficulty in interpreting the plasma concentrations of these basic compounds. TCAs bind to α_1-acid glycoprotein (AAG) with a relatively high affinity but somewhat low capacity. They also bind to serum albumin.[5] Lipoprotein concentrations may be important[6] since the degree of binding for amitriptyline and nortriptyline has been associated with cholesterol and triglyceride concentrations. Elevated concentrations of AAGs in response to certain inflammatory processes alter the plasma binding and potential therapeutic range for the TCAs.[7] It is also difficult to determine whether the alterations in plasma protein-binding for TCAs are due to patient variations or to the collection techniques and the assay methodologies used to determine the unbound drug concentrations. Whereas the plasma protein-binding of the various TCAs is not identical, they all have a free fraction of less than 10%; for most, approximately 5% of the drug in plasma is unbound or free.[5,7,8] Although higher free fractions have been reported,[9,10] it is unclear whether these studies represent actual variations in plasma protein-binding or artifacts in the assay methodology.

The therapeutic range for nortriptyline of 50 to 150 µg/L (ng/mL) is more clearly established than that for other tricyclic agents.[2,3,11] Desipramine has an accepted therapeutic range of approximately 100 to 250 µg/L.[11,12] One study indicated that plasma concentrations above 115 µg/L strongly correlated with positive therapeutic outcomes, while others have suggested that plasma concentrations as low as 75 µg/L were potentially therapeutic.[13,14]

Imipramine is metabolized to desipramine. To date, no one has been able to distinguish a therapeutic difference between these two compounds; therefore, plasma concentration ranges are usually described as the sum of the imipramine and desipramine concentrations. Most studies suggest that the combined concentration range should be at least 150

TABLE 13.1 **Tricyclic Antidepressants**

Drug	Dosage Forms Available
Amitriptyline	10, 25, 50, 75, 100, and 150 mg tablets
	10 mg/mL 10 mL injectable (multidose vial)
Desipramine	10, 25, 50, 75, 100, and 150 mg tablets
Imipramine	10, 25, and 50 mg tablets
	75, 100, 125, and 150 mg capsules (Tofranil-PM)
Nortriptyline	10, 25, 50, and 75 mg capsules
	10 mg/5mL oral solution

μg/L and perhaps as high as 240 μg/L.[11,15] Whereas the therapeutic range of imipramine is somewhat variable depending on the source, many clinicians use a relatively wide range of 180 to 350 μg/L.[11,16]

Amitriptyline is metabolized to an active metabolite, nortriptyline; therefore, its therapeutic range represents the sum of these two compounds. Although the therapeutic range is not clearly established, most clinicians accept a range of 120 to 250 μg/L.[11,17] It is generally believed that concentrations above this range, and especially concentrations > 450 μg/L, are not likely to result in a therapeutic response for patients whose conditions have failed to respond at lower concentrations. Patients can, however, have significant anticholinergic side effects including dry mouth, blurred vision, confusion, and delirium.[18]

Although most clinicians simply monitor the patient's clinical response to TCAs, plasma concentration monitoring is occasionally useful (see Tricyclic Antidepressants: Time to Sample).

BIOAVAILABILITY (F)

Although gastrointestinal absorption of orally administered TCAs is almost complete, the significant first-pass metabolism that occurs as the drugs pass through the liver reduces their bioavailability to less than 50% in most patients. As with most drugs exhibiting significant first-pass metabolism, the bioavailability range is broad and difficult to estimate in any individual patient. Amitriptyline is generally considered to have a bioavailability of approximately 30% to 60%[8,19,20]; desipramine, 30% to 50%;[8,20,21] imipramine, 20% to 70%;[20,22] and nortriptyline, 45% to 70%.[20,23] The rate of absorption is also variable, with peak concentrations occurring 2 to 8 hours following a single dose.[22] In general, the various dosage forms of the TCAs are considered to be bioequivalent and there is little information suggesting that their absorption is altered by drug interactions or food. There may be some differences, however, between oral and parenteral dosage forms. The high liver extraction and metabolic conversion of orally administered tricyclic compound does not occur following parenteral administration. Thus, the parent compound to metabolite ratio may differ when the same drug is given orally and parenterally. This factor could be important if the metabolites and parent compound have different therapeutic effects.[24]

VOLUME OF DISTRIBUTION (V)

TCAs are widely distributed throughout the body; considering their extensive binding to plasma proteins, their tissue binding is impressive. Although estimates for the volume of distribution of the TCAs vary, most values are in the range of 15 to 20 L/kg.[19-21,23] Volume of distribution is a pharmacokinetic parameter that is not used clinically, because loading doses of TCAs are not administered. The large volume of distribution and high plasma protein-binding do indicate that hemodialysis is not likely to remove a significant amount of drug from the body.

CLEARANCE (Cl)

TCAs are cleared almost exclusively by the liver; less than 5% of these compounds are eliminated by the kidney.[22,25] As previously mentioned, metabolites of some TCAs are active and need to be considered when monitoring the plasma concentrations. Clearances estimated for the TCAs reported in the literature vary by up to 3 to 5 times. Average values are usually in the range of 10 mL/kg/min (0.6 L/kg/hr). Some of this variance is due to intra- and interindividual variation in hepatic metabolism and drug interactions. For example, cimetidine decreases the hepatic metabolism of imipramine; this not only reduces its clearance but also increases its bioavailability by decreasing the first-pass effect.[26]

Many compounds and liver disease appear to increase the plasma concentrations of TCAs. Those that decrease hepatic metabolism, such as chloramphenicol, disulfiram, and alcoholic liver disease, are easy to predict. Others, such as haloperidol, fluoxetine, and oral contraceptives, may not come to mind readily as inhibitors of hepatic metabolism but have reportedly increased the plasma concentrations of TCAs.[20,27] Most of the drugs that have been reported to increase the metabolism of TCAs are easy to predict and include carbamazepine, phenytoin, barbiturates, smoking, and chloral hydrate.[20] It is difficult to estimate the clinical significance of any of these drug interactions, because some patients appear to exhibit substantial changes in metabolism while others exhibit relatively little change in TCA concentrations when these agents are added to or deleted from a therapeutic regimen. Because the intrinsic metabolism of TCAs varies widely among patients, and because the magnitude of drug interactions is difficult to predict, all patients should be carefully monitored any time concurrent drug therapy is changed. Although plasma concentration monitoring may help to sort out some of these problems, careful observation of the patient's clinical symptoms is especially warranted.

HALF-LIFE (t½)

As mentioned previously, TCAs have an exceptionally large volume of distribution and a high clearance which results in an average half-life of ≈20 hours.[8,20] As with the volume of distribution and clearance, half-life also has an extremely wide reported range: 9 to > 50 hours. It is difficult to know whether this wide range reflects true alterations in pharmacokinetic parameters or the limitations that exist when attempting to estimate a drug's half-life within a dosing interval that is approximately equal to the drug's half-life. In any case, it is unclear whether the half-life of the drug would be used clinically to establish a dosing interval for the TCAs. The significant lag between the onset of clinical response relative to the time plasma concentrations plateau suggests that the therapeutic response is associated with a more slowly equilibrating deep tissue compartment or some other biochemical change associated with TCA therapy. Therefore, daily changes in drug levels may not be important with regard to therapeutic control of depression but could be an issue with regard to side effects of TCAs.

TIME TO SAMPLE

Several factors should be considered in selecting the appropriate time to sample TCAs. First, unless there are overt signs of clinical toxicity, plasma samples obtained before steady state has been achieved are not recommended because they can be misleading. For this reason, most clinicians wait at least 1 week before obtaining a plasma concentration. Using steady-state concentrations, adjustments in the dosing regimen can be made in proportion to the desired change in plasma concentration. The appropriate time to obtain the sample within a dosing interval, however, is a bit more complex. Peak concentrations obtained a few hours after the dose is administered are unpredictable because the rate of absorption is so variable; trough concentrations are often inconvenient because these agents are normally dosed at bedtime. Therefore, most clinicians attempt to standardize the sampling time at about 12 hours after an oral dose, which is usually in the morning if the TCA is administered at bedtime. Mid-interval plasma concentrations should approximate the average steady-state concentration; thus, any revision of pharmacokinetic parameters will focus on estimates of clearance and bioavailability.

$$\text{Css ave} = \frac{(S)(F)(\text{Dose}/\tau)}{Cl} \qquad \text{[Eq. 13.1]}$$

A large number of techniques have been used to help clinicians select an initial dosing regimen that will achieve a target concentration.[28] One method utilizes the principle of mean residence time (see Part I: Interpretation of Plasma Drug Concentrations, Single-Point Determination of Clearance) and recommends measuring a plasma concentration at a specified point in time (usually 24 to 36 hours after an initial dose).[29-31] As previously discussed, these techniques are most effective when the sampling time occurs at ≈ 1.5 half-lives.

The first question that one should consider is whether plasma concentrations ought to be monitored. Although wide variations in both bioavailability and clearance might make TCAs ideal candidates for therapeutic drug monitoring, most clinicians do not routinely monitor TCA concentrations. Instead, they rely on clinical observations and limit drug level monitoring to specific circumstances. Some have suggested TCA monitoring early in therapy to allow adjustment of the dosing regimen 1 or 2 weeks after initiating therapy. This method should result in a more rapid dose adjustment since clinicians must wait 3 or more weeks to adjust the dose based on the antidepressant clinical response. While this technique is not routinely employed, early drug level monitoring of steady-state concentrations for agents that have a delayed therapeutic benefit makes sense. Drug concentrations also are used to differentiate noncompliant patients from those who are unresponsive to treatment. However, differentiation between noncompliant patients and those who exhibit unusual metabolism or low bioavailability is difficult; this assessment is made most easily when the TCA concentrations are exceedingly low < 30 μg/L). These low levels are unlikely to be due to unusual pharmacokinetic disposition, assuming a dose that would be expected to achieve therapeutic concentrations has been prescribed. Occasionally, TCA levels are used to document suspected drug toxicity; concentrations > 500 μg/L are often associated with side effects, and concentrations > 1,000 μg/L are usually considered inappropriate and warrant withholding the TCA.[18] Many clinicians believe that plasma concentrations should only be measured to support clinically observed side effects such as changes in visual accommodation, dry mouth, and mental changes that include confusion and, potentially, seizures. Cardiovascular side effects also should be considered. Orthostatic hypotension and electrocardiogram (ECG) changes, such as widening QRS intervals or obvious arrhythmias, require adjustment in the TCA dose. Because these agents can exacerbate cardiovascular diseases, some clinicians start patients with preexisting heart disease on minimal doses and slowly adjust their doses upward with careful clinical and drug level monitoring. Other patients who are likely to be susceptible to cardiovascular side effects include the elderly and patients whose concurrent drug therapy is known to influence the pharmacokinetics of TCAs. Age-related or disease-related decreases in renal function may also lead to an increased accumulation of potentially toxic polar metabolites, particularly hydroxylated products from secondary amine TCAs.[32,33]

Question #1. *A.R., a 39-year-old, 65-kg woman, is to be given desipramine for depression. She has no other significant medical history and takes acetaminophen or ibuprofen rarely for headaches. Describe a reasonable starting dose and schedule for increasing her maintenance regimen.*

Because the bioavailability and intrinsic hepatic clearance of TCAs varies over a wide range, most clinicians start therapy with conservative doses in a divided daily schedule. Doses are increased only after the initial dose has achieved steady state and side effects can be evaluated. Because A.R. has no other concurrent illnesses or medications that would be expected to alter her TCA metabolism, a starting desipramine dose of 25 mg twice daily is reasonable. Given the expected half-life of ≈20 hours, steady state should be achieved in approximately 4 days; however, most clinicians would probably wait 5 to 7 days before considering an increase in her maintenance schedule. Although the plasma concentrations of desipramine can be expected to plateau relatively quickly, full therapeutic effects will not be evident for several weeks. If at the end of the first week of therapy A.R. is experiencing no significant side effects, the dose would probably be incrementally increased to a total daily dose of 150 mg, even though the full therapeutic benefit from the initial dose is unlikely to be evident. Maintenance doses are increased before the full therapeutic effect is achieved because an excessively long titration period would accrue if the interval between dose escalation were a month or more. If A.R. begins to experience significant side effects from her desipramine (e.g., central nervous system depression or anticholinergic side effects), future dose increases would probably be withheld. With time, these side effects may diminish somewhat, once again permitting an increase in the daily dose if required.

Question #2. *After 3 weeks of titration, A.R. has been stabilized on 150 mg/day of desipramine for 1 week. She has relatively few side effects, but her depression has improved only minimally. Would plasma levels of desipramine be useful? What would one expect the average steady-state desipramine concentration to be?*

One would not expect to see full therapeutic effects of TCAs within 3 weeks of initiating therapy. Some clinicians believe that early plasma concentration monitoring may help to identify those patients with low plasma concentrations and therefore at higher risk for therapeutic failure. Depending on the severity of A.R.'s depression, one approach would be to continue her current regimen for another few weeks. If a satisfactory response is not obtained, the dose could be increased to ≈200 mg/day in an attempt to achieve adequate control of her depression. It would not be irrational, however, to obtain a plasma concentration from A.R. now to determine if it is anywhere near the therapeutic range (100 to 250 μg/L). If her plasma concentration is low and compliance could be assured, it would be logical to escalate her dose at this time. This saves waiting the additional 3 weeks to evaluate the full therapeutic response and diminishes the total time required to achieve optimal dose titration.

The expected average steady-state desipramine concentrations can be calculated using Equation 13.1.

$$\text{Css ave} = \frac{(S)(F)(\text{Dose}/\tau)}{Cl}$$

Substituting 1.0 and 0.4 for S and F, respectively; 39 L/hr for Cl (0.6 L/kg/hr × 65 kg); and 150,000 μg/24 hr for dose/τ, a value of 64 μg/L (ng/mL) is estimated.

$$\text{Css ave} = \frac{(S)(F)(Dose/\tau)}{Cl}$$

$$= \frac{(1)(0.4)(150,000 \ \mu g/24 \ hr)}{39 \ L/hr}$$

$$= \frac{(2,500 \ \mu g/hr)}{39 \ L/hr}$$

$$= 64.1 \ \mu g/L$$

Question #3. *S.U., a 68-year-old, 70-kg man, is in good health following a mild myocardial infarction (MI) 2 years ago. He has been treated intermittently for the past 20 years for endogenous depression and is now to start taking nortriptyline. His most frequent complaint has been a general lack of interest in his usual activities. What would be a reasonable starting dose? Would plasma concentration monitoring be useful?*

S.U.'s age and history of cardiac disease place him at higher risk for tricyclic toxicity than other patients.[34,35] Therefore, he should be started on the lowest available dose (10 to 25 mg/day). Even though these low doses are unlikely to result in a therapeutic response, concern for both the cardiovascular and other side effects in the elderly is sufficient to warrant caution. Most clinicians would carefully evaluate S.U. weekly and, if no side effects are observed (e.g., changes in visual acuity, dry mouth, orthostatic hypotension, cardiac arrhythmias), increase the dose by approximately 10 to 25 mg until he is stabilized on a dose of 50 to 75 mg/day. If S.U. has not responded adequately after a sufficient time interval and there are no obvious side effects, it will be necessary to decide whether a further increase in dose is appropriate. Many clinicians feel that the elderly and patients with preexisting cardiac disease are candidates for therapeutic drug level monitoring. Thus, it might be appropriate to obtain a plasma nortriptyline level at this point. If the plasma concentrations are low and an adequate therapeutic response has been attained, the dose should not be increased. If, however, low concentrations are associated with a poor therapeutic response, a further escalation of the dose is probably warranted. If nortriptyline concentrations are within the usual therapeutic range (50 to 150 µg/L) and there is an inadequate therapeutic response, a decision to increase the dose would be difficult. As an alternative, a drug with a lower toxicity profile could be considered.

Question #4. *O.N., a 38-year-old, 60-kg woman, is being titrated on increasing doses of desipramine and, for the past month, has been receiving 150 mg at bedtime. In the past she has complained of dry mouth; lately she does not feel this is a problem and has no other symptoms that might be considered side effects of desipramine. She takes no other concurrent medication except for acetaminophen* *occasionally and smokes one pack of cigarettes per day. Estimate her desipramine concentration.*

To calculate O.N.'s steady-state desipramine concentration, it will first be necessary to select a pharmacokinetic model. The average steady-state desipramine concentration can be calculated by using Equation 13.1 below.

$$\text{Css ave} = \frac{(S)(F)(Dose/\tau)}{Cl}$$

When the appropriate values are inserted, S = 1.0, F = 0.4, Dose/τ = 150,000 μg/24 hr, and Cl = 36 L/hr (0.6 L/kg/hr $\times$ 60 kg), an average expected steady-state concentration of $\approx$70 μg/L (ng/mL) is calculated.

$$\text{Css ave} = \frac{(S)(F)(Dose/\tau)}{Cl}$$

$$= \frac{(1)(0.4)(150,000 \ \mu g/24 \ hr)}{36 \ L/hr}$$

$$= \frac{(2,500 \ \mu g/hr)}{36 \ L/hr}$$

$$= 69.44 \ \mu g/L$$

Because the expected half-life of desipramine is $\approx$20 hours and the dosing interval is 24 hours, the continuous infusion model is not appropriate. The intermittent steady-state bolus dose model is appropriate when a non–sustained-release product is used and absorption occurs over a short period relative to the drug half-life.

$$\text{Css min} = \frac{\dfrac{(S)(F)(Dose)}{V}}{1 - e^{-K\tau}}(e^{-K\tau}) \qquad \text{[Eq. 13.2]}$$

By inserting the appropriate parameters as listed above, as well as the usual V of 1200 L (20 L/kg $\times$ 60 kg), K of 0.0347 hr^{-1}, as calculated from Equation 13.3:

$$K = \frac{0.693}{t\frac{1}{2}} \qquad \text{[Eq. 13.3]}$$

$$= \frac{0.693}{20 \text{ hr}}$$

$$= 0.0347 \text{ hr}^{-1}$$

and τ of 24 hours, the predicted steady-state trough concentration would be $\approx$40 μg/L.

$$\text{Css min} = \frac{\dfrac{(S)(F)(Dose)}{V}}{1 - e^{-K\tau}}(e^{-K\tau})$$

$$= \frac{\dfrac{(1)(0.4)(150,000 \ \mu g)}{1,200 \text{ L}}}{1 - e^{-(0.0347 \text{ hr}^{-1})(24 \text{ hr})}}(e^{-(0.0347 \text{ hr}^{-1})(24 \text{ hr})})$$

$$= \frac{50 \ \mu g/L}{(1 - 0.435)}(0.435)$$

$$= 38.4 \ \mu g/L$$

Although there are differences between the calculated average steady-state and trough concentrations, they are somewhat similar. If the measured concentrations differ from the predicted levels, it will be difficult to explain. For example, if a measured trough concentration is reported to be 60 μg/L, one could revise the bioavailability, clearance, or volume of distribution since all these parameters can vary significantly. However, while V is a variable, it would require an exceedingly large V to increase the trough concentration to 60 μg/L when the average concentration is expected to be 69.4 μg/L (see Part I: Interpretation of Plasma Drug Concentrations, Sensitivity Analysis and Bayesian Analysis). Therefore, the most common approach would be to adjust the clearance value, because this parameter is thought to be more variable than either bioavailability or volume of distribution for most of the TCAs. However, hepatic clearance and the first-pass effect are the predominant reasons for the low bioavailability; thus, if a patient has a lower-than-average clearance, one should anticipate an increase in bioavailability.

Question #5. *O.N. did not respond well to her therapy, and a trough desipramine level was obtained. The laboratory reported a value of 68 ng/mL (µg/L). Because she is not responding, the physician plans to increase O.N.'s desipramine concentration to 100 to 150 ng/mL. What dose adjustment is likely to achieve this goal?*

One approach is to calculate a new set of pharmacokinetic parameters as described in Part I: Interpretation of Plasma Drug Concentrations: Choosing a Model for Revision of Clearance at Steady State. As outlined, the peak concentration would first be estimated by adding the observed trough concentration to the expected change associated with the dose.

$$\text{Css max} = [\text{Css min}] + \left[\frac{(S)(F)(Dose)}{V} \right] \qquad \text{[Eq. 13.4]}$$

Again, by substituting the appropriate values, a maximum concentration of approximately 118 µg/L can be calculated.

$$\text{Css max} = [\text{Css min}] + \left[\frac{(S)(F)(Dose)}{V} \right]$$

$$= [68\ \mu g/L] + \left[\frac{(1)(0.4)(150,000\ \mu g)}{1,200\ L} \right]$$

$$= 118\ \mu g/L$$

Using Equation 13.5 below, the revised elimination rate constant (K) of 0.023 hr^{-1} can be calculated:

$$K = \frac{\ln\left(\frac{\text{Css max}}{\text{Css min}}\right)}{\tau} \qquad \text{[Eq. 13.5]}$$

$$= \frac{\ln\left(\frac{118\ \mu g/L}{68\ \mu g/L}\right)}{24\ hr}$$

$$= 0.023\ hr^{-1}$$

and using Equation 13.6 the K value of 0.023 hr^{-1} corresponds to a half-life of approximately 30 hours.

$$t\frac{1}{2} = \frac{0.693}{K}$$ [Eq. 13.6]

$$= \frac{0.693}{0.023 \text{ hr}^{-1}}$$

$$= 30 \text{ hr}$$

These data can then be used along with Equation 13.7 and the assumed values of S, F, and V to calculate a dose. Assuming the Css min is a trough value, τ would be 24 hours and the calculated dose would be $\approx$300 mg.

$$\text{Dose} = \frac{(\text{Css min})(V)(1 - e^{-K\tau})}{(S)(F)(e^{-K\tau})}$$ [Eq. 13.7]

$$= \frac{(150 \text{ } \mu\text{g/L})(1,200 \text{ L})(1 - e^{-(0.023 \text{ hr}^{-1})(24 \text{ hr})})}{(1)(0.4)(e^{-(0.023 \text{ hr}^{-1})(24 \text{ hr})})}$$

$$= \frac{(180,000 \text{ } \mu\text{g})(1 - 0.576)}{(1)(0.4)(0.576)}$$

$$= 331,250 \text{ } \mu\text{g or} \approx 300 \text{ mg}$$

It is unlikely that the maintenance dose would be increased by this amount, because it is a large percentage increase in dose (although consistent with the desired increase in plasma concentration) and because the new dose is approaching or exceeding the maximum recommended dose. While it may be necessary to increase O.N.'s dose to the range of 300 mg/day to achieve a plasma concentration of 150 µg/L, most clinicians would probably increase O.N.'s maintenance dose by approximately 25 to 50 mg/day and observe her for clinical improvement and side effects as described previously. This step-wise approach is more rational because some patients respond at lower plasma concentrations and the chances of side effects are substantial with larger doses.

Question #6. *N.H., a 27-year-old man, has been stabilized on imipramine 100 mg/day (50 mg twice) with good response to his depression. Two weeks ago his physician prescribed 100 mg capsules (Tofranil PM) at bedtime to simplify the regimen. Unfortunately, N.H. continued to take two capsules a day (2 × 100 mg) at bedtime and now presents with confusion, dry mouth, and blurred vision. Would a drug plasma level be useful to establish a course of action for N.H. and an apparent imipramine toxicity?*

Some clinicians believe that cases of suspected tricyclic toxicity are indications for obtaining plasma concentrations. Plasma levels help the clinician distinguish tricyclic-induced dementia from other potential causes.[36,37] However, the relationship between TCA concentrations and side effects is variable and cannot be relied on as an absolute indicator. Many clinicians believe that any plasma concentration > 500 μg/L is reason to withhold or reduce the maintenance dose and that concentrations > 1,000 μg/L warrant withholding the drug and monitoring the patient for cardiovascular side effects.[20] In N.H.'s case, the diagnosis is not in question; therefore, the use of a plasma concentration for this purpose is not warranted. If an imipramine plasma concentration could be rapidly obtained, it might provide the clinician with enough information to determine if N.H.'s side effects could be treated in an outpatient setting. This would also depend on the severity of the side effects. One could also obtain a plasma concentration for medical-legal reasons, even if it will not alter the immediate care of the patient.

REFERENCES

1. Hammer W, Sjoqvist F. Plasma levels of monomethylated tricyclic antidepressants during treatment with imipramine-like compounds. Life Sci 1967;6:1895–1903.

2. Kragh-Sorensen P, et al. Self-inhibiting action of nortriptyline's antidepressant effect at high plasma levels. Psychopharmacology 1976;45:305–314.

3. Perry PJ, et al. Two prospective dosing methods for nortriptyline. Clin Pharmacokinet 1984;9:555–563.

4. Gram LF, et al. Drug level monitoring in psychopharmacology: usefulness and clinical problems, with special reference to tricyclic antidepressants. Ther Drug Monit 1982; 4:17–25.

5. Piafsky KM, Borga O. Plasma binding of basic drugs II: importance of α_1-acid glycoprotein for interindividual variation. Clin Pharmacol Ther 1977;22:545–549.

6. Pike E, Skuterud B. Plasma binding variations of amitriptyline and nortriptyline. Clin Pharmacol Ther 1982;32:228–234.

7. Freilich DL, Giardina E-GV. Imipramine binding to α_1-acid glycoprotein in normal subjects and cardiac patients. Clin Pharmacol Ther 1984;35:670–674.

8. Thummel KE, Shen DD. Appendix II: design and optimization of dosage regimen: pharmacokinetic data. In: Hardman JG, et al., eds. Goodman and Gilman's The Pharmacologic Basis of Therapeutics. 10th Ed. New York: McGraw-Hill, Medical Publishing Division, 2001:1917–2023.

9. Potter WZ, et al. Binding of imipramine to plasma protein and to brain tissue: relationship to CSF tricyclic levels in man. Psychopharmacology 1979;63:187–192.

10. Weder HJ, Bickel MH. Interactions of drugs with proteins. I. Binding of tricyclic thymoleptics to human and bovine plasma proteins. J Pharm Sci 1970;59:1505–1507.

11. Pollock BG, Perel JM. Tricyclic antidepressants: contemporary issues for therapeutic practice. Can J Psychiatry 1989;34:609–671.

12. Jarvis MR. Clinical pharmacokinetics of tricyclic antidepressant overdose. Psychopharmacol Bull 1991;27:541–550.

13. Nelson JC, et al. Desipramine plasma concentration and antidepressant response. Arch Gen Psychiatry 1982;39:1419–1422.

14. Friedel RO, et al. Desipramine plasma levels and clinical response in depressed outpatients. Commun Psychopharmacol 1979;2:81–87.

15. Costa D, et al. Endogenous depression and imipramine levels in the blood. Psychopharmacology 1980;70:291–294.

16. Glassman AH, et al. Tricyclic antidepressant blood level measurements and clinical outcome. Am J Psychiatry 1985;142:155–163.

17. Breyer-Pfaff U, et al. Validation of a therapeutic plasma level range in amitriptyline treatment of depression. J Clin Psycholpharmacol 1989;9:116–121.

18. Preskorn SH, Irwin HA. Toxicity of tricyclic antidepressants-kinetics, mechanism, intervention: a review. J Clin Psychiatry 1982;43:151–156.

19. Jorgensen A, Hanson V. Pharmacokinetics of amitriptyline infused intravenously in man. Eur J Clin Pharmacol 1976;10:337–341.

20. DeVane CL, Jarecke CR. Cyclic antidepressants. In: Evans WE et al., eds. Applied Pharmacokinetics: Principles of Therapeutic Drug Monitoring. 3rd Ed. Vancouver: Applied Therapeutics, 1992:33:4.

21. DeVane CL, et al. Desipramine and 2-hydroxy-desipramine pharmacokinetics in normal volunteers. Eur J Clin Pharmacol 1981;19:61–64.

22. Sutfin TA, et al. The analysis and disposition of imipramine and its active metabolites in man. Psychopharmacology 1984;82:310–317.

23. Alexanderson B. Pharmacokinetics of desmethylimipramine and nortriptyline in man after single and multiple oral doses: a cross-over study. Eur J Clin Pharmacol 1972;5:1–10.

24. Randup A, Braestrup C. Uptake inhibition of biogenic amines by newer antidepressant drugs: relevance to the dopamine hypothesis of depression. Psychopharmacology 1977;53:309–314.

25. Potter WZ, Calil HM. Metabolites in tricyclic antidepressants. Biological activity and clinical implications. In: Usdin E, et al., eds. Clinical Pharmacology in Psychiatry. New York: Elsevier, 1981:311–324.

26. Abernethy DR, et al. Imipramine-cimetidine interaction: impairment of clearance and enhanced absolute bioavailability. J Pharmacol Exp Ther 1984;229:702–705.

27. Ciraulo DA, Shader RL. Fluoxetine drug-drug interactions. J Clin Psychopharmacol 1990;10:48–50, 213–217.

28. Nelson JC, Jatlow PI. Nonlinear desipramine kinetics: prevalence and importance. Clin Pharmacol Ther 1987;41:666–670.

29. Dawling S, et al. Nortriptyline therapy in elderly patients: dosage prediction after single dose pharmacokinetic study. Eur J Pharmacol 1980;18:147–150.

30. Potter WZ, et al. Single-dose kinetics predict steady-state concentrations of imipramine and desipramine. Arch Gen Psychiatry 1980;37:314–320.

31. Cooper TB, et al. Prediction of steady-state plasma and saliva levels of desmethylimipramine using a single dose, single time point procedure. Psychopharmacology 1981;74:115–121.

32. Preskorn SH. Pharmacokinetics of antidepressants: why and how they are relevant to treatment. J Clin Psychiatry 1993;54(Suppl):14–34.

33. Linder MW, Keck PE. Standards of laboratory practice: antidepressant drug monitoring. Clin Chem 1998;44(5):1073–1084.

34. Nelson JC, et al. Major adverse reactions during desipramine treatment. Arch Gen Psychiatry 1982;39:1055–1061.

35. Glassman AH, Bigger JT. Cardiovascular effects of therapeutic doses of tricyclic antidepressants. Arch Gen Psychiatry 1981;38:815–820.

36. Crome P, Braithwaite RA. Relationship between clinical features of tricyclic antidepressant poisoning and plasma concentrations in children. Arch Dis Child 1978;53:902–905.

37. Pederson OL, et al. Overdosage of antidepressants: clinical and pharmacokinetic aspects. Eur J Clin Pharmacol 1982;23:513–521.

14

VALPROIC ACID

Michelle M. Wheeler and Michael E. Winter

Valproic acid is currently used to treat various seizure disorders, to prevent migraines, and to treat a variety of psychiatric disorders such as bipolar disorder, anxiety, depression, psychosis, substance-abuse withdrawal, and other behavioral disturbances.[1-4] The mechanism of action for valproic acid is uncertain; it purportedly increases the brain concentrations of gamma aminobutyric acid (GABA), an inhibitory neurotransmitter in the central nervous system. The usual dose for prevention of migraines is 500 mg daily for 7 days followed by 1000 mg daily thereafter.[5] The extended-release version (Depakote ER) is limited to this indication because of a lack of experience in patients when used for seizure control.[4] The usual initial dose of valproic acid for treatment of seizures is 15 mg/kg/day. Many patients receive doses of 30 mg/kg/day, and in a few cases daily doses as high as 60 mg/kg/day have been used.[1-3] Valproic acid is interesting from a pharmacokinetic point of view for several reasons. First, valproic acid is known to influence the pharmacokinetics of a number of other drugs. The metabolism of phenobarbital and the major metabolite of carbamazepine appear to be inhibited by valproic acid.[1-3,6,7] The metabolism of phenytoin also appears to be inhibited; however, this interaction is difficult to evaluate accurately because valproic acid also displaces phenytoin from its binding sites on serum albumin.[8,9] In addition, valproic acid is highly bound to serum albumin, and at therapeutic plasma concentrations, saturates plasma protein binding sites.[1-4,10]

THERAPEUTIC AND TOXIC PLASMA CONCENTRATIONS

Valproic acid's therapeutic range for seizure control is 50 to 100 mg/L;[1-3,11] however, valproic acid concentrations in excess of 100 mg/L are often required in patients with partial seizures. When used in the treatment of bipolar psychiatric disorders the usually accepted therapeutic range is 50 to 125 mg/L.[12-14] There is some evidence that the therapeutic effect of valproic acid lags behind the attainment of steady-state plasma concentrations. This observation is consistent with the fact that some patients continue to experience persistent side effects for several days after the drug has been discontinued.[15] In most cases, the dose-limiting side effects are gastrointestinal (e.g., nausea, vomiting, diarrhea, and abdominal cramps). Sedation and drowsiness do occur but may, in part, be due to the interaction between valproic acid and other concomitant anticonvulsant therapy. Other infrequent side effects include alopecia, a benign essential tremor, thrombocytopenia, pancreatitis, hyperammonemic encephalopathy, and hepatotoxicity. Although not clearly established, elevated levels of valproic acid have been associated with hepatotoxicity.[1-4,16,17] Whereas the hepatotoxicity associated with valproic acid is rare, it is a serious complication of therapy and should be considered in any patient with elevated liver enzymes. Patients at higher risk include those who are young, developmentally delayed, have metabolic disorders, and are receiving polyanticonvulsant therapy. Children younger than 2 years of age have the greatest risk of hepatotoxicity, especially when they are taking other anticonvulsants along with valproic acid. It is believed that hepatotoxicity from valproic acid is due to low concentrations of l-carnitine in the body. The use of intravenous l-carnitine has been shown to halt the progression of liver toxicity once it occurs and should be considered when patients are diagnosed with liver toxicity.[18,19]

A fixed dose is often prescribed when extended-release valproic acid is used in the treatment of migraine headaches.[4,5] Therefore, plasma levels of valproic acid are not routinely recommended for these patients. However, some clinicians will monitor patients receiving long-term therapy and adjust the dose of valproic acid to achieve the same concentration range as is used in the treatment of seizure disorders.

KEY PARAMETERS: Valproic Acid	
Therapeutic Plasma Concentration	50–100 mg/L

F
    Extended release tablets
    All other forms
	
	80–90%
	100%

S	1.0
V[a]	0.14 (0.1–0.5) L/kg

Cl[a,b]
    Children
    Adults
	
	13 mL/kg/hr
	8 mL/kg/hr

t½
    Children
    Adults
	
	6–8 hours
	10–12 hours

[a]V and Cl may be increased in patients with end-stage renal disease, hypoalbuminemia, or valproic acid levels > 50 mg/L because of altered plasma protein binding.
[b]Cl may be in increased in patients receiving other anticonvulsant drug therapy.

BIOAVAILABILITY (F)

Both sodium valproate and valproic acid appear to be rapidly and completely absorbed. Plasma valproate concentrations usually peak 1 to 3 hours after oral administration when fasting.[20] Meals, however, appear to slow the rate of absorption of valproic acid; serum concentrations peak as late as 6 to 8 hours after oral administration when taken with food.[21] The intravenous formulation has a more consistent peak which occurs at the end of the 1-hour infusion. The amount of sodium valproate in the oral solution formulation and the amount of valproic acid in the capsule preparation are labeled in mg of valproic acid. Consequently, both the bioavailability (F) and the salt form (S) are 1.0 for the intravenous product, oral solution, and capsules, with the exception of the extended-release tablets for which the bioavailability is 80% to 90%.[1-4,22]

Enteric-coated valproic acid tablets are not sustained in their release characteristics, but absorption is delayed and is significantly influenced by the timing of meals.[23] The bead-filled capsule (Depakote Sprinkles) does appear to have a more sustained plasma profile and more closely approximates a continuous infusion model.[24] The extended-release tablets also approximate the continuous infusion model. Valproic acid oral solution has been diluted with equal parts water and administered rectally with apparently good absorption.[25]

VOLUME OF DISTRIBUTION (V)

The apparent volume of distribution for valproic acid is variable and ranges from 0.1 to 0.5 L/kg.[1-4,22,26,27] Alterations in plasma protein binding (e.g., in patients with low serum albumin or end-stage renal disease) as well as the capacity-limited binding to plasma protein by this drug account for the variable volume of distribution of valproic acid. Valproic acid's binding to serum albumin appears to become saturated when valproic acid concentrations exceed 50 mg/L.[28] For most patients with valproic acid concentrations in the range of 25 to 50 mg/L, an average volume of distribution of 0.14 L/kg is a reasonable value to use for pharmacokinetic calculations, assuming the patient has normal serum albumin concentrations and normal renal function.

CLEARANCE (Cl)

Valproic acid is almost entirely eliminated from the body through hepatic metabolism; less than 5% of the drug is eliminated by the renal route.[1-4,10,22,26] The usual clearance values for valproic acid are 6 to 10 mL/kg/hr with an average value of 8 mL/kg/hr. In pediatric patients and in patients receiving additional antiepileptic drugs, the clearance values may be substantially higher (10 to 13 mL/kg/hr).[29] In addition, capacity-limited plasma protein binding may result in nonlinear changes in the plasma concentration of valproic acid, especially when concentrations exceed 50 mg/L. As long as the trough concentrations are ≤ 50 mg/L, the changes in trough concentrations should be reasonably proportional to the dose. Therefore, a one-compartment linear model can be used to describe the valproic trough concentrations for most patients in the clinical setting. When the intravenous dosage form is administered as an intermittent infusion, there is likely to be more fluctuation in the plasma concentrations because of a shorter input time for the intravenous versus oral routes of absorption. For that reason the dosing interval should not exceed 6 hours unless it can be clearly documented that the peak and trough concentrations are acceptable with more extended dosing intervals.

HALF-LIFE (t½)

The half-life for valproic acid ranges from 4 to 17 hours, with an average value of 10 to 12 hours. In children and patients receiving other antiepileptic drugs, the half-life of valproate is reduced. Because the usual half-life is relatively short, valproic acid plasma concentrations appear to plateau within 24 to 48 hours after therapy is initiated. Loading doses are usually not given. The short half-life, coupled with the dosing interval of 8 to 12 hours, results in wide fluctuations in plasma concentrations within a dosing interval.[1-4,10,22,27,30,31]

TIME TO SAMPLE

Due to wide fluctuations in plasma valproate concentrations within a dosing interval, monitoring both the peak and trough concentrations of this drug would seem to be desirable. Nevertheless, only trough concentrations are routinely monitored because of the uncertainty about the time at which peak plasma concentrations will occur and the difficulty evaluating significantly elevated valproic acid concentrations given its capacity-limited plasma protein binding. In general, valproic acid concentrations in plasma are monitored within 2 to 4 days following 1) initiation of therapy, 2) change in a dosing regimen, or 3) addition of other antiepileptic drugs to the patient's regimen. Valproic acid concentrations are also measured whenever the patient's clinical course has changed (e.g., a decrease in seizure control or laboratory or physical findings consistent with valproic acid toxicity). As stated previously, there is some evidence that even though valproic acid concentrations may plateau relatively rapidly, increased therapeutic effects may continue to be observed for some time following the achievement of steady-state valproic acid concentrations.

Question #1. *A.H., an 8-year-old, 25-kg male, is receiving 250 mg of valproic acid every 12 hours for absence seizures. Although seizure frequency has declined with this therapy, he is still experiencing one to two absence seizures per day. A.H. has experienced no obvious side*

*effects from the valproic acid therapy and has normal renal and he-
patic function. What is the expected trough concentration for A.H.
with his current regimen?*

First, the clearance for A.H. can be calculated by using an average
valproic acid clearance for children of 13 mL/kg/hr. Then, A.H.'s volume
of distribution can be calculated by using the average volume of distribution value of 0.14 L/kg (see Key Parameters: Valproic Acid). According to
the calculations shown below, A.H. would have a valproic acid clearance
of 0.325 L/hr and a volume of distribution of 3.5 L.

$$Cl = (13 \text{ mL/kg/hr})(25 \text{ kg})$$

$$= 325 \text{ mL/hr } or \text{ 0.325 L/hr}$$

$$V = (0.14 \text{ L/kg})(25 \text{ kg})$$

$$= 3.5 \text{ L}$$

Using these values for clearance and volume of distribution,
Equations 14.1 and 14.2 can be used as follows to calculate A.H.'s elimination rate constant of 0.093 hr^{-1} and the corresponding half-life of 7.5
hours.

$$K = \frac{Cl}{V} \qquad \text{[Eq. 14.1]}$$

$$= \frac{0.325 \text{ L/hr}}{3.5 \text{ L}}$$

$$= 0.093 \text{ hr}^{-1}$$

$$t\frac{1}{2} = \frac{0.693}{K} \qquad \text{[Eq. 14.2]}$$

$$= \frac{0.693}{0.093 \text{ hr}^{-1}}$$

$$= 7.5 \text{ hr}$$

Assuming steady state has been achieved and the salt form and
bioavailability are 1.0, Equation 14.3 can be used to calculate the expected
steady-state trough concentration of ≈35 mg/L as follows:

$$\text{Css min} = \frac{\dfrac{(S)(F)(Dose)}{V}}{(1 - e^{-KT})} e^{-KT} \qquad \text{[Eq. 14.3]}$$

$$= \frac{\dfrac{(1)(1)(250 \text{ mg})}{3.5 \text{ L}} e^{-(0.093 \text{ hr}^{-1})(12 \text{ hr})}}{(1 - e^{-(0.093 \text{ hr}^{-1})(12 \text{ hr})})}$$

$$= 34.8 \text{ mg/L or } \approx 35 \text{ mg/L}$$

Question #2. *A.H. had a measured trough concentration of 25 mg/L. Because of the inadequate seizure control and the lack of apparent side effects, it is decided to increase the trough concentration to 50 mg/L. What dose will be required to achieve the target trough concentration of 50 mg/L if the dosing interval is decreased from every 12 hours to every 8 hours?*

If the dosing interval had remained unchanged (12 hours), the trough concentration would have changed in proportion to the maintenance dose. The trough concentration will not be directly proportional to the dose, however, because the dosing interval is to be decreased. Therefore, it will be necessary to estimate A.H.'s apparent pharmacokinetic parameters. If the serum concentration of valproic acid of 25 mg/L represents a steady-state trough value, Equation 14.4 can be used to estimate a peak concentration of $\approx$96 mg/L as shown below.

$$\text{Css max} = [\text{Css min}] + \left[\frac{(S)(F)(Dose)}{V} \right] \qquad \text{[Eq. 14.4]}$$

$$= [25 \text{ mg/L}] + \left[\frac{(1)(1)(250 \text{ mg})}{3.5 \text{ L}} \right]$$

$$= [25 \text{ mg/L}] + [71.4 \text{ mg/L}]$$

$$= 96.4 \text{ mg/L}$$

By substituting the peak concentration of 96.4 mg/L for C_1, the measured trough concentration of 25 mg/L for C_2, and the dosing interval of 12 hours for t, Equation 14.5 can be used to estimate an elimination rate constant (K) of 0.112 hr^{-1}.

$$K = \frac{\ln\left(\dfrac{C_1}{C_2}\right)}{t}$$ [Eq. 14.5]

$$= \frac{\ln\left(\dfrac{96.4 \text{ mg/L}}{25 \text{ mg/L}}\right)}{12 \text{ hr}}$$

$$= 0.112 \text{ hr}^{-1}$$

This K value can be used in Equation 14.2 to estimate a half-life of 6.2 hours as follows:

$$t\frac{1}{2} = \frac{0.693}{K}$$

$$= \frac{0.693}{0.112 \text{ hr}^{-1}}$$

$$= 6.2 \text{ hr}$$

The assumed volume of distribution of 3.5 L and the calculated elimination rate constant of 0.112 hr^{-1} then can be used in Equation 14.6 to calculate a clearance of 0.39 L/hr (15.6 mL/kg/hr).

$$Cl = (K)(V)$$ [Eq. 14.6]

$$= (0.112 \text{ hr}^{-1})(3.5 \text{ L}) = 0.392 \text{ L/hr}$$

Equation 14.3 for Css min:

$$\text{Css min} = \frac{\dfrac{(S)(F)(\text{Dose})}{V}}{(1 - e^{-K\tau})} e^{-K\tau}$$

can be rearranged so that the dose required to achieve a desired trough concentration can be calculated.

$$\text{Dose} = \frac{(\text{Css min})(V)(1 - e^{-K\tau})}{(S)(F)(e^{-K\tau})}$$ [Eq. 14.7]

By making the appropriate substitutions for the steady-state drug level, elimination rate constant, dosing interval, and volume of distribution, the dose required to achieve a trough concentration of 50 mg/L would be ≈250 mg given every 8 hours:

$$Dose = \frac{(50 \text{ mg/L})(3.5 \text{ L})(1 - e^{-(0.112 \text{ hr}^{-1})(8 \text{ hr})})}{(1)(1)(e^{-(0.112 \text{ hr}^{-1})(8 \text{ hr})})}$$

$$= 253 \text{ mg or} \approx 250 \text{ mg}$$

The actual measured trough concentration, however, may not coincide with the calculations for a number of reasons. First, the volume of distribution of 3.5 L (0.14 L/kg) is an assumed value and may not correspond to A.H.'s actual volume of distribution. Second, the target concentration of 50 mg/L is approaching the range where capacity-limited plasma protein binding may be observed. If the plasma protein binding sites become saturated, the measured or total drug concentration may be lower than calculated. Sampling at the trough concentration helps to avoid this capacity-limited binding problem, because the measured drug levels are at their lowest concentration and are least likely to be at a concentration range where protein binding can become saturated.

Question #3. *S.N., a 23-year-old, 70-kg woman, is receiving phenobarbital 60 mg BID and phenytoin 300 mg QD. The steady-state plasma drug concentrations are 18 mg/L for phenobarbital and 10 mg/L for phenytoin. Because of poor seizure control, valproic acid 500 mg every 8 hours was added to this drug treatment regimen. Two months later, S.N. complained of increased drowsiness. At that time, plasma drug concentrations were measured and reported as follows: phenobarbital 30 mg/L, phenytoin 6 mg/L, and valproic acid 75 mg/L. How can the increased phenobarbital concentration and decreased phenytoin concentration be explained?*

Valproic acid decreases the clearance of phenobarbital by approximately 40%.[7,32] The increase in plasma phenobarbital concentration from 18 mg/L to 30 mg/L 60 days after valproic acid was added is consistent with a 40% decrease in the phenobarbital clearance. If the original steady-state phenobarbital concentration of 18 mg/L is desired, the daily phenobarbital dose should be decreased by about 40%.

The decline in the plasma phenytoin concentration from 10 mg/L to 6 mg/L is probably the result of competition for plasma protein binding between valproic acid and phenytoin. In patients with normal serum albumin concentrations and normal renal function, valproic acid (at a concentration of ≈70 mg/L) produces a 30% to 40% decline in phenytoin plasma concentrations.[28,33,34] This acute decline in the plasma concentration of phenytoin is due to a decrease in the bound concentration. The unbound or therapeutically active plasma phenytoin concentration appears to remain unchanged because any bound phenytoin that is displaced re-equilibrates with the large tissue compartment. Since the tissue space is large, the increased tissue concentrations will be negligible (also see

Phenytoin: Alterations in Plasma Protein Binding, Drug Displacement). There is less well-documented evidence that chronic valproic acid therapy increases the unbound phenytoin concentration; this may be caused by inhibition of phenytoin metabolism. To minimize the impact of competitive plasma protein binding on the assessment of drug concentrations, both phenytoin and valproic acid samples should be obtained when valproic acid concentrations are at their lowest (i.e., at trough or just before the next dose).

Question #4. *C.B., a 10-year-old, 32-kg female, is receiving valproic acid sprinkles 250 mg (2 × 125 mg) PO every 8 hours for her seizure disorder. Calculate her valproic acid level at steady state.*

Because C.B. is receiving valproic acid as the sprinkle product, one would not expect a great deal of fluctuation within the dosing interval. For this reason, Equation 14.8 is a reasonable model to use to predict her valproic acid concentration.

$$\text{Css ave} = \frac{(S)(F)(Dose/\tau)}{Cl} \qquad \text{[Eq. 14.8]}$$

Assuming the average value of 13 mL/kg/hr for clearance of valproic acid, C.B.'s clearance would be 0.416 L/hr:

$$Cl = (13 \text{ mL/kg/hr})(32 \text{ kg})$$

$$= 416 \text{ mL/hr } or \text{ } 0.416 \text{ L/hr}$$

Assuming S and F to be 1.0 and inserting the appropriate dose, dosing interval, and assumed clearance, C.B.'s valproic acid concentration should be ≈75 mg/L.

$$= \frac{(1)(1)(250 \text{ mg/8 hr})}{0.416 \text{ L/hr}}$$

$$= 75.1 \text{ mg/L}$$

This predicted valproic acid concentration is within the usually accepted therapeutic range of 50 to 100 mg/L. However, plasma concentration monitoring would be useful to confirm this prediction if satisfactory therapeutic effects are not achieved or toxicities occur.

Question #5. *C.B. comes back in 3 weeks and is to undergo elective surgery and will not be able to take anything orally. The doctors would like to switch her from oral to intravenous valproic acid. Her valproate level at this time is 60 mg/L. Can the doctors use the same* *dosing schedule with the intravenous form as with the oral form? What would be an appropriate intravenous dose and dosing interval?*

The intravenous formulation has only been studied using a dosing interval of 6 hours. C.B. is on an 8-hour schedule using a sustained-release product and has had valproic acid concentrations measured. Pharmacokinetic calculations need to be performed to help guide therapy. One simple approach might be to take the total daily dose (750 mg) and divide it equally into 4 doses to be given every 6 hours. This approach should result in the same Css ave because the dosing rate is the same for both the oral and intravenous regimens. However, with the new intravenous regimen, the drug will be absorbed (infused) over a short time every 6 hours, resulting in a higher Css peak and a lower Css min than her current sustained-release oral regimen.

Another approach might be to use C.B.'s current regimen, which is on a formulation that has little fluctuation within the dosing interval and the measured Css ave of 60 mg/L to calculate C.B's patient specific valproate clearance. Using Equation 14.9, C.B.'s valproic acid clearance of 0.52 L/hr can be calculated.

$$Cl = \frac{(S)(F)(Dose/\tau)}{Css\ ave} \qquad [Eq.\ 14.9]$$

$$= \frac{(1)(1)(250\ mg/8\ hr)}{60\ mg/L}$$

$$= \frac{31.25\ mg/hr}{60\ mg/L}$$

$$= 0.52\ L/hr$$

Using this patient-specific valproate clearance and our average assumed value of 0.14 L/kg for V or 4.5 L for this 32 kg patient, we can calculate the expected elimination rate constant using Equation 14.1

$$K = \frac{Cl}{V}$$

$$= \frac{0.52\ L/hr}{4.5\ L}$$

$$= 0.116\ hr^{-1}$$

and the corresponding $t\frac{1}{2}$ using Equation 14.2.

$$t\tfrac{1}{2} = \frac{0.693}{K}$$

$$= \frac{0.693}{0.116 \text{ hr}^{-1}}$$

$$= 6 \text{ hr}$$

At this point we have two choices. We can choose the usual dosing interval of 6 hours for the intravenous dosage form and a reasonable dose in Equation 14.3 to calculate the expected Css min:

$$\text{Css min} = \frac{\dfrac{(S)(F)(Dose)}{V}}{(1 - e^{-K\tau})} e^{-K\tau}$$

Or use the dosing interval of 6 hours and a target trough concentration in Equation 14.7 to calculate a corresponding dose.

$$\text{Dose} = \frac{(\text{Css min})(V)(1 - e^{-K\tau})}{(S)(F)(e^{-K\tau})}$$

We would use the second approach if our major concern is to ensure that Css min does not fall below our previous Css ave. A dose designed to maintain a Css min of 60 mg/L can be calculated using Equation 14.7. Assuming F and S to be 1, a dosing interval of 6 hours, an elimination rate constant of 0.116 hr^{-1}, and a volume of distribution of 4.5 L, the dose would be calculated as follows:

$$\text{Dose} = \frac{(\text{Css min})(V)(1 - e^{-K\tau})}{(S)(F)(e^{-K\tau})}$$

$$= \frac{(60 \text{ mg/L})(4.5 \text{ L})(1 - e^{-(0.116 \text{ hr}^{-1})(6 \text{ hr})})}{(1)(1)(e^{-(0.116 \text{ hr}^{-1})(6 \text{ hr})})}$$

$$= \frac{(270 \text{ mg})(1 - 0.5)}{(1)(1)(0.5)}$$

$$= 270 \text{ mg}$$

Our calculations indicate that a dose of approximately 270 mg given by the intravenous route would be necessary to maintain a trough concentration of 60 mg/L. We could also estimate the expected peak concentration using Equation 14.4:

$$\text{Css max} = [60 \text{ mg/L}] + \left[\frac{(1)(1)(270 \text{ mg})}{4.5 \text{ L}} \right]$$

$$= [60 \text{ mg/L}] + [60 \text{ mg/L}]$$

$$= 120 \text{ mg/L}$$

The actual concentration at the end of the valproic acid infusion is likely to be greater than 120 mg/L because of the two-compartment modeling that is almost always seen with intravenous drug administration. However, there is no evidence that these transiently elevated concentrations are at equilibrium with the central nervous system; therefore, we do not expect excessive toxicities.

Question #6. *C.B's mother is having migraines and saw a television commercial about the use of valproic acid as prophylactic treatment. She is wondering if it is the same product her daughter uses for seizures and would she have to be monitored in the same manner if she began to take it?*

The valproic acid recommended on television (Depakote ER) has the same active ingredient, but is an extended-release tablet with absorption characteristics that are different from the product her daughter takes. These extended-release tablets are used primarily to treat migraines. Assuming that her neurologist agrees that a trial of valproic acid is warranted, valproic acid levels would not be routinely drawn because the dosing is usually fixed and not guided by serum level measurement. Although some clinicians do adjust valproic acid therapy to achieve the target levels used for seizure disorders, there is little evidence that this approach is superior to the fixed dosage regimen. The standard dose is 500 mg once daily for 1 week, then, if tolerated, increase to 1,000 mg once daily. If either of the doses are not tolerated, the maintenance dose can be decreased. C.B's mother would still require the other laboratory tests that are performed in her daughter's case to monitor the side effects of the drug.

REFERENCES

1. Abbott Laboratories. Depakote (divalproex sodium) delayed-release tablets package insert. North Chicago, IL: Abbott Laboratories, April 2002.
2. Abbott Laboratories. Depacon (valproate sodium) injection package insert. North Chicago, IL: Abbott Laboratories, April 2002.
3. Abbott Laboratories. Depakote (divalproex sodium) sprinkle capsules package insert. North Chicago, IL: Abbott Laboratories, April 2002.
4. Abbott Laboratories. Depakote ER (divalproex sodium) extended-release tablets package insert. North Chicago, IL: Abbott Laboratories, April 2002.
5. Freitag FG, et al. A randomized trial of divalproex sodium extended-release tablets in migraine prophylaxis. Neurology 2002;58:1652–1659.
6. Levy RH, et al. Carbamazepine/valproic acid interaction in man and rhesus monkey. Epilepsia 1984;25:338–345.
7. Patel IH, Levy RH, Cutler RE. Phenobarbital–valproic acid interaction. Clin Pharmacol Ther 1980;27:515–521.
8. Cramer JA, Mattson RH. Valproic acid: in vitro plasma protein binding and interaction with phenytoin. Ther Drug Monit 1979;1:105–116.
9. Haidukewych D, Rodin EA, Zielinski JJ. Derivation and evaluation of an equation for prediction of free phenytoin concentration in patients co-medicated with valproic acid. Ther Drug Monit 1989;11:134–139.

10. Gugler R, Schell A, Eichelbaum M, Froscher W, Schulz HU. Disposition of valproic acid in man. Eur J Clin Pharmacol 1977;12:125–132.

11. Gram L, Flachs H, Wurtz-Jorgensen A, Parnas J, Andersen B. Sodium valproate, serum level and clinical effect in epilepsy: a controlled study. Epilepsia 1979;20:303–311.

12. Stoner SC, Worrel JA, Vlach D, Jones MT, Ramlatchman LV. Retrospective analysis of serum valproate levels and need for an antidepressant drug. Pharmacotherapy 2001;21:850–854.

13. Davis LL, Ryan W, Adinoff B, Petty F. Comprehensive review of the psychiatric uses of valproate. J Clin Psychopharmacol 2000;20:1S–17S.

14. De Leon OA. Antiepileptic drugs for the acute and maintenance treatment of bipolar disorder. Harv Rev Psychiatry 2001;9:209–222.

15. Lockard JS, Levy RH. Valproic acid: reversibly acting drug? Epilepsia 1976;17:477–479.

16. Donat JF, Bocchini JA Jr, Gonzalez E, Schwendimann RN. Valproic acid and fatal hepatitis. Neurology 1979;29:273–274.

17. Suchy FJ, et al. Acute hepatic failure associated with the use of sodium valproate. N Engl J Med 1979;300:962–966.

18. DeVivo DC. Effect of L-carnitine treatment for valproate-induced hepatotoxicity. Neurology 2002;58:507–508.

19. Bohan TP, et al. Effect of L-carnitine treatment for valproate-induced hepatotoxicity. Neurology 2001;56:1405–1409.

20. Klotz U, Antonin KH. Pharmacokinetics and bioavailability of sodium valproate. Clin Pharmacol Ther 1977;21:736–743.

21. Chun AH, Hoffman DJ, Friedmann N, Carrigan PJ. Bioavailability of valproic acid under fasting/nonfasting regimens. J Clin Pharmacol 1980;20:30–36.

22. Abbott Laboratories. Depakene (valproic acid) capsules and syrup package insert. North Chicago, IL: Abbott Laboratories, April 2002.

23. Carrigan PJ, Brinker DR, Cavanaugh JH, Lamm JE, Cloyd JC. Absorption characteristics of a new valproate formulation: divalproex sodium-coated particles in capsules (Depakote Sprinkle). J Clin Pharmacol 1990;30:743–747.

24. Cloyd JC, et al. Comparison of sprinkle versus syrup formulations of valproate for bioavailability, tolerance, and preference. J Pediatr 1992;120:634–638.

25. Cloyd JC, Brundage RC. Valproic acid. In: Taylor WJ, et al. A Text for Clinical Drug Monitoring. Irving: Abbott Laboratories Diagnostics Division, 1986:269–280.

26. Gugler R, von Unruh GE. Clinical pharmacokinetics of valproic acid. Clin Pharmacokinet 1980;5:67–83.

27. Mihaly GW, Vajda FJ, Miles JL, Louis WJ. Single and chronic dose pharmacokinetic studies of sodium valproate in epileptic patients. Eur J Clin Pharmacol 1979;16:23–29.

28. Monks A, Richens A. Effect of single doses of sodium valproate on serum phenytoin levels and protein binding in epileptic patients. Clin Pharmacol Ther 1980;27:89–95.

29. Cloyd JC, Fischer JH, Kriel RL, Kraus DM. Valproic acid pharmacokinetics in children. IV. Effects of age and antiepileptic drugs on protein binding and intrinsic clearance. Clin Pharmacol Ther 1993;53:22–29.

30. Pinder RM, Brogden RN, Speight TM, Avery GS. Sodium valproate: a review of its pharmacological properties and therapeutic efficacy in epilepsy. Drugs 1977;13:81–123.

31. Cloyd JC, Kriel RL, Fischer JH, Sawchuk RJ, Eggerth RM. Pharmacokinetics of valproic acid in children: I. Multiple antiepileptic drug therapy. Neurology 1983;33:185–191.

32. Bruni J, Wilder BJ, Perchalski RJ, Hammond EJ, Villarreal HJ. Valproic acid and plasma levels of phenobarbital. Neurology 1980;30:94–97.

33. Friel PN, Leal KW, Wilensky AJ. Valproic acid-phenytoin interaction. Ther Drug Monit 1979;1:243–248.

34. Perucca E, et al. Interaction between phenytoin and valproic acid: plasma protein binding and metabolic effects. Clin Pharmacol Ther 1980;28:779–789.

15

VANCOMYCIN

Peter J. Ambrose and Michael E. Winter

Vancomycin is an antibiotic with a gram-positive spectrum of activity that is effective in the treatment of nafcillin- or methicillin-resistant *Staphylococcus aureus* (NRSA or MRSA). It is also an alternative to penicillin in patients who have a history of serious penicillin allergy.[1-6] Vancomycin is bactericidal for most gram-positive organisms, except against enterococci, and it is synergistic with gentamicin against most strains of *S. aureus* and enterococci.[5,7] It is not an effective agent for gram-negative bacteria. There has been a resurgence in the use of vancomycin because of the increased prevalence of nafcillin-resistant staphylococcus.

Vancomycin is poorly absorbed orally and has been used to treat gastrointestinal overgrowths of gram-positive bacteria. When used to treat systemic infections, vancomycin must be given by the intravenous route or intraperitoneally for those patients receiving continuous ambulatory peritoneal dialysis (CAPD). The usual adult dose, in patients with normal renal function, is 1 g (10 to 15 mg/kg) administered intravenously over 60

KEY PARAMETERS: Vancomycin

Therapeutic Plasma Concentration[a]
  Peak
  Trough
	< 40–50 mg/L
	≈ 10 ± 5 mg/L

F (Oral)	< 5%
V [b,c]	V(L) = 0.17 (age in years) + 0.22 (TBW in kg) + 15
Cl [c]	Equal to Cl_{Cr}
$t_{1/2}$	6–7 hours

[a]A peak concentration of approximately 30 mg/L is a reasonable target; however, to ensure efficacy, trough concentrations should be maintained at or above 5 mg/L.
[b]The average volume of distribution for vancomycin is approximately 0.7 L/kg, and TBW represents total body weight including any excess adipose and/or third-space fluid weight.
[c]For adult patients (older than 18 years of age).

minutes every 12 hours.[4-6] Although 2 g/day (20 to 30 mg/kg/ day) of vancomycin had been recommended in the past, this dose can be excessive,
particularly in the elderly and in patients with diminished renal function.
Generally in these individuals, doses should be adjusted. Vancomycin is
not administered intramuscularly because it is painful and causes local ir-
ritation and a histamine reaction.

THERAPEUTIC AND TOXIC PLASMA CONCENTRATIONS

The ideal vancomycin dosing regimen is one that results in peak vancomycin plasma concentrations that are less than 40 to 50 mg/L and
trough concentrations that are in the range of 5 to 15 mg/L.[1,2,5,6,8-13] Peak
concentrations greater than 50 mg/L have been associated with ototoxicity; however, vancomycin-induced ototoxicity has been primarily reported
in patients with vancomycin concentrations > 80 mg/L.[1,3,14]

Although the above concentrations are widely accepted, there is
some controversy about their validity and the necessity for routinely monitoring plasma vancomycin concentrations.[15,16] Vancomycin exhibits con-
centration-independent killing, and specific peak plasma concentrations
have not been correlated with efficacy. Another confounding issue is the
fact that peak concentrations are often obtained at different times relative
to the end of the infusion. Furthermore, the minimum inhibitory concentration (MIC) for sensitive bacteria is < 5 mg/L and there is a limited
postantibiotic effect of 0.5 to 3 hours,[5,17] making it difficult to establish exactly when and how long over the dosing interval plasma concentrations
should exceed 5 mg/L. Certainly, the patients most likely to require vancomycin plasma concentration monitoring are those at highest risk for
therapeutic failure or potential drug toxicity. These include pediatric patients because they have high clearances and short half-lives; consequently, their trough concentrations are frequently well below 5 mg/L. It
also seems prudent to monitor plasma vancomycin concentrations in patients with poor renal function who are receiving empiric dosages, because
they are at greater risk of toxicity from vancomycin concentrations that
significantly exceed those required for efficacy.

A relatively high incidence of adverse effects was initially associated
with vancomycin. However, it is believed that some of these adverse reactions were due to impurities in the original products; the current formulations are more pure.[1] Other major side effects associated with vancomycin
therapy include phlebitis and a histamine reaction that presents as flushing, tachycardia, and hypotension. To minimize the histamine response,
vancomycin should be infused slowly over 60 minutes. Even at this rate of
infusion, some patients will experience flushing and tachycardia.[18,19] As a
single agent, vancomycin is associated with a low incidence of nephrotoxicity; however, when it is combined with aminoglycoside antibiotics,
the incidence may be as high as 30%.[14] It is difficult to know whether this

high incidence of nephrotoxicity is a result of the patient population se-lected (i.e., critically-ill patients) or a synergistic nephrotoxicity caused by the concurrent use of vancomycin and aminoglycosides.

The MIC for most strains of staphylococcus is less than 5 mg/L; therefore, trough concentrations should be maintained in the range of 5 to 15 mg/L. Some clinicians recommend maintaining plasma trough con-centrations above 10 mg/L because there is evidence of increased efficacy in patients with endocarditis and there is no known increased risk of tox-icity at these concentrations.[8,10,11,20]

BIOAVAILABILITY (F)

Vancomycin is poorly absorbed following oral administration (i.e., < 5%); as a result, parenteral or intraperitoneal administration is necessary for the treatment of systemic infections. Vancomycin's limited oral bioavailability has been used advantageously to treat enterocolitis.[1,4-6] Oral vancomycin and metronidazole are commonly used to treat *Clostridium difficile*-produced pseudomembranous colitis, a clinical condition that can be pre-cipitated by the use of broad-spectrum antibiotics. However, metronida-zole is usually recommended as the drug of choice in the treatment of *C. difficile* as it appears to be as effective and is much less expensive for a course of treatment.

VOLUME OF DISTRIBUTION (V)

The volume of distribution for vancomycin ranges between 0.5 and 1 L/kg.[21-23] In clinical practice, an average value of 0.7 L/kg is often used; however, age and gender may also influence the distribution of van-comycin.[22,23] The following method of estimating V for vancomycin in adults (i.e., those older than 18 years of age) incorporates both total body weight (TBW) and patient age: [22]

$$V(L) = 0.17(\text{age in years}) + 0.22(\text{TBW in kg}) + 15 \qquad \text{[Eq. 15.1]}$$

A two- or three-compartment model best describes the distribution of vancomycin. The complexity of this model can be problematic when peak plasma samples are obtained during the distribution phase. In clini-cal practice, a one-compartment model is frequently used.[13,22,24]

CLEARANCE (Cl)

Vancomycin is eliminated primarily by the renal route; approximately 5% of the dose is metabolized.[21,25] The clearance of vancomycin approximates that of creatinine clearance[22-24]:

$$Cl_{cr} \text{ for males (mL/min)} = \frac{(140 - \text{Age})(\text{Weight in kg})}{(72)(SCr_{ss})} \qquad [\text{Eq. 15.2}]$$

$$Cl_{cr} \text{ for females (mL/min)} = (0.85)\frac{(140 - \text{Age})(\text{Weight in kg})}{(72)(SCr_{ss})} \qquad [\text{Eq. 15.3}]$$

$$\text{Vancomycin } Cl \approx Cl_{cr} \qquad [\text{Eq. 15.4}]$$

For issues that should be considered when estimating creatinine clearance (e.g., whether SCr should be normalized to 1.0 mg/dL), see Part I: Creatinine Clearance.

Very little vancomycin is cleared by standard hemo- or peritoneal dialysis.[10,26,27] In patients undergoing continuous ambulatory peritoneal dialysis (CAPD), the small but continuous drug loss due to peritoneal dialysis exchanges is significant. The usual approach is to replace vancomycin with intermittent intravenous injections on a somewhat more frequent basis than is usually done for patients with end-stage renal disease (in some cases as often as every 3 to 5 days), or to instill vancomycin directly into the peritoneal space to treat peritonitis and achieve systemic concentrations of vancomycin.[28,29] Some caution should be used in evaluating plasma concentrations in patients with end-stage renal disease. Some immunoassays that use polyclonal antibodies overestimate actual vancomycin concentrations due to an accumulation of pseudometabolites (crystalline degradation products) that cross-react with the assay.[30,31] In patients undergoing high-flux or high-efficiency hemodialysis, a significant amount of vancomycin can be removed. Early studies estimated that as much as 30% of vancomycin was removed during high-flux hemodialysis; recent reports indicate only 17% of vancomycin is removed during these procedures. Early investigators did not recognize that a redistribution of vancomycin occurs after the completion of dialysis.[32,33]

HALF-LIFE (t½)

The usual serum half-life of vancomycin is 5 to 10 hours; in patients with end-stage renal disease the half-life may approach 7 days.[10,21,22,25] This wide range in the serum half-life partially explains the variability in the dose and dosing intervals used for vancomycin. Patients with normal renal function may receive the drug every 8 to 12 hours, whereas those with end-stage renal disease may receive a dose once a week.[10,26]

NOMOGRAMS

Dosing nomograms for vancomycin are available.[10,34] However, an understanding of the desired therapeutic range and the pharmacokinetic parameters of vancomycin provides the clinician more flexibility to tailor doses and dosing intervals which meet the specific needs of the patient. For example, using pharmacokinetic parameters allows targeting plasma vancomycin concentrations above a specific MIC, which is particularly advantageous when treating infections with vancomycin-intermediate-sensitive bacteria.

TIME TO SAMPLE

Wide fluctuations in vancomycin plasma concentrations within a normal dosing interval suggest that both peak and trough concentrations should be monitored. In general, however, steady-state trough concentrations appear to be adequate in most cases. As a general rule, vancomycin is dosed with an interval of approximately one half-life. Assuming an average volume of distribution, peak concentrations can be estimated with reasonable accuracy based on the dose administered, an estimate of the volume of distribution, and a measured trough concentration. This is especially true in patients with diminished renal function and a long vancomycin half-life. Although the bulk of the literature suggests that both peak and trough concentrations are appropriate, the concept of using only trough concentrations is supported by both the pharmacokinetic and clinical characteristics of the drug.[16,35] However, for patients in whom the pharmacokinetic parameters may be difficult to estimate with confidence (e.g., very overweight or underweight patients), monitoring both peak and trough concentrations is advisable, particularly for seriously-ill patients.

If the highest expected peak concentration is below 40 to 50 mg/L for a dose that produces a trough concentration of 5 to 15 mg/L, the dose is acceptable. If the trough concentration is known, the peak concentration (Css max) can be approximated using Equation 15.5.

$$\text{Css max} = [\text{Css min}] + \left[\frac{(S)(F)(Dose)}{V} \right] \qquad \text{[Eq. 15.5]}$$

The $\frac{(S)(F)(Dose)}{V}$ represents the change in concentration (ΔC) following a dose.

As described in Part I, the use of the above equation requires that several conditions be met. They are as follows:

1. Steady state has been achieved.
2. The measured plasma concentration is a trough concentration.
3. The bolus dose is an acceptable model.

In the clinical setting, trough concentrations are often obtained slightly before the true trough. Because vancomycin has a relatively long half-life, most plasma concentrations obtained within 1 hour of the true trough can be assumed to have met condition 2 above.

Since vancomycin follows a multicompartmental model, it is difficult to avoid the distribution phase when obtaining peak plasma concentrations.[36] If peak levels are to be measured, samples should be obtained at least 1 or possibly 2 hours after the end of the infusion period. It is difficult to evaluate the appropriateness of a dosing regimen that is based on plasma samples obtained before steady state. Additional plasma concentrations are required to more accurately estimate a patient's apparent clearance and half-life, and to ensure that any dosing adjustments based on a nonsteady-state trough concentration actually achieve the targeted steady-state concentrations.

Question #1. *B.C., a 65-year-old, 45-kg man with a serum creatinine concentration of 2.2 mg/dL, is being treated for a presumed hospital-acquired, nafcillin-resistant S. aureus infection. Design a dosing regimen that will produce peak concentrations less than 40 to 50 mg/L and trough concentrations of 5 to 15 mg/L.*

The first step in calculating an appropriate dosing regimen for B.C. is to estimate his pharmacokinetic parameters (i.e., volume of distribution, clearance, elimination rate constant, and half-life).

The volume of distribution for B.C. can be calculated by using Equation 15.1 (see Key Parameters: Vancomycin). According to the calculations shown below, B.C.'s expected volume of distribution would be 36.0 L.

$$V(L) = 0.17(65 \text{ yrs}) + 0.22(45 \text{ kg}) + 15 = 36.0 \text{ L}$$

Using Equations 15.2 and 15.4, B.C.'s creatinine clearance and vancomycin clearance are estimated to be approximately 21.3 mL/min, as shown:

$$Cl_{cr} \text{ for males (mL/min)} = \frac{(140 - \text{Age})(\text{Weight in kg})}{(72)(SCr_{ss})}$$

$$= \frac{(140 - 65 \text{ yrs})(45 \text{ kg})}{(72)(2.2 \text{ mg/dL})}$$

$$= 21.3 \text{ mL/min}$$

Using Equation 15.4, the corresponding vancomycin clearance for B.C. is 1.28 L/hr.

$$\text{Vancomycin Cl} \approx Cl_{cr}$$

$$= 21.3 \text{ mL/min}$$

or

$$= 21.3 \text{ mL/min} \times \frac{60 \text{ min/hr}}{1000 \text{ mL/L}}$$

$$= 1.28 \text{ L/hr}$$

The calculated vancomycin clearance of 1.28 L/hr and the volume of distribution of 36.0 L then can be used to estimate the elimination rate constant of 0.036 hr^{-1}.

$$K = \frac{Cl}{V} \qquad \text{[Eq. 15.6]}$$

$$= \frac{1.28 \text{ L/hr}}{36 \text{ L}}$$

$$= 0.036 \text{ hr}^{-1}$$

and the corresponding vancomycin half-life can be calculated using Equation 15.7.

$$t\frac{1}{2} = \frac{(0.693)(V)}{Cl} \qquad \text{[Eq. 15.7]}$$

$$= \frac{(0.693)(36.0 \text{ L})}{1.28 \text{ L/hr}}$$

$$= 19.5 \text{ hr}$$

In clinical practice, loading doses of vancomycin are seldom administered. This is probably because most clinicians prescribe about 15 mg/kg as their maintenance dose. Using Equation 15.8, our patient's weight, and the volume of distribution of 36 L that we calculated above, and substituting the usual maintenance dose as mg/kg for the dose, it can be seen that the initial plasma concentration should be approximately 20 mg/L.

$$C° = \frac{(S)(F)(\text{Loading Dose})}{V} \qquad \text{[Eq. 15.8]}$$

$$C° = \frac{(1)(1)(15 \text{ mg/kg} \times 45 \text{ kg})}{36 \text{ L}}$$

$$= 18.8 \text{ mg/L} \approx 20 \text{ mg/L}$$

Although this value is below the usual targeted peak concentration of about 30 mg/L, it is well above that needed for efficacy (5 to 15 mg/L). If one wanted to calculate an initial dose, Equation 15.9 and the assumed volume of distribution of 36.0 L could be used. The salt form and bioavailability are assumed to be 1.0 when vancomycin is administered intravenously. Using an initial target of 30 mg/L, the loading dose would be approximately 1,000 mg.

$$\text{Loading Dose} = \frac{(V)(C)}{(S)(F)} \qquad \text{[Eq. 15.9]}$$

$$= \frac{(36.0 \text{ L})(30 \text{ mg/L})}{(1)(1)}$$

$$= 1080 \text{ mg or} \approx 1000 \text{ mg}$$

There are no known renal or ototoxicities associated with elevated vancomycin levels that occur during the distribution phase. However, to minimize the cardiovascular effects associated with rapid administration, the initial and subsequent doses should be administered over approximately 60 minutes. In addition, if peak concentrations are measured, samples should be drawn at least 1 to 2 hours after completion of the infusion period to avoid the distribution phase.

The maintenance dose can be calculated by a number of methods. One approach might be to first approximate the hourly infusion rate required to maintain the desired average concentration. Then, the hourly infusion rate can be multiplied by an appropriate dosing interval to calculate a reasonable dose to be given on an intermittent basis. For example, if an average concentration of 20 mg/L is selected (approximately halfway between the desired peak concentration of ≈30 mg/L and trough concentration of ≈10 mg/L), the hourly administration rate would be 25.6 mg/hr (Equation 15.10).

$$\text{Maintenance Dose} = \frac{(Cl)(Css \text{ ave})(\tau)}{(S)(F)} \qquad \text{[Eq. 15.10]}$$

$$= \frac{(1.28 \text{ L/hr})(20 \text{ mg/L})(1 \text{ hr})}{(1)(1)}$$

$$= 25.6 \text{ mg/hr}$$

Although a number of dosing intervals could be selected, 24 hours is reasonable because it is a convenient interval and approximates B.C.'s half-life for vancomycin of 19.5 hours. A dosing interval of approximately 1 half-life should result in peak concentrations that are below 40 to 50 mg/L and trough concentrations that are within the 5 to 15 mg/L range, in this case. If an interval of 24 hours is selected, the dose would be approximately 600 mg.

$$\text{Maintenance Dose} = \frac{(1.28 \text{ L/hr})(20 \text{ mg/L})(24 \text{ hr})}{(1)(1)}$$

$$= 614 \text{ or} \approx 600 \text{ mg}$$

This method assumes that the average concentration is halfway between the peak and trough. As mentioned in Part I, this is approximately correct as long as the dosing interval is less than or approximately equal to the drug's half-life. When dosing intervals greatly exceed the half-life, the true average concentration is much lower than halfway between peak and trough levels.

A second approach that can be used to calculate the maintenance dose is to select a desired peak and trough concentration that is consistent with the therapeutic range and B.C.'s vancomycin half-life. For example, if steady-state peak concentrations of 30 mg/L are desired, it would take approximately two half-lives for that peak level to fall to 7.5 mg/L (a level of 30 mg/L declines to 15 mg/L in one half-life and to 7.5 mg/L in the second half-life). Since the vancomycin half-life in B.C. is approximately 1 day, the dosing interval would be 48 hours. The dose to be administered every 48 hours can be calculated using Equation 15.11.

$$\text{Dose} = \frac{(V)(\text{Css max} - \text{Css min})}{(S)(F)} \qquad \text{[Eq. 15.11]}$$

$$= \frac{(36.0 \text{ L})(30 \text{ mg/L} - 7.5 \text{ mg/L})}{(1)(1)}$$

$$= 810 \text{ mg or} \approx 800 \text{ mg}$$

The peak and trough concentrations that are expected using this dosing regimen can be calculated by using Equations 15.12 and 15.14, respectively:

$$\text{Css max} = \frac{\dfrac{(S)(F)(\text{Dose})}{V}}{1 - e^{-KT}} \qquad \text{[Eq. 15.12]}$$

$$= \frac{\dfrac{(1)(1)(800 \text{ mg})}{36.0 \text{ L}}}{(1 - e^{-(0.036 \text{ hr}^{-1})(48 \text{ hr})})}$$

$$= 27.0 \text{ mg/L}$$

Note that although 27 mg/L is an acceptable peak, the actual clinical peak would normally be obtained approximately 1 hour after the end of a 1-hour infusion, or 2 hours after this calculated peak concentration, and would be about 25 mg/L, as calculated by Equation 15.13.

$$C_2 = C_1(e^{-Kt}) \qquad \text{[Eq. 15.13]}$$

$$= 27.0 \text{ mg/L } (e^{-(0.036 \text{ hr}^{-1})(2 \text{ hr})})$$

$$= 27.0 \text{ mg/L } (0.93)$$

$$= 25.1 \text{ mg/L}$$

The calculated trough concentration would be about 5 mg/L (Equations 15.14 and 15.15).

$$Css \ min = \frac{\dfrac{(S)(F)(Dose)}{V}}{1 - e^{-K\tau}}(e^{-K\tau}) \qquad \text{[Eq. 15.14]}$$

$$Css \ min = (Css \ max)(e^{-K\tau}) \qquad \text{[Eq. 15.15]}$$

$$= (27 \text{ mg/L})(e^{(-0.036 \text{ hr}^{-1})(48 \text{ hr})})$$

$$= (27 \text{ mg/L})(0.178)$$

$$= 4.8 \text{ mg/L}$$

This process of checking the expected peak and trough concentrations is most appropriate when the dose or the dosing interval has been changed from a calculated value (e.g., twice the half-life) to a practical value (e.g., 8, 12, 18, 24, 36, or 48 hours). Many institutions generally prefer not to use dosing intervals of 18 or 36 hours, because the time of day when the next dose is to be given changes, potentially resulting in dosing errors. If different plasma vancomycin concentrations are desired, Equations 15.12 and 15.14 can be used to target specific vancomycin concentrations by adjusting the dose and/or the dosing interval. For example, a dosage regimen of 1,000 mg every 48 hours would result in calculated peak and trough concentrations of 33.8 mg/L and 6.0 mg/L, respectively. Alternatively, 800 mg every 36 hours would result in an expected peak concentration of 30.6 mg/L and a trough concentration of 8.4 mg/L, at steady state.

A third alternative is to rearrange Equation 15.14:

$$Css \ min = \frac{\dfrac{(S)(F)(Dose)}{V}}{1 - e^{-K\tau}}(e^{-K\tau})$$

such that the dose can be calculated.

$$\text{Dose} = \frac{(\text{Css min})(V)(1 - e^{-K\tau})}{(S)(F)(e^{-K\tau})}$$ [Eq. 15.16]

Note that it is the Css min or trough concentration that is used to solve for dose. This is because it is the trough concentration that has been associated with efficacy and therefore is the primary target for dosing. Making the appropriate substitutions for the parameters indicated in Equation 15.16 and choosing a target trough concentration of 10 mg/L and a dosing interval of 24 hours, a dose of approximately 500 mg is calculated.

$$\text{Dose} = \frac{(10 \text{ mg/L})(36.0 \text{ L})(1 - e^{-(0.036 \text{ hr}^{-1})(24 \text{ hr})})}{(1)(1)(e^{-(0.036 \text{ hr}^{-1})(24 \text{ hr})})}$$

$$= \frac{(10 \text{ mg/L})(36.0 \text{ L})(1 - 0.42)}{(1)(1)(0.42)}$$

$$= 497 \text{ mg} \approx 500 \text{ mg}$$

Alternatively, doses could have been calculated for dosing intervals of 36 or 48 hours if those intervals were deemed to be appropriate.

Question #2. *E.K., a 60-year old, 50-kg woman with a serum creatinine of 1.0 mg/dL, has been empirically started on 500 mg of vancomycin every 8 hours for treatment of a hospital-acquired staphylococcal infection. What are the expected peak and trough vancomycin concentrations for E.K.?*

To calculate the peak and trough concentrations, E.K.'s volume of distribution, clearance, and elimination rate constant (or half-life) need to be estimated. Using Equation 15.1, the expected volume of distribution for E.K. is 36.2 L.

$$V(L) = 0.17(60 \text{ yrs}) + 0.22(50 \text{ kg}) + 15 = 36.2 \text{ L}$$

E.K.'s creatinine clearance can be calculated using Equation 15.3, and Equation 15.4 can be used to calculate her vancomycin clearance of 2.83 L/hr, as shown below.

$$\text{Cl}_{cr} \text{ for females (mL/min)} = (0.85)\frac{(140 - \text{Age})(\text{Weight in kg})}{(72)(\text{SCr}_{ss})}$$

$$= (0.85)\frac{(140 - 60 \text{ yrs})(50 \text{ kg})}{(72)(1.0 \text{ mg/dL})}$$

$$= 47.2 \text{ mL/min}$$

Using Equation 15.4 to calculate vancomycin clearance:

$$\text{Vancomycin Cl} \approx \text{Cl}_{cr}$$

$$\text{Vancomycin Cl} = 47.2 \text{ mL/min}$$

or

$$= (47.2 \text{ mL/min})\left(\frac{60 \text{ min/hr}}{1000 \text{ mL/L}}\right)$$

$$= 2.83 \text{ L/hr}$$

Equation 15.6 can now be used to calculate E.K.'s elimination rate constant and Equation 15.7 to calculate the corresponding half-life.

$$K = \frac{Cl}{V}$$

$$= \frac{2.83 \text{ L/hr}}{36.2 \text{ L}}$$

$$= 0.078 \text{ hr}^{-1}$$

$$t\frac{1}{2} = \frac{(0.693)(V)}{Cl}$$

$$= \frac{(0.693)(36.2 \text{ L})}{2.83 \text{ L/hr}}$$

$$= 8.9 \text{ hr}$$

Equations 15.12 and 15.15 can be used to calculate the expected peak and trough concentrations for E.K.

$$\text{Css max} = \frac{\dfrac{(S)(F)(\text{Dose})}{V}}{1 - e^{-KT}}$$

$$= \frac{\dfrac{(1)(1)(500 \text{ mg})}{36.2 \text{ L}}}{(1 - e^{-(0.078 \text{ hr}^{-1})(8 \text{ hr})})}$$

$$= 29.8 \text{ mg/L}$$

To calculate the clinical peak concentration, which is usually sampled 2 hours after the start of a vancomycin infusion (1 hour after the end of a 1-hour infusion), the Css max could be decayed for 2 hours using Equation 15.13.

$$C_2 = C_1(e^{-Kt})$$

$$= 29.8 \text{ mg/L } (e^{-(0.078 \text{ hr}^{-1})(2 \text{ hr})})$$

$$= 29.8 \text{ mg/L } (0.86)$$

$$= 25.6 \text{ mg/L (2 hours after starting infusion)}$$

Css min can be calculated using Equation 15.15 and the dosing interval of 8 hours.

$$\text{Css min} = (\text{Css max})(e^{-K\tau})$$

$$= (29.8 \text{ mg/L})(e^{(-0.078 \text{ hr}^{-1})(8 \text{ hr})})$$

$$= (29.8 \text{ mg/L})(0.536)$$

$$= 16.0 \text{ mg/L}$$

Although the expected peak concentration of ≈30 mg/L is not above the usually accepted range for peak concentrations, the trough concentration of 16 mg/L is slightly above the usual targeted range of 5 to 15 mg/L, which is required for efficacy. This suggests that decreasing the dose and/or increasing the dosing interval, as well as monitoring plasma concentrations of vancomycin, would be appropriate.

Question #3. *A steady-state trough concentration of 35 mg/L was obtained for E.K. Design a dosing regimen that will produce lower therapeutic vancomycin concentrations for E.K.*

To design such a regimen, E.K.'s pharmacokinetic parameters should first be revised so that they are consistent with the observed trough concentration of 35 mg/L. Some assumptions will have to be made. Because the measured trough concentration is much higher than predicted, her half-life is much longer than the estimate of 8.9 hours. For E.K., the percent fluctuation between peak and trough concentrations should be relatively small at steady state because her dosing interval of 8 hours is much shorter than her apparent half-life. Therefore, the best approach is to use the literature estimate for volume of distribution and then calculate the corresponding elimination rate constant and clearance values.

If E.K.'s volume of distribution is assumed to be 36.2 L (see calculation above using Equation 15.1) and the observed trough concentration of 35 mg/L is used, a peak concentration of approximately 49 mg/L can be calculated by using Equation 15.5, as follows:

$$\text{Css max} = [\text{Css min}] + \left[\frac{(S)(F)(\text{Dose})}{V}\right]$$

$$\text{Css max} = [35 \text{ mg/L}] + \left[\frac{(1)(1)(500 \text{ mg})}{36.2 \text{ L}}\right]$$

$$\approx 49 \text{ mg/L}$$

Using the observed trough concentration of 35 mg/L and the predicted peak concentration of 49 mg/L, an elimination rate constant (K) can be calculated using Equation 15.17, where C_1 is the peak concentration of 49 mg/L, C_2 is the trough concentration of 35 mg/L, and the interval between those two concentrations, t, is the dosing interval of 8 hours.

$$K = \frac{\ln\left(\dfrac{C_1}{C_2}\right)}{t} \qquad \text{[Eq. 15.17]}$$

$$= \frac{\ln\left(\dfrac{49 \text{ mg/L}}{35 \text{ mg/L}}\right)}{8 \text{ hr}}$$

$$= 0.042 \text{ hr}^{-1}$$

This apparent elimination rate constant of 0.042 hr^{-1} corresponds to a half-life of approximately 16.5 hours (Equation 15.18) as shown below.

$$t\tfrac{1}{2} = \frac{0.693}{K} \qquad \text{[Eq. 15.18]}$$

$$= \frac{0.693}{0.042 \text{ hr}^{-1}}$$

$$= 16.5 \text{ hr}$$

The apparent elimination rate constant of 0.042 hr^{-1} and the assumed volume of distribution of 36.2 L can be used in Equation 15.19 to calculate E.K.'s vancomycin clearance.

$$Cl = (K)(V) \qquad \text{[Eq. 15.19]}$$

$$= (0.042 \text{ hr}^{-1})(36.2 \text{ L})$$

$$= 1.52 \text{ L/hr}$$

Because the revised t$\tfrac{1}{2}$ is $\geq \tau$, we expect Css ave to be halfway between Css max and Css min. Therefore, clearance could have been approximated by assuming Css ave is approximately equal to:

$$Css \text{ ave} = Css \text{ min} + \left(\frac{1}{2}\right)\frac{(S)(F)(Dose)}{V} \qquad \text{[Eq. 15.20]}$$

and then calculating clearance by using Equation 15.21.

$$Cl = \frac{(S)(F)(Dose/\tau)}{Css\ ave} \qquad [Eq.\ 15.21]$$

(See Part I: Choosing a Model to Revise or Estimate a Patient's Clearance at Steady State.)

The maintenance dose can then be calculated by using Equation 15.16. Because the apparent half-life is approximately 16 hours, the most logical dosing interval and Css min would be 24 hours and 10 mg/L, respectively.

$$Dose = \frac{(Css\ min)(V)(1 - e^{-K\tau})}{(S)(F)(e^{-K\tau})}$$

$$Dose = \frac{(10\ mg/L)(36.2\ L)(1 - e^{-(0.042\ hr^{-1})(24\ hr)})}{(1)(1)(e^{-(0.042\ hr^{-1})(24\ hr)})}$$

$$= 630\ mg\ or \approx 600\ mg\ every\ 24\ hours$$

This dosing regimen of 600 mg every 24 hours should result in a steady-state peak concentration of approximately 26 mg/L by using Equation 15.12:

$$Css\ max = \frac{\dfrac{(S)(F)(Dose)}{V}}{1 - e^{-K\tau}}$$

$$= \frac{\dfrac{(1)(1)(600\ mg)}{36.2\ L}}{(1 - e^{-(0.042\ hr^{-1})(24\ hr)})}$$

$$= 26.1\ mg/L$$

A trough concentration of 9.5 mg/L can be calculated by using Equation 15.15:

$$Css\ min = (Css\ max)(e^{-K\tau})$$

$$= (26.1\ mg/L)(e^{(-0.042\ hr^{-1})(24\ hr)})$$

$$= (26.1\ mg/L)(0.365)$$

$$= 9.5\ mg/L$$

The target trough concentration of approximately 10 mg/L should be acceptable because the goal is to maintain trough concentrations in the therapeutic range (5 to 15 mg/L).

Question #4. *A.C., a 50-year-old, 60-kg woman with end-stage renal disease and a serum creatinine of 9 mg/dL, is undergoing standard intermittent hemodialysis treatments 3 times a week and currently has an apparent shunt infection which is to be treated with vancomycin. Calculate an appropriate dose for A.C.*

Vancomycin is extensively cleared by the kidneys; consequently, patients with end-stage renal disease have prolonged half-lives that average 5 to 7 days. This extended half-life is consistent with a residual vancomycin clearance of 3 to 4 mL/70 kg/min (0.18 to 0.24 L/70 kg/hr) and an average volume of distribution. Depending on A.C.'s residual renal function, the half-life may be shorter or longer than this general range. Note that for dialysis patients it is not appropriate to use their SCr to estimate creatinine clearance with Equation 15.2 or 15.3, because the SCr is not at steady state. The duration and frequency of A.C.'s hemodialysis is not a factor in vancomycin dosing, because the amount of vancomycin cleared during standard hemodialysis is negligible.

The usual approach to the use of vancomycin in patients receiving intermittent hemodialysis is to administer 1 gm every 5 days to 2 weeks. Using Equation 15.1 to estimate the volume of distribution:

$$V(L) = 0.17(50 \text{ yrs}) + 0.22(60 \text{ kg}) + 15 = 36.7 \text{ L}$$

Then one can see from Equation 15.8 that the first 1 gm dose should result in an initial peak concentration of 27 mg/L .

$$C^\circ = \frac{(S)(F)(\text{Loading Dose})}{V}$$

$$C^\circ = \frac{(1)(1)(1000 \text{ mg})}{36.7 \text{ L}}$$

$$= 27.2 \text{ mg/L}$$

For a dose of 1 gm administered weekly, a steady-state peak and trough levels of approximately 44 mg/L and 17 mg/L, respectively, can be calculated using an average vancomycin clearance of 3.5 mL/min (0.21 L/hr), a volume of distribution of 36.7 L, and a corresponding elimination rate constant of 0.00572 hr^{-1} (Equations 15.12 and 15.15):

$$\text{Css max} = \frac{\dfrac{(S)(F)(Dose)}{V}}{1 - e^{-K\tau}}$$

$$= \frac{\dfrac{(1)(1)(1000 \text{ mg})}{36.7 \text{ L}}}{(1 - e^{-(0.00572 \text{ hr}^{-1})(24 \text{ hr/day})(7 \text{ days})})}$$

$$= 44.1 \text{ mg/L} \approx 44 \text{ mg/L}$$

$$\text{Css min} = (\text{Css max})(e^{-K\tau})$$

$$= [44.1 \text{ mg/L}][e^{(-0.00572 \text{ hr}^{-1})(24 \text{ hr/day})(7 \text{ days})}]$$

$$= (44.1 \text{ mg/L})(0.383)$$

$$= 16.9 \text{ mg/L} \approx 17 \text{ mg/L}$$

If the 1 gm dose had been administered every 2 weeks, the expected peak and trough vancomycin concentrations would have been approximately 32 mg/L and 5 mg/L, respectively. However, because of the long half-life of vancomycin in renal failure (approximately 1 week) and a usual course of therapy of 2 weeks, steady state would not be achieved. Alternatively, if a dose of 500 mg was given weekly for a prolonged period, the expected steady-state peak and trough concentrations would have been approximately 22 mg/L and 9 mg/L, respectively. When the same average dosing rate (SFDose/τ) is administered as a smaller dose given more frequently, the steady-state peak concentration is lower, the steady-state trough concentration is higher, but the average steady-state concentration is the same, as demonstrated by Equation 15.22 (also see Part I: Interpretation of Plasma Drug Concentrations).

$$\text{Css ave} = \frac{(S)(F)(Dose/\tau)}{Cl} \qquad \text{[Eq. 15.22]}$$

$$= \frac{(1)(1)(1000 \text{ mg})/(14 \text{ days})(24 \text{ hr/day})}{0.21 \text{ L/hr}}$$

$$= 14.2 \text{ mg/L}$$

versus

$$= \frac{(1)(1)(500 \text{ mg})/(7 \text{ days})(24 \text{ hr/day})}{0.21 \text{ L/hr}}$$

$$= 14.2 \text{ mg/L}$$

If an extended course of therapy is anticipated, it is probably advisable to obtain vancomycin plasma levels to make certain that A.C.'s actual plasma levels are within an acceptable range. In seriously-ill patients it might be appropriate to obtain an initial vancomycin level 3 to 5 days after the initiation of therapy. The purpose is to ensure that the patient's actual clearance is not unusually large, resulting in vancomycin levels that are below the desired therapeutic range.

If A.C. had been receiving CAPD as her method of dialysis, it is probable that the vancomycin would be administered via her peritoneal dialysis fluid. The usual approach is to place 15 to 30 mg/kg of vancomycin (approximately 1 to 2 gm for A.C.) into an initial dialysate exchange, which should result in approximately 50% of that dose being absorbed during the usual 4- to 6-hour dwell time. Her maintenance dose would then be administered in one of two ways. An additional 15 to 30 mg/kg dose could be administered in single exchanges every 3 to 5 days such that her pre-dose trough vancomycin concentration would be maintained at ≈10 mg/L. A less common, alternative method for maintenance therapy is to place in each dialysis exchange enough vancomycin to achieve a dialysate concentration of 15 to 20 mg/L (30 to 40 mg in a 2 L exchange). This technique of placing vancomycin in each exchange results in an average steady-state plasma concentration approximately equal to the concentration of vancomycin in the dialysate fluid, after multiple exchanges (i.e., 15 to 20 mg/L).[28,29]

Question #5. *Suppose A.C. was given an initial 1 gm dose and 3 days later she underwent high-flux hemodialysis for 2 hours. Calculate a replacement dose after the dialysis session.*

Although the amount of vancomycin removed by standard hemodialysis is negligible, high-flux hemodialysis has been reported to remove approximately 17% over 2 hours.[33] Assuming the initial plasma concentration is 27.2 mg/L and using the estimated K of 0.00572 hr⁻¹, as calculated above for A.C, the pre-dialysis concentration can be determined by using Equation 15.13.

$$C_2 = C_1(e^{-Kt})$$

$$= 27.2 \text{ mg/L } (e^{-(0.00572 \text{ hr}^{-1})(72 \text{ hr})})$$

$$= 27.2 \text{ mg/L } (0.66)$$

$$= 18.0 \text{ mg/L (pre-dialysis concentration)}$$

If the plasma concentration declines by approximately 17% due to high-flux hemodialysis, then the post-dialysis plasma concentration will be 83% of the pre-dialysis concentration. This ignores any additional elimination from the intrinsic clearance during the 2-hour dialysis period, since it is negligible.

$$C_{Post-Dialysis} = 18.0 \text{ mg/L } (0.83)$$

$$= 14.9 \text{ mg/L}$$

If a replacement dose is desired at this point, the dose can be calculated by using Equation 15.23.

$$\text{Dose} = \frac{(V)(\Delta C)}{(S)(F)} \qquad \text{[Eq. 15.23]}$$

$$= \frac{(36.7 \text{ L})(27.2 \text{ mg/L} - 14.9 \text{ mg/L})}{(1)(1)}$$

$$= 451 \text{ mg} \approx 450 \text{ mg}$$

A similar approach can be used in a step-wise fashion to determine dosing needs on any particular day and dialysis schedule. The amount of actual drug loss will depend on the intrinsic Cl, V, time of decay (t), duration of hemodialysis, and efficiency of the dialysis treatment.

Question #6. *K.G., a 50-year-old, 70-kg man with a serum creatinine of 1.2 mg/dL, is receiving vancomycin 1000 mg IV every 12 hours at 10:00 a.m. and 10:00 p.m. for a nafcillin-resistant S. aureus (NSRA) infection. A steady-state vancomycin level was drawn at 6:00 a.m. and was reported to be 18 mg/L. (Note: This level was drawn 8 hours after the start of the vancomycin infusion and is 4 hours before the trough.) Based on this information, estimate K.G.'s vancomycin Cl and K values and the true trough concentration.*

Because this level was drawn 4 hours early, Equation 15.5 should not be used to estimate the peak concentration because Css min is not yet known.

$$\text{Css max} = [\text{Css min}] + \left[\frac{(S)(F)(\text{Dose})}{V} \right]$$

Instead, an iterative search technique must be used to determine K.G.'s pharmacokinetic parameters. The usual technique is to use Equation 15.24 where t_1 is 8 hours from the start of the infusion and to assume K.G. has an average volume of distribution of 38.9 L, using Equation 15.1.

$$V(L) = 0.17(\text{age in years}) + 0.22(\text{TBW in kg}) + 15$$

$$= [0.17][50 \text{ yr}] + [0.22][70 \text{ kg}] + 15$$

$$= 38.9 \text{ L}$$

Then, by trial and error, solve for the elimination-rate constant (K) that predicts a plasma concentration equal to the observed value of 18 mg/L. For example, if a K of 0.113 hr^{-1} is inserted into the equation (the initial K is calculated from population V and Cl), a concentration of 14.0 mg/L is calculated. This value is lower than the observed concentration of 18 mg/L and therefore does not satisfy the equation. By trial and error, one can discover that an elimination rate constant of 0.0935 hr^{-1} calculates a concentration of approximately 18 mg/L.

$$Css_1 = \frac{\dfrac{(S)(F)(Dose)}{V}}{1 - e^{-K\tau}}(e^{-Kt_1}) \qquad [Eq.\ 15.24]$$

$$Css_1 = \frac{\dfrac{(1)(1)(1000\ mg)}{38.9\ L}}{1 - e^{-K(12\ hr)}}(e^{-K(8\ hr)})$$

$$= \frac{\dfrac{(1)(1)(1000\ mg)}{38.9\ L}}{1 - e^{-(0.113\ hr^{-1})(12\ hr)}}(e^{-(0.113\ hr^{-1})(8\ hr)})$$

$$= \frac{25.7\ mg/L}{(1 - 0.26)}(0.405)$$

$$= 14.0$$

and subsequently

$$Css_1 = \frac{\dfrac{(1)(1)(1000\ mg)}{38.9\ L}}{1 - e^{-(0.0935\ hr^{-1})(12\ hr)}}(e^{-(0.0935\ hr^{-1})(8\ hr)})$$

$$= \frac{25.7\ mg/L}{(1 - 0.326)}(0.473)$$

$$= 18.0$$

It can be reasonably assumed, then, that this elimination rate constant of 0.0935 hr^{-1} is the value that would be most appropriate for K.G. When this K is coupled with Equations 15.18 and 15.19, a revised half-life and vancomycin clearance can be calculated for K.G.

$$t_{1/2} = \frac{0.693}{K}$$

$$= \frac{0.693}{0.0935 \text{ hr}^{-1}}$$

$$= 7.4 \text{ hr}$$

$$Cl = (K)(V)$$

$$= (0.0935 \text{ hr}^{-1})(38.9 \text{ L})$$

$$= 3.64 \text{ L/hr}$$

Others may use the iterative method by adjusting the clearance value and calculating the corresponding K. This approach emphasizes that clearance is the independent pharmacokinetic parameter that is being revised. However, the outcome is the same using either technique and is a matter of personal preference and experience.

In addition, Equation 15.13 can be used to calculate the expected trough concentration (12 hours after the dose was administered) by decaying the reported value at 8 hours an additional 4 hours.

$$C_2 = C_1(e^{-Kt})$$

$$= 18 \text{ mg/L } (e^{-(0.0935 \text{ hr}^{-1})(4 \text{ hr})})$$

$$= 18 \text{ mg/L } (0.688)$$

$$= 12.4 \text{ mg/L}$$

This concentration is reasonable considering the usual target trough concentrations are 5 to 15 mg/L. If the estimated trough concentration was not acceptable, then the revised half-life and clearance coupled with the assumed volume of distribution for K.G. could be used to establish a new dosing regimen.

Question #7. *C.U. is a 40-year-old, 5-foot 7-inch, 105-kg man with a serum creatinine of 1.2 mg/dl. He has a penicillin allergy history and for that reason, vancomycin is being considered for empiric therapy. Should the dosing regimen of vancomycin be based on C.U.'s total or ideal body weight?*

The volume of distribution of vancomycin is greater in obese subjects than in non-obese subjects. The apparent volume of distribution for vancomycin tends to correlate best with actual (total) body weight, although there is a fair degree of variability.[9,22,23,37,38] Whereas some investigators have reported higher vancomycin clearances in obese patients, others have observed that vancomycin clearance is still essentially equivalent to creatinine clearance.[9,22,23,37,38] Owing to the wide variability in the pharmacokinetic parameters, monitoring serum vancomycin concentrations in very obese patients is advisable.

The approach used here (Equations 15.2, 15.3, and 15.4) to estimate vancomycin clearance has been shown to correlate better with ideal rather than total body weight in obese subjects.[22]

To calculate the expected pharmacokinetic parameters for C.U., first estimate ideal body weight and creatinine clearance using Equations 15.25 and 15.2, respectively.

$$\frac{\text{Ideal Body Weight}}{\text{for males in kg}} = 50 + (2.3)(\text{Height in inches} > 60) \qquad \text{[Eq. 15.25]}$$

$$= 50 + (2.3)(7 \text{ inches})$$

$$= 66 \text{ kg}$$

$$\text{Cl}_{cr} \text{ for males (mL/min)} = \frac{(140 - \text{Age})(\text{Weight in kg})}{(72)(\text{SCr}_{ss})}$$

$$= \frac{(140 - 40 \text{ yrs})(66 \text{ kg})}{(72)(1.2 \text{ mg/dL})}$$

$$= 76.4 \text{ mL/min}$$

Use Equation 15.4 to calculate vancomycin clearance:

$$\text{Vancomycin Cl} \approx \text{Cl}_{cr}$$

$$\text{Vancomycin Cl} = 76.4 \text{ mL/min}$$

or

$$= (76.4 \text{ mL/min})\left(\frac{60 \text{ min/hr}}{1000 \text{ mL/L}}\right)$$

$$= 4.58 \text{ L/hr}$$

Equation 15.1 can be used to calculate C.U.'s volume of distribution of 44.9 L:

$$V(L) = 0.17(\text{age in years}) + 0.22(\text{TBW in kg}) + 15$$

$$= 0.17(40 \text{ yrs}) + 0.22(105 \text{ kg}) + 15$$

$$= 44.9 \text{ L}$$

and Equation 15.6 can be used with the clearance of 4.58 L/h and the volume of distribution of 44.9 L to calculate an elimination rate constant of 0.102 hr⁻¹.

$$K = \frac{Cl}{V}$$

$$= \frac{4.58 \text{ L/hr}}{44.9 \text{ L}}$$

$$= 0.102 \text{ hr}^{-1}$$

Finally, using Equation 15.7 the vancomycin t½ can be estimated to be 6.8 hour.

$$t\frac{1}{2} = \frac{(0.693)(V)}{Cl}$$

$$= \frac{(0.693)(44.9 \text{ L})}{4.58 \text{ L/hr}}$$

$$= 6.8 \text{ hr}$$

Given the half-life and the desire to choose a dosing interval that is between 1 and 2 half-lives for vancomycin, a logical approach would be to use a convenient dosing interval of 12 hours, a trough concentration of 10 mg/L and Equation 15.16 to solve for a dose.

$$\text{Dose} = \frac{(Css \text{ min})(V)(1 - e^{-K\tau})}{(S)(F)(e^{-K\tau})}$$

$$\text{Dose} = \frac{(10 \text{ mg/L})(44.9 \text{ L})(1 - e^{-(0.102 \text{ hr}^{-1})(12 \text{ hr})})}{(1)(1)(e^{-(0.102 \text{ hr}^{-1})(12 \text{ hr})})}$$

$$= 1078 \text{ mg} \approx 1000 \text{ mg every 12 hours}$$

This dose would usually be rounded off to a reasonable amount, and 1,000 mg would probably be given every 12 hours. The steady-state peak and trough concentrations on this new dose could be confirmed by using Equations 15.12 and 15.15 and inserting the appropriate values.

$$\text{Css max} = \frac{\frac{(S)(F)(\text{Dose})}{V}}{1 - e^{-K\tau}}$$

$$= \frac{\frac{(1)(1)(1000\ \text{mg})}{44.9\ \text{L}}}{(1 - e^{-(0.102\ \text{hr}^{-1})(12\ \text{hr})})}$$

$$= 31.5\ \text{mg/L}$$

$$\text{Css min} = (\text{Css max})(e^{-K\tau})$$

$$= (31.5\ \text{mg/L})(e^{(-0.102\ \text{hr}^{-1})(12\ \text{hr})})$$

$$= (31.5\ \text{mg/L})(0.294)$$

$$= 9.3\ \text{mg/L}$$

Alternatively, the expected trough concentration could have been calculated by simply using a ratio of the new dose to the old dose.

$$\text{Css Desired} = \frac{\text{Desired Dose}}{\text{Current Dose}} \times \text{Css Current} \qquad [\text{Eq. 15.26}]$$

$$= \frac{1000\ \text{mg}}{1078\ \text{mg}} \times 10\ \text{mg/L}$$

$$= 0.928 \times 10\ \text{mg/L}$$

$$= 9.3\ \text{mg/L}$$

This technique of using a ratio of doses to calculate the new steady-state concentration is appropriate as long as the dosing interval and time of sampling has not changed for a drug that exhibits stable linear pharmacokinetics.

Note that any difference between the plasma concentrations calculated by the two methods is due to rounding-off errors and not to any other assumptions.

REFERENCES

1. Alexander MB. A review of vancomycin. Drug Intell Clin Pharm 1974;8:520.
2. Kirby WMM, et al. Treatment of staphylococcal septicemia with vancomycin. N Engl J Med 1960;262:49.
3. Banner WN Jr, Ray CG. Vancomycin in perspective. Am J Dis Child 1984;183:14.
4. Cunha BA, Ristuccia AM. Clinical usefulness of vancomycin. Clin Pharm 1983;2:417.
5. Wilhelm MP, Estes L. Vancomycin. Mayo Clin Proc 1999;74:928.

6. Lundstrom TS, Sobel JD. Antibiotics for gram-positive bacterial infections: vancomycin, teicoplanin, quinupristin/dalfopristin, and linezolid. Infect Dis Clin North Am 2000; 14:463.

7. Watanakunakom C, Tisone JC. Synergism between vancomycin and gentamicin or tobramycin for methicillin-susceptible and methicillin-resistant *Staphyloccus aureus* strains. Antimircob Agents Chemother 1982;22:903.

8. Rotschafer JC, et al. Pharmacokinetics of vancomycin: observations in 28 patients and dosage recommendations. Antimicrob Agents Chemother 1982;22:391.

9. Blouin RA, et al. Vancomycin pharmacokinetics in normal and morbidly obese subjects. Antimicrob Agents Chemother 1982;21:575.

10. Mollering RC, et al. Vancomycin therapy in patients with impaired renal function: a nomogram for dosage. Ann Intern Med 1981;94:343.

11. Zimmermann AE, Katona BG, Plaisance KI. Association of vancomycin serum concentrations with outcomes in patients with gram-positive bacteremia. Pharmacotherapy 1995;15:85.

12. Mulhern JG, et al. Trough serum vancomycin levels predict the relapse of gram-positive peritonitis in peritoneal dialysis patients. Am J Kidney Dis 1995;25:611.

13. Welty TE, Copa AK. Impact of vancomycin therapeutic drug monitoring on patient care. Ann Pharmacother 1994;28:1335.

14. Farber BF, Mollering RC Jr. Retrospective study of the toxicity of preparations of vancomycin from 1974 to 1981. Antimicrob Agents Chemother 1983;23:138.

15. Edwards DJ, Pancrobo S. Routine monitoring of serum vancomycin concentrations: waiting for proof of its value. Clin Pharm 1987;6:652.

16. Fitzsimmons WE, Postelnick MJ. Rational use of vancomycin serum concentrations: update on infectious disease for the hospital pharmacist. Florham Park, NJ: Macmillan Health Care Information, 1988;2:1.

17. Aeschlimann JR, Hershberber E, Rybak MJ. Analysis of vancomycin population susceptibility profiles, killing activity, and postantibiotic effect against vancomycin-intermediate staphylococcus aureus. Antimicrob Agents Chemother 1999;43:1914.

18. Newfield P, Roizen MF. Hazards of rapid administration of vancomycin. Ann Intern Med 1979;91:581.

19. Cook FV, Farrar WE. Vancomycin revisited. Ann Intern Med 1978;88:813.

20. Karchmer WA. Staphylococcal endocarditis: laboratory and clinical basis for antibiotic therapy. Am J Med 1985;78:116.

21. Krogstad DJ, et al. Single dose kinetics of intravenous vancomycin. J Clin Pharm 1980;20:197.

22. Rushing TA, Ambrose PJ. Clinical application and evaluation of vancomycin dosing in adults. J Pharm Technol 2001;17:33.

23. Ducharme MP, Slaughter RL, Edwards DJ. Vancomycin pharmacokinetics in a patient population: effect of age, gender, and body weight. Ther Drug Monit 1994;16:513.

24. Leonard AE, Boro MS. Vancomycin pharmacokinetic parameters in middle-aged and elderly men. Am J Hosp Pharm 1994;51:798.

25. Nielsen HE, et al. Renal excretion of vancomycin in kidney disease. Acta Med Scand 1975;197:261.

26. Lindholm DD, Murray JS. Persistence of vancomycin in the blood during renal failure and its treatment by hemodialysis. N Engl J Med 1966;274:1047.

27. Ayus JC, et al. Peritoneal clearance and total body elimination of vancomycin during chronic intermittent peritoneal dialysis. Clin Nephrol 1979;11:129.

28. Paton TW, et al. Drug therapy in patients undergoing peritoneal dialysis: clinical pharmacokinetic considerations. Clin Pharmacokinet 1985;10:404.

29. Morse GD, et al. Comparative study of intraperitoneal and intravenous vancomycin pharmacokinetics during continuous ambulatory peritoneal dialysis. Antimicrob Agents Chemother 1987;31:173.

30. Morse GD, et al. Overestimate of vancomycin concentrations utilizing fluorescence polarization immunoassay in patients on peritoneal dialysis. Ther Drug Monit 1987;9:212.

31. Smith PF, Morse GD. Accuracy of measured vancomycin serum concentrations in patients with end-state renal disease. Ann Pharmacother 1999;33:1329.

32. Lanese DM, et al. Markedly increased clearance of vancomycin during hemodialysis using polysulfone dialyzers. Kidney Int 1989;35:1409.

33. Pollard TA, et al. Vancomycin redistribution: dosing recommendations following high-flux hemodialysis. Kidney Int 1994;45:232.

34. Karam CM, et al. Outcome assessment of minimizing vancomycin monitoring and dosing adjustments. Pharmacotherapy 1999;19:257.

35. Freeman CD, et al. Vancomycin therapeutic drug monitoring: is it necessary? Ann Pharmacother 1993;27:594.

36. Schadd UB, et al. Clinical pharmacology and efficacy of vancomycin in pediatric patients. Pediatr Pharmacol Ther 1980;96:119.

37. Vance-Bryan K, et al. Effect of obesity on vancomycin pharmacokinetics as determined by a Bayesian forecasting technique. Antimicrob Agents Chemother 1993;37:436.

38. Bearden DT, Rodvold KA. Dosage adjustments for antibacterials in obese patients: applying clinical pharmacokinetics. Clin Pharmacokinet 2000;38:415.

Nomogram for Calculating the Body Surface Area of Adults[a]

Height	Surface Area	Weight

Height (cm / in): cm 100–79 in scale
Surface Area: 2.80 m² – 0.90 m²
Weight: kg 150 / 330 lb – kg 30 / 66 lb

[a] From the formula of DuBois and DuBois. Arch Intern Med. 1916;17:863: $S = W^{0.425} \times H^{0.725} \times 71.84$, or $\log S = 0.425 \log W + 0.725 \log H + 1.8564$, where S = Body surface area in cm², W = Weight in kg, H = Height in cm. Reprinted with permission from the publisher. Lontmer C., ed. Geigy Scientific Tables. 8th edition. Volume 1: Basle: Ciba-Geigy. 1981:226-27.

NOMOGRAMS FOR CALCULATING BODY SURFACE AREA

Nomogram for Calculating the Body Surface Area of Children[a]

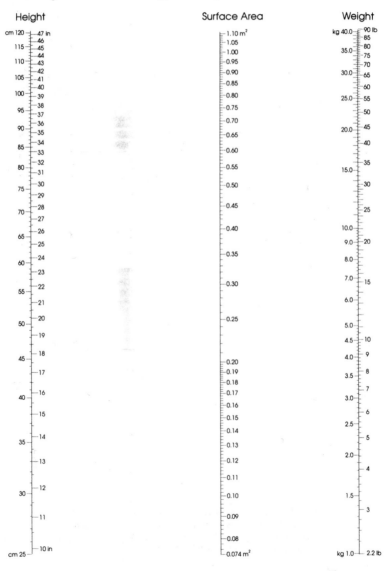

[a] From the formula of DuBois and DuBois. Arch Intern Med. 1916;17:863: $S = W^{0.425} \times H^{0.725} \times 71.84$, or $\log S = 0.425 \log W + 0.725 \log H + 1.8564$, where S = Body surface area in cm^2, W = Weight in kg, H = Height in cm.

COMMON EQUATIONS USED THROUGHOUT THE TEXT

The following is a list of equations that are frequently used in pharmaco-kinetic calculations. They are grouped together according to specific dosing situations. For a complete discussion, refer to the text and figures cited next to each equation. Although some of the equations may appear complicated, most are simple rearrangements of basic equations that can be broken down into one or more of the following components:

$\dfrac{(S)(F)(Dose)}{V}$ — The change in plasma concentration following a dose (ΔCp).

$\dfrac{(S)(F)(Dose/\tau)}{Cl}$ — Average steady-state concentration.

(e^{-Kt}) — Fraction remaining after time of decay (t).

$(1 - e^{-Kt})$ — Fraction lost during decay phase *or* fraction of steady state achieved during infusion.

SINGLE DOSE (ABSORPTION TIME OR $t_{in} \leq \frac{1}{6} t_{1/2}$)

$$\text{Loading Dose} = \frac{(V)(C)}{(S)(F)}$$

Part I:
Equation 11;
Figure 21

$$\frac{\text{Incremental}}{\text{Loading Dose}} = \frac{(V)(C \text{ desired} - C \text{ initial})}{(S)(F)}$$

Part I:
Equation 12

$$C = \frac{(S)(F)(\text{Loading Dose})}{(V)}$$

Part I:
Equation 49;
Figure 21

$$= (\text{Change in Concentration})$$

$$C_1 = \frac{(S)(F)(\text{Loading Dose})}{V} (e^{-Kt_1})$$

$$= \left(\begin{array}{c}\text{Change in}\\\text{Concentration}\end{array}\right)\left(\begin{array}{c}\text{Fraction Remaining}\\\text{After Time of Decay } t_1\end{array}\right)$$

Part I:
Equation 50;
Figure 21

HALF-LIFE ($t\frac{1}{2}$) AND ELIMINATION RATE CONSTANT (K)

$$K = \frac{Cl}{V}$$

Part I:
Equation 29

$$t\frac{1}{2} = \frac{(0.693)(V)}{Cl}$$

Part I:
Equation 32

$$K = \frac{0.693}{t\frac{1}{2}}$$

Part II:
Ch 8: Methotrexate,
Equation 8.8

$$t\frac{1}{2} = \frac{0.693}{K}$$

Part I:
Equation 31

$$K = \frac{\ln\left(\dfrac{C_1}{C_2}\right)}{t}$$

Part I:
Equation 30

SINGLE DOSE (ABSORPTION OR $t_{in} > \frac{1}{6} t\frac{1}{2}$)

$$C_2 = \frac{(S)(F)(\text{Dose}/t_{in})}{Cl} (1 - e^{-Kt_{in}})(e^{-Kt_2})$$

Part I:
Equation 54;
Figure 24

$$= \left(\begin{array}{c}\text{Average}\\\text{Steady-State}\\\text{Concentration}\end{array}\right)\left(\begin{array}{c}\text{Fraction of}\\\text{Steady State}\\\text{Achieved After}\\\text{Time of Infusion } t_{in}\end{array}\right)\left(\begin{array}{c}\text{Fraction Remaining}\\\text{After } t_2\\\text{Time of Decay}\end{array}\right)$$

$$= \left(\begin{array}{c}\text{Change in}\\\text{Concentration}\\\text{at the End of a}\\\text{Short Infusion}\end{array}\right)\left(\begin{array}{c}\text{Fraction Remaining}\\\text{After } t_2\\\text{Time of Decay}\end{array}\right)$$

CONTINUOUS INFUSION

At Steady State

$$\text{Maintenance Dose} = \frac{(Cl)(Css\ ave)(\tau)}{(S)(F)}$$

Part I:
Equation 16

$$Css\ ave = \frac{(S)(F)(Dose/\tau)}{Cl}$$

= Average Steady State Concentration

Part I:
Equation 35;
Figure 22

Decay From Steady State

$$C_2 = \frac{(S)(F)(Dose/\tau)}{Cl}\ (e^{-Kt_2})$$

Part I:
Equation 52;
Figure 22

$$= \left(\begin{array}{c} \text{Average} \\ \text{Steady-State} \\ \text{Concentration} \end{array} \right) \left(\begin{array}{c} \text{Fraction Remaining} \\ \text{After } t_2 \\ \text{Time of Decay} \end{array} \right)$$

NonSteady State

$$C_1 = \frac{(S)(F)(Dose/\tau)}{Cl}\ (1 - e^{-Kt_1})$$

Part I:
Equation 37;
Figure 19

$$= \left(\begin{array}{c} \text{Average} \\ \text{Steady-State} \\ \text{Concentration} \end{array} \right) \left(\begin{array}{c} \text{Fraction of} \\ \text{Steady State} \\ \text{Achieved } t_1 \text{ Time} \\ \text{After Starting Infusion} \end{array} \right)$$

Decay From NonSteady State

$$C_2 = \frac{(S)(F)(Dose/\tau)}{Cl}\ (1 - e^{-Kt_1})(e^{-Kt_2})$$

Part I:
Equation 41;
Figure 19

$$= \left(\begin{array}{c} \text{Average} \\ \text{Steady-State} \\ \text{Concentration} \end{array} \right) \left(\begin{array}{c} \text{Fraction of} \\ \text{Steady State} \\ \text{Achieved } t_1 \\ \text{Time After} \\ \text{Starting Infusion} \end{array} \right) \left(\begin{array}{c} \text{Fraction} \\ \text{Remaining} \\ \text{After } t_2 \\ \text{Time of Decay} \end{array} \right)$$

MULTIPLE DOSE
(CONSISTENT τ AND DOSE): STEADY STATE

Absorption or $t_{in} \leq \frac{1}{6} t\frac{1}{2}$

$$Css_1 = \frac{\frac{(S)(F)(Dose)}{V}}{1 - e^{-Kt}} (e^{-Kt_1})$$

Part I:
Equation 48;
Figure 26

$$= \left(\frac{\text{Change in Concentration}}{\binom{\text{Fraction Lost in}}{\text{Dosing Interval}}}\right) \left(\begin{array}{c}\text{Fraction} \\ \text{Remaining} \\ \text{After } t_1 \\ \text{Time of Decay}\end{array}\right)$$

$$= \left(\begin{array}{c}\text{Steady-State} \\ \text{Peak} \\ \text{Concentration}\end{array}\right) \left(\begin{array}{c}\text{Fraction Remaining} \\ \text{After } t_1 \\ \text{Time of Decay}\end{array}\right)$$

Absorption or $t_{in} > \frac{1}{6} t\frac{1}{2}$

$$Css_2 = \frac{\frac{(S)(F)(Dose/t_{in})}{Cl}(1 - e^{-Kt_{in}})}{1 - e^{-K\tau}} (e^{-Kt_2})$$

Part I:
Equation 58
Part II: Ch 1:
Aminoglycoside
Antibiotics,
Equation 1.20,
Figure 1.1

$$= \frac{\left(\begin{array}{c}\text{Average} \\ \text{Steady-State} \\ \text{Concentration}\end{array}\right) \left(\begin{array}{c}\text{Fraction of} \\ \text{Steady State} \\ \text{Achieved After } t_{in} \\ \text{Time of Infusion}\end{array}\right)}{\left(\begin{array}{c}\text{Fraction} \\ \text{Lost in a} \\ \text{Dosing Interval}\end{array}\right)} \left(\begin{array}{c}\text{Fraction} \\ \text{Remaining} \\ \text{After } t_2 \\ \text{Time of Decay}\end{array}\right)$$

$$= \left(\begin{array}{c}\text{Steady-State} \\ \text{Peak Concentration} \\ \text{at End of Short Infusion}\end{array}\right) \left(\begin{array}{c}\text{Fraction Remaining} \\ \text{After } t_2 \text{ Time of Decay}\end{array}\right)$$

MULTIPLE DOSE
(CONSISTENT τ AND DOSE): NONSTEADY STATE

Absorption or $t_{in} \leq \frac{1}{6} t\frac{1}{2}$

$$C_2 = \frac{\frac{(S)(F)(Dose)}{V}}{(1 - e^{-K\tau})}(1 - e^{-K(N)\tau})(e^{-Kt_2})$$

Part I:
Equation 56

$$= \left(\begin{array}{c} \text{Change in} \\ \text{Concentration} \\ \hline \text{Fraction Lost in} \\ \text{Dosing Interval} \end{array}\right) \left(\begin{array}{c} \text{Fraction of} \\ \text{Steady State} \\ \text{Achieved} \\ \text{After N Doses} \end{array}\right) \left(\begin{array}{c} \text{Fraction} \\ \text{Remaining} \\ \text{After } t_2 \text{ Time} \\ \text{of Decay} \end{array}\right)$$

$$= \left(\begin{array}{c} \text{Steady-State} \\ \text{Peak} \\ \text{Concentration} \end{array}\right) \left(\begin{array}{c} \text{Fraction of} \\ \text{Steady State} \\ \text{Achieved} \\ \text{After N Doses} \end{array}\right) \left(\begin{array}{c} \text{Fraction} \\ \text{Remaining} \\ \text{After } t_2 \text{ Time} \\ \text{of Decay} \end{array}\right)$$

MASS BALANCE

$$\frac{(S)(F)(Dose/\tau) - \frac{(C_2 - C_1)V}{t}}{C\ ave} = Cl$$

Part I:
Equation 65

CREATININE CLEARANCE (Cl$_{cr}$)

$$\frac{Cl_{cr} \text{ for males}}{\text{(mL/min)}} = \frac{(140 - Age)(Weight)}{(72)(SCr_{ss})}$$

Part I:
Equation 70

$$\frac{Cl_{cr} \text{ for females}}{\text{(mL/min)}} = (0.85)\frac{(140 - Age)(Weight)}{(72)SCr_{ss}}$$

Part I:
Equation 71

where: Age in Years, Weight in kg, SCr_{ss} in mg/dL

$$\frac{Cl_{cr} \text{ for children}}{\text{(mL/min/1.73 m}^2)} = \frac{(0.48)(\text{Height in cm})}{SCr_{ss}}$$

Part I:
Equation 76

$$\frac{Cl_{cr} \text{ for children}}{\text{(mL/min)}} = (Cl_{cr} \text{ mL/min/1.73 m}^2)\left(\frac{BSA}{1.73 \text{ m}^2}\right)$$

Part I:
Equation 77

$$BSA \text{ in m}^2 = \left(\frac{\text{Patient's Weight in kg}}{70 \text{ kg}}\right)^{0.7}(1.73 \text{ m}^2)$$

Part I:
Equation 17

NONLINEAR EQUATIONS (PHENYTOIN)

$$(S)(F)(Dose/\tau) = \frac{(Vm)(Css\ ave)}{Km + Css\ ave}$$

Part II:
Ch 10: Phenytoin
Equation 10.14

$$Css = \frac{(Km)[(S)(F)(Dose/\tau)]}{Vm - [(S)(F)(Dose/\tau)]}$$

Part II:
Ch 10: Phenytoin
Equation 10.15

Time Required to Achieve 90% of Steady State ($t_{90\%}$)

$$t_{90\%} = \frac{(Km)(V)}{[Vm - (S)(F)(Dose/day)]^2}[(2.3\ Vm) \\ - (0.9)(S)(F)(Dose/day)]$$

Part II:
Ch 10: Phenytoin
Equation 10.23

Has Steady State Been Achieved?

$$90\%\ t = \frac{[115 + (35)(C)][C]}{(S)(F)(Dose/day)}$$

Part II:
Ch 10: Phenytoin
Equation 10.24

Days on current maintenance regimen must exceed 90% t value to assure that steady state has been achieved. Dose is in mg/day normalized to 70 kg.

ADJUSTMENT FOR PLASMA PROTEIN BINDING (PHENYTOIN)

Adjustment For Serum Albumin If $Cl_{cr} > 25$ mL/min

$$\frac{\text{Phenytoin Concentration}}{\text{Normal Plasma Binding}} = \frac{\text{Patient's Phenytoin Concentration With Altered Plasma Binding}}{\left[0.9 \times \dfrac{\text{Patient's Serum Albumin}}{4.4\ gm/dL}\right] + 0.1}$$

Part II:
Ch 10: Phenytoin
Equation 10.2

Adjustment For Serum Albumin If $Cl_{cr} < 10$ mL/min

$$\frac{\text{Phenytoin Concentration}}{\text{Normal Plasma Binding}} = \frac{\text{Dialysis Patient's Phenytoin Concentration With Altered Plasma Binding}}{\left[(0.9)(0.48)\left(\dfrac{\text{Patient's Serum Albumin}}{4.4\ gm/dL}\right)\right] + 0.1}$$

Part II:
Ch 10: Phenytoin
Equation 10.3

ALGORITHM FOR EVALUATING AND INTERPRETING PLASMA CONCENTRATIONS

Step 1. Initial Data Collection

Before one can interpret the patient's pharmacokinetic parameters or plasma drug concentrations, appropriate information must be collected so that factors which may influence drug absorption and disposition can be considered.

Relevant Physical Data, Medical and Surgical History:

Height, weight, age, sex, race, current diseases and symptoms.

Relevant Laboratory Data:

Renal Function: SCr, BUN, Cl_{Cr} (Is the collection complete?)

Hepatic Function:
Serum albumin, bilirubin, prothrombin time, serum enzymes.

Protein Binding: Plasma protein concentration. Acidic drugs—Albumin. Basic drugs—?Globulins. Evaluate displacing factors such as other drugs or presence of uremia

Thyroid function

Drug Administration History:

Collect dosing data (dose, frequency, and route) for 3–5 half-lives. In acute Care Settings consider history prior to admissions as well as during hospital stay.

It is critical to determine the *exact* time of administration for those doses taken just prior to drug level sampling.

Time of Sampling Relative to the Last Dose:

The best time to sample is usually just prior to the next dose. For drugs with a short half-life, peak and trough levels may be appropriate. Avoid absorption and distribution phase when peak levels are obtained.

(Continued on next page)

Step 2. Evaluation of Reported Plasma Concentrations

Has the patient been receiving constant dosing for more than 3 to 4 half-lives prior to obtaining the plasma sample?

Yes

No ↓

Nonsteady State Plasma Concentration

The plasma concentration must be evaluated by considering the contribution of each dose at the time the plasma sample was obtained. Use Equation 50 for each bolus dose or Equation 54 for each short infusion. If several different sustained infusion rates have been used during the accumulation period, Equations 37 or 41 should be used for each infusion rate.

C is greater than expected:

See List A.

V may be less than expected.

Sample may have been obtained during distribution phase.

C is less than expected:

See List B.

V may be greater than expected.

Sample may have been obtained too soon after the dose was administered and absorption was not yet complete.

List A

When drug concentrations are greater than expected, consider:

1. Increased bioavailability. This is only important if the drug s bioavailability is usually low.
2. Nonadherence. Intake is greater than prescribed.
3. Decreased clearance.
4. Increased plasma protein binding. Changes in plasma protein binding will be most important if fu is ≤ 0.1 and are unlikely to be signi icant if fu is > 0.5. Increased plasma protein binding will also decrease the volume of distribution and clearance of most drugs.

List B

When drug concentrations are less than expected, consider:

1. Decreased bioavailability.
2. Nonadherence. Intake is less than prescribed.
3. Increased clearance.
4. Decreased plasma protein binding. Changes in plasma protein binding will be most important if fu is ≤ 0.1. It is unlikely to be significant if fu is > 0.5. Decreased plasma binding will also increase the volume of distribution and the clearance of most drugs.

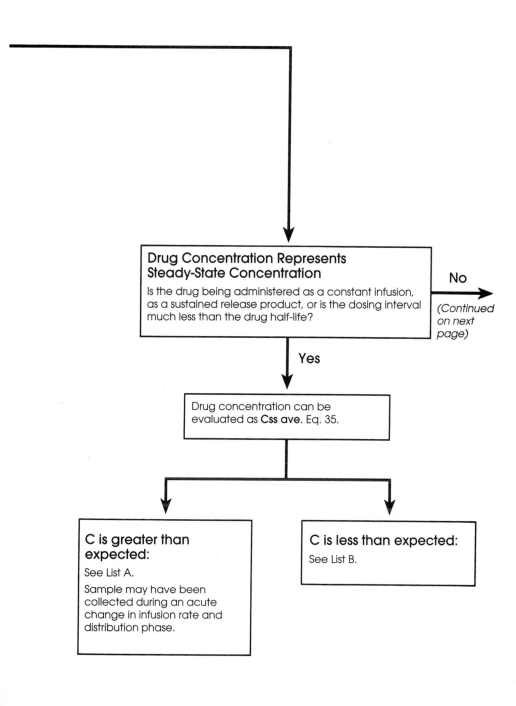

Drug Concentration Represents Steady-State Concentration

Is the drug being administered as a constant infusion, as a sustained release product, or is the dosing interval much less than the drug half-life?

No

(Continued on next page)

Yes

Drug concentration can be evaluated as **Css ave**. Eq. 35.

C is greater than expected:

See List A.

Sample may have been collected during an acute change in infusion rate and distribution phase.

C is less than expected:

See List B.

Step 2. Evaluation of Reported Plasma Concentrations
(Continued)

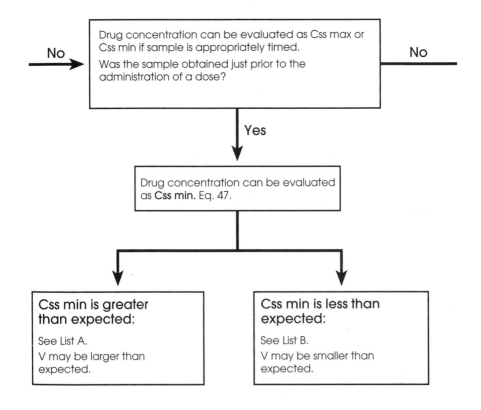

No

Drug concentration can be evaluated as Css max or Css min if sample is appropriately timed.

Was the sample obtained just prior to the administration of a dose?

No

Yes

Drug concentration can be evaluated as **Css min**. Eq. 47.

Css min is greater than expected:

See List A.
V may be larger than expected.

Css min is less than expected:

See List B.
V may be smaller than expected.

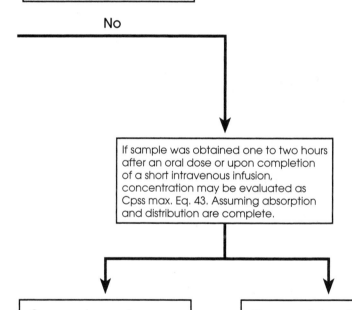

List A

When drug concentrations are greater than expected, consider:

1. Increased bioavailability. This is only important if the drug s bioavailability is usually low.
2. Nonadherence. Intake is greater than prescribed.
3. Decreased clearance.
4. Increased plasma protein binding. Changes in plasma protein binding will be most important if fu is ≤ 0.1 and are unlikely to be significant if fu is > 0.5. Increased plasma protein binding will also decrease the volume of distribution and clearance of most drugs.

List B

When drug concentrations are less than expected, consider:

1. Decreased bioavailability.
2. Nonadherence. Intake is less than prescribed.
3. Increased clearance.
4. Decreased plasma protein binding. Changes in plasma protein binding will be most important if fu is ≤ 0.1. It is unlikely to be significant if fu is > 0.5. Decreased plasma binding will also increase the volume of distribution and the clearance of most drugs.

No

If sample was obtained one to two hours after an oral dose or upon completion of a short intravenous infusion, concentration may be evaluated as Cpss max. Eq. 43. Assuming absorption and distribution are complete.

Css max is greater than expected:

See List A.

Sample may have been obtained during the distribution phase.

V may be smaller than expected.

Css max is less than expected:

See List B.

V may be larger than expected.

Absorption of dose delayed or slower than expected.

GLOSSARY OF TERMS AND ABBREVIATIONS

Ab: See Amount of Drug in the Body.

Accumulation Factor: $1/1-e^{-k\tau}$ or the degree to which a maintenance dose will accumulate when steady state is achieved.

Adjusted Body Weight: A weight for dosing drugs in obese patients that is between ideal body weight and total body weight.

Administration Rate (R_A): The average rate at which a drug is administered to the patient.

Alpha (α): The initial half-life in a two compartment model, usually representing distribution (see Figure 9).

Amount of Drug in the Body (Ab): The total amount of active drug that is in the body at any given time.

Average Steady-State Concentration (Css ave): The average plasma drug concentration at steady state.

Beta (β): Second decay half-life in a two compartment model, usually representing elimination.

Bioavailability (F): The fraction of an administered dose that reaches the systemic circulation.

Body Surface Area (BSA): The surface area of a patient, as determined by weight and height (see Appendix I).

Bolus Dose: A model for rapid input of a dose into the body or an individual dose usually given by intravenous injection.

BSA: See Body Surface Area.

CAPD: See Continuous Ambulatory Peritoneal Dialysis.

Cl: See Clearance

Cl$_{adjusted}$: Clearance of a patient that has been adjusted or altered for the presence of a disease state such as renal failure or heart failure.

Cl$_{CAPD}$: Drug clearance by peritoneal dialysis.

Cl$_{Cr}$: See Creatinine Clearance.

Cl$_{CRRT}$: Drug clearance by CRRT (See CRRT).

Cl$_{dial}$: Drug clearance by dialysis.

Cl$_m$: See Clearance, metabolic.

Cl_{pat}: Drug clearance of patient, usually associated with decreased renal function.

Cl_r: See Clearance, renal.

Clearance (Cl_t or Cl): Total body clearance is a measure of how well a patient can metabolize or eliminate drug. It is used to calculate maintenance doses or average steady-state plasma concentrations.

Clearance, metabolic (Cl_m): A measure of how well the body can metabolize drugs. The major metabolic organ is usually the liver.

Clearance, renal (Cl_r): A measure of how well the kidneys can excrete unchanged or unmetabolized drug. It is usually assumed to be proportional to creatinine clearance.

C: See Plasma Concentration.

C′: Plasma concentration measured in patients with altered plasma protein binding.

C_1: The initial plasma concentration at the beginning of a decay phase, usually following a loading dose.

C_2: The drug concentration at the end of a decay phase.

ΔC: Change in plasma concentration resulting from a single dose.

C desired: Plasma concentration desired following an incremental loading dose.

C free: Unbound or free plasma concentration.

$C_{Normal\ Binding}$: Plasma concentration that would be observed or measured if patient's plasma protein binding is normal.

$C_{initial}$: Plasma concentration present in patient before an incremental loading dose.

C_{tin}: Plasma concentration at the end of a short infusion or at the end of absorption.

Css ave: Average plasma concentration at steady state.

Css max: The maximum or peak concentration at steady state, when a constant dose is administered at a constant dosing interval.

Css min: The minimum or trough concentration at steady state, when a constant dose is administered at a constant dosing interval.

Continuous Renal Replacement Therapy: A type of hemodialysis that is continuous versus intermittent.

Creatinine Clearance (Cl_{Cr}): A measure of the kidney's ability to eliminate creatinine from the body. Total renal function is usually assumed to be proportional to creatinine clearance.

CRRT: See Continuous Renal Replacement Therapy.

Dosing Interval (τ): The time interval between doses when a drug is given intermittently.

Dry Weight: Weight of patient before excessive 3rd space fluid weight gain.

Dwell Time (T_D): The time between instillation and removal of a peritoneal dialysis exchange volume.

e^{-Kt}: Fraction remaining at the end of a time interval.

$1-e^{-Kt}$: a) Fraction lost during a dosing interval at steady state, if $t = \tau$.
b) Fraction of steady state achieved during a constant infusion "t" hours after starting the infusion.

Elimination Rate Constant (K): The fractional rate of drug loss from the body or the fraction of the volume of distribution that is cleared of drug during a time interval.

Elimination Rate (R_E): The amount of drug eliminated from the body during a time interval.

Extraction Ratio: Fraction of drug that is removed from the blood or plasma as it passes through the eliminating organ.

F: See Bioavailability.

First-Pass: Drug removed from the blood or plasma, following absorption from the gastrointestinal tract, before reaching the systemic circulation.

First-Order Elimination: A process whereby the amount or concentration of drug in the body diminishes logarithmically over time. The rate of elimination is proportional to the drug concentration.

fu: Fraction of total plasma concentration that is free or unbound.

Half-Life ($t\frac{1}{2}$): Time required for the plasma concentration to be reduced to one-half of the original value.

Half-life, alpha ($\alpha\ t\frac{1}{2}$): Initial decay half-life usually representing distribution of drug into the tissue or slowly equilibrating second compartment in a two-compartmental model.

Half-life, beta ($\beta\ t\frac{1}{2}$): Second decay half-life; usually represents the elimination half-life. Half-life, beta for most drugs can be calculated using the elimination rate constant.

IBW: See Ideal Body Weight.

Ideal Body Weight: Body weight used as an estimate of non-obese weight.

Incremental Loading Dose: An adjusted loading dose required to achieve a desired plasma concentration (C desired) when a preexisting plasma concentration (C observed) is present.

Initial Volume of Distribution (Vi): Initial volume into which the drug rapidly equilibrates following an intravenous bolus dose injection.

Iterative Search: A trial and error process to determine patient-specific pharmacokinetic parameters when direct solutions are not possible due to the nature of the pharmacokinetic model.

K: See Elimination Rate Constant.

$K_{adjusted}$: Elimination rate constant that has been adjusted or altered for the presence of a disease state such as renal failure.

K_{dial}: Elimination rate constant representing both the patient's drug clearance and the drug clearance by dialysis.

Km (Michaelis-Menten Constant): Plasma concentration at which the rate of metabolism is half the maximum rate.

$K_{metabolic}$ (K_m): The elimination rate constant calculated from the metabolic clearance and the volume of distribution (Cl_m/V).

K_{renal} (K_r): The elimination rate constant calculated from the renal clearance and the volume of distribution (Cl_r/V).

Linear Pharmacokinetics: Assumes the elimination rate constant is not affected by plasma drug concentration and that the rate of drug elimination is directly proportional to the concentration of drug in plasma.

ln: Natural logarithm using the base 2.718 rather than 10, which is used for the common logarithm or log.

Loading Dose: Initial total dose required to rapidly achieve a desired plasma concentration.

Maintenance Dose: The dose required to replace the amount of drug lost from the body so that a desired plasma concentration can be maintained.

Mass Balance: The process of comparing drug administration rate (R_A) to the rate of change of drug in the body ((ΔC)(V)/t) in order to estimate drug elimination rate (R_E).

(N): The number of doses that have been administered at a fixed-dosing interval.

One-Compartment Model: Assumes that drug distributes rapidly and equally to all areas of the body. Most drugs can be modeled this way if sampling during the initial distribution phase is avoided.

P_{NL} or P′: Plasma protein concentration. P_{NL} refers to the normal plasma protein concentration and P′ refers to the plasma protein concentration of the specific patient.

Pharmacokinetics: Study of the absorption, distribution, metabolism, and excretion of a drug and its metabolites in the body.

Plasma Concentration (C): Concentration of drug in plasma. Usually refers to the total drug concentration and includes both the bound and unbound or free drug concentration.

R_A: See Administration Rate.
R_E: See Elimination Rate.

S: See Salt Form.
Salt Form (S): Fraction of administered salt or ester form of the drug that is the active moiety.

Sensitivity Analysis: The practice of examining the relationship between a change in either clearance or volume of distribution and the corresponding change in the calculated plasma concentration. (See Part I: Interpretation of Plasma Drug Concentrations: Sensitivity Analysis.)

SrCr: Serum Creatinine Concentration.

Steady State: Steady state is achieved when the rate of drug administration is equal to the rate of drug elimination.

t½: See Half-Life.

t$_{90\%}$: Time required to achieve 90% of steady state for phenytoin on a fixed dosing regimen in a patient with known values of V, Vm, and Km.

Tau (τ): See Dosing Interval.

$\tau - t_{in}$: Time from end of infusion to trough concentration when using a short infusion model.

TBW: See Total Body Weight.

T$_d$: Time of dialysis for intermittent hemodialysis.

T$_D$: See dwell time.

T$_{in}$: Time required for drug to be infused or absorbed.

Tissue Concentration (C$_t$): Concentration of drug in the tissue.

Tissue Volume of Distribution (Vt): Apparent volume into which the drug appears to distribute following rapid equilibration with the initial volume of distribution.

Total Body Weight: Total weight of a patient usually used for obese patients.

Two-Compartment Model: Comprised of an initial, rapidly equilibrating volume of distribution (Vi) and an apparent second, more slowly equilibrating volume of distribution (Vt).

Unbound V: Volume of distribution based on the free or unbound plasma concentration.

V: See Volume of Distribution.

Vi: See Initial Volume of Distribution.

Vm: Maximum rate at which metabolism can occur.

Vt: See Tissue Volume of Distribution

Volume of Distribution (V): The apparent volume required to account for all the drug in the body if it were present throughout the body in the same concentration as in the sample obtained from the plasma.

90% t: Duration of therapy on a fixed dosing regimen that must be exceeded to assure that a measured phenytoin concentration represents steady state.

INDEX

Page numbers in *italics* denote figures; those followed by t denote tables

initial dose of, 430–431, 431
key parameters of, 424t, 426–429
maintenance dose of, 429–430,
434–435
and newer antidepressants, usage,
424
plasma concentration(s) of
monitoring, efficacy of, 423,
430–431, 431, 435–436
steady-state, expected, 430–431
steady-state, pharmacokinetic
modeling, 431–433
therapeutic, 424t, 425–426
time to sample, 428–429
toxic, 425–426, 431, 435–436
sampling timing for, 428–429
toxicity of, 425–426, 431, 435–436
volume of distribution of, 426–427
Trileptal (*see* Oxcarbazepine)
Two-compartment computer models,
26
Two-compartment modeling, of
volume of distribution, 23–26,
24, 494
loading dose and plasma drug
concentration in, 23–25
and offset of drug effect evaluation,
25
significant and non significant,
25–26

Unbound plasma concentration (*see*
Fraction unbound)
Uremic patients
clearance in, 33–35
decreased tissue binding of drugs in,
22
free drug plasma concentration in,
16
phenytoin pharmacokinetics in,
15–16, 22 (*see also under*
Phenytoin)
Urine creatinine evaluation, 108–110
Valproic acid, 438–449
bioavailability of, 440
fu value, 14t
clearance of, 440–441
in children, 442–443
drug interaction with, 445–446
extended-release, 439
for migraines, 449

formulations of, 439, 440, 446, 449
half-life of, 441
intravenous, appropriate dose and
dosing interval, 446–449
key parameters of, 439t, 440–441
maintenance dose of, 438
increasing, 443–445
oral to intravenous dosing of,
conversion, 446–449
pharmacodynamics of, 438
plasma concentration(s) of, 10
dosing interval effect on, 443–445
steady-state, using sprinkle
formulation, 446
therapeutic, 438–439, 439t
time to sample, 441
toxic, 438–439
trough, expected, 441–443
trough, increasing, 443–445
sampling timing for, 441
sprinkle formulation of, 440, 446
volume of distribution of, 440

Vancomycin, 451–474
administration of, 451–452
bioavailability of, 453
fu value, 14t
clearance of, 453–454
in dialysis, 454
patient specific, estimating,
463–465
dialysis of, 454, 466–468, 468–469
dosing nomograms for, 454–455
dosing regimen of, 451–452
adjusting, 463–465
in end-stage renal disease,
466–468
in high-flux hemodialysis, 468–469
in obese patients, 471–474
patient specific, 456–461
replacement, after dialysis,
468–469
half-life of, 454
key parameters of, 451t, 453–454
patient specific, estimating,
456–461, 469–471, 471–474
maintenance dose of, 451–452
multicompartmental modeling of,
456
pharmacodynamics of, 451–452
plasma concentration(s) of